Natural Toxic Compounds *of* Foods

Formation *and* Change During Processing *and* Storage

Edited by

Jiří Davídek, Ph.D., D.Sc.
Professor of Food Science
Department of Food Chemistry and Analysis
Faculty of Food and Biochemical Technology
Institute of Chemical Technology
Prague, Czech Republic

CRC

CRC Press
Boca Raton Ann Arbor London Tokyo

Library of Congress Cataloging-in-Publication Data

Natural toxic compounds of foods : formation and change during processing and storage / edited by Jiri Davidek.
p. cm.
Includes bibliographical references and index.
ISBN 0-8493-4623-1
1. Food--Toxicology--Health aspects. 2. Food industry and trade--Health aspects. 3. Food--Storage--Health aspects. 4. Food--Microbiology.
I. Davidek, Jiri, 1932-.
RA1258.N37 1995
615.9'54--dc20

94-32289
CIP

International Standard Book Number 0-8493-4623-1
Library of Congress Card Number 94-32289
Printed in the United States of America 2 3 4 5 6 7 8 9 0
Printed on acid-free paper

PREFACE

Without doubt, the nutritional influence on the health status of the population, and hence food composition and the quality of consumed food, are very important.

Our knowledge of food chemistry is growing very rapidly. Research in the last five decades has revealed many basic findings, which let us understand many positive, as well as negative, changes that occur not only during processing and storage of foodstuffs, but also during home preparation of meals.

The goal of the food industry is to produce products that are of the highest quality not only from the nutritional, sensorial, but also from the hygienic, points of view. All attributes of quality are very important, but the hygienic ones can in some cases be the *most* important. This is valid especially in cases when foodstuffs contain higher concentrations of undesirable compounds (above legislation limits) that can harm human health. Harmful compounds can occur in foodstuffs as contaminants (from environmental pollution, agricultural activity, etc.), or they can be present as natural constituents in raw material, they can be formed by microbiological activity, or they can be due to biochemical and chemical interaction of food components during food processing and storage.

Recently, much attention has been paid to contaminants due to the increase of environmental pollution and the occurrence of higher quantities of toxic compounds in foodstuffs. We are now more concerned about the danger from natural toxic components that are present in some raw material or that can be formed due to the microbiological acitivity or chemical reactions during food processing and storage. The level of some toxic compounds in material of plant and animal origin are known and many reviews have been published, but the frequency of their occurence in foodstuffs and their changes during cooking, food processing, and storage are not well documented.

This book is intended to summarize our knowledge in the field of naturally occurring toxic and antinutritive compounds of foods, i.e., compounds present because of the inherent genetic characteristics of the plant or animal from which the foods are derived. The guiding principle is to include those plants and animals that are of value or potentially of value for human nutrition, either by direct consumption or indirect consumption because they may serve as feed for domestic animals. No attempt has been made to cover intentional food additives; toxic compounds that could become part of the food as a result of human activities in agriculture, during processing, etc., or unwanted contaminants resulting from careless handling, spoilage, or some other uncontrolled or uncontrollable circumstances. Futhermore, no attempt has been made to provide comprehensive coverage of the vast number of plants that are of primarily pharmaceutical interest or that produce toxic effects if *accidentally* ingested by humans or animals.

The main attention in all chapters is focused on the changes during processing and storage. Information about the chemistry, toxic effects, and occurrence of these compounds in raw materials and foods are reduced to a minimum, but are necessary for understanding reactions that take place during the formation and change of toxic and antinutritive compounds during processing and storage. Besides toxic and antinutritive compounds that are present as natural constituents in raw materials and foodstuffs, toxic and antinutritive compounds that are formed from food components during processing and storage are also included.

We tried to fulfill our task to include in this book all necessary information from this field. Our readers will judge to what extent we have succeeded.

Jiří Davídek
Prague, February 1994

THE EDITOR

Jiří Davídek, Ph.D., D.Sc., is a Professor of Food Science in the Faculty of Food and Biochemical Technology and is a member of the Department of Food Chemistry and Analysis, Institute of Chemical Technology, Prague, Czech Republic.

Dr. Davídek received his M.Sc. degree from the Institute of Chemical Technology, Faculty of Food and Biochemical Technology in 1954. He obtained his Ph.D. in 1969 from that same Institute under the direction of Prof. Dr. G. Janíček. After doing postdoctoral work with Dr. J. Fragner at the Research Institute of Food Industry in Prague and with Dr. A. W. Khan at the National Research Council, Division of Biosciences in Ottawa, Canada, he was appointed Assistant Professor of Food Chemistry and Analysis at the Faculty of Food and Biochemical Technology, Institute of Chemical Technology, Prague in 1960, and became a full Professor there in 1970.

Dr. Jiří Davídek is a member of the Czech Chemical Society and is on its Committee for Food and Agricultural Chemistry. He is a national representative of the Working Party of Food Chemistry, European Chemical Society and is a member of the Czech Biochemical Society, the American Institute of Food Technologists, and numerous other scientific societies. He is also a member of the editorial board of the *Czech Journal of Food Science* and of Germany's *Zeitschrift für Lebensmittel-Untersuchung und Forschung.* In 1972 he received the State Prize for Research, and in 1982 he was awarded both the Gold Medal from the Czechoslovak Academy of Agriculture and the Silver Medal from the Czechoslovak Academy of Science.

Dr. Davídek has published over 300 papers and is the author or co-author of 15 books published variously in Czech, English, German, and Polish. He has also delivered more than 300 lectures at seminars and symposiums. He often works as a chairman or a member at the international meetings organized by the Working Party of Food Chemistry, European Chemical Society (EURO FOOD, Chemical Reactions in Foods, etc.). His research interests focus on Maillard reactions, formation of sensory active compounds, food additives, and natural toxic compounds and contaminants.

CONTRIBUTORS

Jiří Čulík, Ph.D.
Department of Special Analyses
Research Institute of Brewing and Malting
Prague, Czech Republic

Jiří Davídek, Ph.D., D.Sc.
Department of Food Chemistry and Analysis
Faculty of Food and Biochemical Technology
Institute of Chemical Technology
Prague, Czech Republic

Tomáš Davídek, Ph.D.
Department of Food Chemistry and Analysis
Faculty of Food and Biochemical Technology
Institute of Chemical Technology
Prague, Czech Republic

Jana Dostálová, Ph.D.
Department of Food Chemistry and Analysis
Faculty of Food and Biochemical Technology
Institute of Chemical Technology
Prague, Czech Republic

Jana Hajšlová, Ph.D.
Department of Food Chemistry and Analysis
Faculty of Food and Biochemical Technology
Institute of Chemical Technology
Prague, Czech Republic

Zuzana Jehličková, Ph.D.
Department of Food Chemistry and Analysis
Faculty of Food and Biochemical Technology
Institute of Chemical Technology
Prague, Czech Republic

Pavel Kalač, Ph.D.
Department of Chemistry
Faculty of Agriculture
University of South Bohemia
Budějovice, Czech Republic

Vladimír Kellner, Ph.D.
Department of Special Analyses
Research Institute of Brewing and Malting
Prague, Czech Republic

Richard Koplík, Ph.D.
Department of Food Chemistry and Analysis
Faculty of Food and Biochemical Technology
Institute of Chemical Technology
Prague, Czech Republic

Jan Pánek, Ph.D.
Department of Food Chemistry and Analysis
Faculty of Food and Biochemical Technology
Institute of Chemical Technology
Prague, Czech Republic

Jan Pokorný, Ph.D., D.Sc.
Department of Food Chemistry and Analysis
Faculty of Food and Biochemical Technology
Institute of Chemical Technology
Prague, Czech Republic

Alexander Príbela, Ph.D., D.Sc
Department of Saccharides and Food Preservation
Faculty of Chemical Technology
Slovak Technical University,
Bratislava, Slovak Republic

Jaroslav Prugar, Ph.D., D.Sc
Department of Plant Quality
Research Institute of Crop Production
Prague, Czech Republic

Pavel Rauch, Ph.D., D.Sc
Department of Biochemistry and Microbiology
Faculty of Food and Biochemical Technology
Institute of Chemical Technology
Prague, Czech Republic

Hana Rauchová, Ph.D.
Institute of Physiology
Czech Academy of Sciences
Prague, Czech Republic

Terézia Šinková, Ph.D.
Food Research Institute
Bratislava, Slovak Republic

Jan Velíšek, Ph.D., D.Sc
Department of Food Chemistry and Analysis
Faculty of Food and Biochemical Technology
Institute of Chemical Technology
Prague, Czech Republic

Michal Voldřich, Ph.D., D.Sc
Department of Preservation Technology
Faculty of Food and Biochemical Technology
Institute of Chemical Technology
Prague, Czech Republic

CONTENTS

Section I
Natural Toxic Compounds of Food

Section II
Toxic and Antinutritive Compounds Formed During Food Processing and Storage

ACKNOWLEDGMENTS

This work could not have been presented without the contributions and cooperation of the numerous authors. I am grateful for their efforts.

The editor and the authors are also most grateful to Dr. M. Saxby for his valuable help and suggestions during the preparation of the English manuscript.

Section I
NATURAL TOXIC COMPOUNDS OF FOOD

This section will be devoted to natural toxic compounds in food, which means substances that occur in raw materials of plant and animal origin and in food produced from these raw materials. Natural toxic compounds are considered those compounds present because of the inherent genetic characteristics of the plant or animal from which foods are derived or that are formed during processing and storage of food. No attention will be paid to toxic compounds that can occur in raw materials and foods due to contamination.

Chapter 1

Food Intolerance-Inducing Compounds

Pavel Rauch and Hana Rauchová

Food intolerance has been the subject of confusion and controversy. There are several different types of individual adverse reactions to foods generally termed food allergies by both physicians and the public. The incidence of food allergy has been estimated at between 0.3 to 7.5% of the population. The mechanisms that result in food sensitivity are varied and should carry descriptive terms.[1] Although there has been an effort to develop common language concerning adverse reactions to foods and food additives, a set of definitions has not been universally accepted.[2,3] Food intolerance can be defined as any abnormal physiological response occurring among a minority of consumers that is attributed to the ingestion of a food or food additive. Food intolerances may be divided into two broad groups:

- Immunogenic compounds, which can be split into:
  - Food allergens (immunoglobulin E [IgE]-mediated response)
  - Food allergens (non-IgE-mediated response)
- Other compounds (nonimmunological response)

Part A
Immunogenic Compounds (Food Allergens)

FOOD ALLERGY — IgE-MEDIATED RESPONSE

The term food allergy should only be used to identify true immunologically based adverse reactions caused by allergens. By definition, food allergens must be capable of stimulating IgE production. In theory, any food protein has the potential for stimulating IgE production and sensitizing an individual to become allergic to that protein. In practice, surprisingly few categories of foods are associated with the vast majority of food allergies. The properties peculiar to the allergenic proteins in these foods that are responsible for their ability to stimulate IgE production are not well understood.

The immunogenicity of a protein is related, in general, to its amino acid sequence and its three-dimensional (secondary and tertiary) structure. It is also related to its perceived degree of foreignness to the host. These concepts, especially as related to IgE production, are not well understood.

Few food allergens have been purified and characterized. They are usually water-soluble glycoproteins, with molecular weights between 10,000 and 70,000 Da. The upper limit on the molecular weight of an allergen may be limited by the constraints of intestinal permeability. Allergens must be resistant to peptic-tryptic digestion and be stable in acid if they are to reach the intestinal mucosa in an immunogenic form. Proteins larger than a upper molecular weight limit are less likely to be efficiently absorbed through the intestinal mucosal membranes and to obtain access to the IgE-producing cells of the body.[4]

0-8493-4623-1/95/$0.00+$.50

Table 1 Possible Treatments of Foods Containing Allergens

Food	Treatment	Ref.
Cow's milk	Enzymatic hydrolysis	10,12
	Heat treatment	10,11,14
	Fermentation	7
	Homogenization	8
	Ultrafiltration	9,13
	Change of pH	14
	Increase of calcium concentration	14
	Ion-exchange chromatography	15
	Chemical modification	16
Legumes	Enzymatic hydrolysis	17
	Heat treatment	17,18
	Disruption of -S-S- bonds	46
	Interaction of protein–saccharide	18
	Interaction of protein–lipid	19
Cereals	Heat treatment	20
	Enzymatic hydrolysis	21
	Carbonate, glyceryl monooleate	
	Treatment	21
Sesame	Heat treatment	24

Unfortunately, allergenic molecules tend to be heat and acid stable and thus resist digestion. Therefore is difficult to change their antigenic and thus also their allergenic behavior. The overview of the successful treatments is shown in Tables 1 and 2. Allergenic food proteins often retain their allergenicity through various food processing treatments.[1,3]

COW'S MILK PROTEINS

Some commonly allergenic foods, such as cow's milk, are complex mixtures of allergens. Cow's milk contains a total protein level of 30 to 35 g.dm^{-3}. The major protein classes are caseins (α, and β), α- and β-lactoglobulins, and α-lactalbumins. Numerous studies have evaluated the allergenicity of these proteins in allergic individuals by skin testing and oral challenges. From these studies, it can be seen that multiple allergens exist in both the casein and whey fractions of cow's milk, and the major proteins are the major allergens, with β-lactoglobulin and casein being the most prevalent ones. Generally, there are three main ways to decrease allergenicity of milk:

- Enzymatic digestion of milk proteins
- Heat denaturation of milk proteins
- Combined effect of digestion and denaturation

Enzymatic digestion of casein leading to fragments with molecular weights smaller than 1000 Da has been shown to be satisfactory to some extent in lowering the sensitizing capacity of casein. However, the severe enzymatic digestion of the protein by a combination of several proteases leads to a low palatability, bitterness, and off-flavors. Thus casein hydrolysis should not be stronger than necessary to lose the antigenicity and hence allergenicity. Although it is quite impossible to specify general and precise limits of molecular weights for peptide immunogenicity, generally the peptides with molecular weight smaller than 5000 Da tend to be weakly immunogenic. Usually, pepsin, trypsin, and chymotrypsin are used, because these three proteases are major endoproteases in the

Table 2 Possible Treatments of Foods Containing Compounds Causing Nonimmunological Adverse Reactions

Compound	Treatment	Ref.
Lactose	Fermentation	37–39
	Enzymatic hydrolysis	36
	Ultrafiltration	40
Vicine, convicine	Soaking, blanching	44,45

gastrointestinal tract of humans. The recovery of peptides was highest and the bitterness was lowest in the chymotrypsin digest. All peptide preparations drastically reduced the antigenicity, in terms of reactivity with immunoglobulin G (IgG) antibody to intact whole casein. On the other hand, it is well known that the usefulness of the *in vitro* techniques, such as enzyme-linked immunosorbent assay (ELISA), is limited by a poor correlation between the results obtained by the *in vitro* tests and provocation tests in patients.[5] The hydrolysates showed a decreased but partially conserved immunogenic/allergenic potency, when tested on children, compared with original milk.[6]

Not only hydrolyzed milk proteins but also fermented milk products using probiotic starter cultures can be used. The use of oils other than milk fat in milk-based products combined with cheese in a ripening process can be used to produce a low allergenic, cheese-flavored product in dairy markets.[7] The full-fat homogenized milk was considerably more allergenic than a corresponding nonhomogenized sample.[8] Finally, a hypoallergenic milk product with the flavor and odor of natural whole milk is produced. It is preferably made with ultrafiltrated permeate of cow's milk, which is substantially free of milk protein and fat. The permeate is supplemented with hypoallergenic protein and fat to meet the minimal daily nutritional requirements for milk.[9]

In recent years, the attitude toward whey proteins has changed. They are no longer considered waste products, but rather valuable nutrients that can be used by the food industry. However, this use is dependent on, among other factors, the possibility of tailoring whey proteins for specific end uses and recovering them with intact functional properties, such as for the production of hypoallergenic infant milk formulas. The reduction of whey allergenicity has usually been made by means of selective enzyme hydrolysis and heat treatment. During enzymatic hydrolysis, cleavage of the polypeptide chain at specific sites leads to a collapse of the antigen architecture of protein molecules. Epitopes depending on conformation are rapidly collapsing, while sequential epitopes may survive the initial stage of hydrolysis. The breakdown of protein antigenicity can be followed with immunochemical methods (Figure 1). It appeared that both β-lactoglobulin and α-lactalbumin antigenicity decreased by three orders of magnitude within the first hour of hydrolysis.[10]

Heat stability is a very favorable property of the hydrolysate during further processing, because it facilitates in-line heat treatments that are required to complete reduction of antigenicity. Some cow's-milk allergens (serum albumin and immunoglobulins) are heat labile; however, some others can retain their allergenicity for 15 min at 120°C (caseins), and α-, and β-lactoglobulins are stable at 100°C. To reduce the more heat-labile but enzyme-resistant whey antigens down to the desired level, heating at 80 and 90°C was required for up to 30 min. It was observed that β-lactoglobulin heat denaturation was reached within 2000 s at 90°C and approximately 200 s at 125°C. In industrial practice, continuous heating in the ultra-high-temperature (UHT) range will be preferred to prolonged heating at lower temperatures with excessively long heating and cooling periods. On the

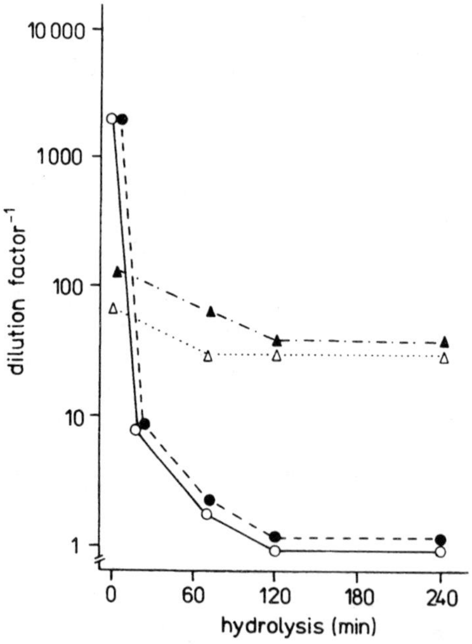

Figure 1 Decrease in different whey antigens during tryptic hydrolysis of protein-upgraded, demineralized whey, as analyzed by double immunodiffusion. The undiluted substrate or hydrolysate consisted of 100 mg dry matter (24 mg protein) ml^{-1}. Each experimental point was obtained by stopping the reaction by addition of trypsin inhibitor. ●, β-Lactoglobulin, ○, α-lactalbumin, △, serum albumin, ▲, immunoglobulin (IgG). (From Jost, R., Monti, J. C., and Pahud, J. J., *Food Technol.*, 41, 118, 1987. With permission.)

other hand, in the UHT range, the danger of lysine blockage, in which lysine complexes with lactose to form a derivative with reduced nutritional properties, increases considerably (page 200). Therefore this parameter has to be kept under control.[11]

Difficulties encountered with whey-predominant formulas upon rehydration led manufacturers to reduce heat treatments to maintain high protein solubility of the product, but these conditions lead to incomplete denaturation of whey proteins in the formula. Formulas developed by combining selective hydrolysis by specific proteases with preceding or subsequent heat treatment appear promising. The main problems associated with decreasing of allergenicity of whey proteins are to choose the appropriate enzymes and control the reaction conditions to limit bitterness and achieve the greatest possible homogeneity of molecular size. These two strategies allow us to make extensive use of whey.[12]

In view of industrial application, the intact whey proteins remaining in the hydrolysates should be eliminated. This could be achieved by modifying the enzymatic system (using immobilized enzymes) and/or by removing allergenic components from the hydrolysate by ultrafiltration.[13] By using the combined effect of heat treatment, different pH, and calcium concentration, it is possible to reduce antigenicity of whey proteins to 0.1% of the initial value.[14] The main allergic protein, β-lactoglobulin, can be extracted from whey by ion-exchange chromatography.[15] Finally, β-lactoglobulin could be chemically modified by covalent attachment of different levels of stearic acid (0.3 to 13.1 moles of fatty acids per mole of lysine) and thus decrease allergenicity of this protein.[16]

LEGUMES

Adverse reactions to soy products have been reported increasingly over the past few years. Soy protein has been consistently one of the five major foods implicated in causing hypersensitivity in over 90% of children with documented adverse food reactions. Several allergens, with subunit molecular weights of 50,000 to 60,000 Da, were found using the sera of adult subjects with histories of adverse reactions to both soybeans and peanuts. A major allergen with a molecular weight of approximately 20,000 Da was identified with the sera of patients who were sensitive only to soybeans. As in the case of milk proteins, the allergenicity of food proteins can be eliminated by heat treatment and enzymatic hydrolysis. Unfortunately, a heat-stable component exists in raw soybean that may possibly induce an allergy. Enzymatic hydrolysis following heat treatment could be effective in producing a hypoallergenic soybean protein hydrolysate.[17] A new possibility to reduce allergenicity is the disruption of the disulfide bonds with *N*-acetylcysteine, which causes a major change in antigenic determinants. Under relatively mild conditions of heating, carbohydrates can reduce the antigenicity of the protein and possibly modify sites known to elicit allergenic responses.[18] Thus, chemical and structural modification during food processing could be at least part of the basis for the observation that allergenic proteins (e.g., from milk, soybean, etc.) are less antigenic *in vivo* after such treatments. On the other hand, interaction of soybean proteins with oxidized lipids greatly increased allerginicity of these complexes, even though oxidized soybean oil itself did not show any allergic response.[19]

Peanuts are a major allergenic food because they contain multiple allergens, but most of them remain unidentified. Both of the major protein fractions of the peanut, arachin and conarachin, possess allergenic activity. An acidic glycoprotein, a major peanut allergen, is heat stable, and usual processing does not destroy allergenicity.[3]

CEREALS

Cereal grains are not a particularly common cause of allergic response.

Three kinds of proteins binding to the IgE antibody of allergic individuals were isolated from buckwheat seeds (*Polygonum fagopyrum*). These proteins were essentially homogeneous and their immunoreactivity was quite stable to heating at 100°C for 1 h.[20]

Atopic dermatitis is a type of allergic skin disease caused by rice allergen (most patients are sensitive also to wheat and barley). A method has been proposed to produce hypoallergenic rice for patients with rice allergy. Newly harvested rice grains were dipped in carbonate (pH 9) containing glyceryl monooleate and Actinase AS (protease produced by Kaken Kagaku, Japan) and then the mixture was exposed to a reduced pressure for degassing. The degassed mixture was incubated at 37°C for 24 h to hydrolyze proteins. The process produced rice grains in which the major allergenic globulin was decomposed. The product was evaluated by the radioallergosorbent test (RAST), as well as clinically administered to patients with atopic dermatitis, and no allergic reaction was observed.[21]

Baker's asthma, an allergy to inhalation of cereal flours, is a widespread disease affecting a considerable number of people involved in flour manipulation. Although this has been known for many years, little progress has been made in the identification of major flour allergens. Recently, allergens from barley and wheat were described.[22] Both barley and wheat allergens have molecular weights around 15,000 Da and they are from a family of cereal endosperm α-amylase inhibitors. No data concerning the stability of these allergens during the processing of foods are available.

OTHER ALLERGENS

Allergenic proteins have also been found in a wide variety of seeds including green peas, castor beans, cottonseeds, and rapeseeds. These allergens are frequently low-molecular-weight proteins with a high cystine content, but information on their biochemical and structural properties is still scarce. Among those cruciferous plants that are suspected to be allergenic, mustards are the most prevalent. The albumin fraction of the yellow mustard seeds contains the major allergen. This protein shows some biochemical properties also found in other allergens, such as low molecular weight, resistance to proteolytic treatments, and high cystine content. The primary structure of this allergen shows a certain degree of similarity with other plant proteins such as a proline-rich zein or a wheat gliadin.[23]

Sesame seeds must be regarded as very potent allergens. They can cause severe adverse reactions in allergic individuals. The allergens in sesame seeds may be inactivated or destroyed through heating. No allergy was observed with heat-extracted sesame seed oil, nor with the sesame seeds usually found on burger buns.[24]

DECREASING ALLERGENICITY

The authors, as mentioned above, used mainly enzymatic hydrolysis and heat treatment for decreasing allergenicity. New antiallergic treatments have now been found. Pectin shows an inhibitory effect on hyaluronidase (EC 3.2.1.35). Hyaluronidase has been suggested as one of the target enzymes controlling the allergic response, so the inhibitory effect on this enzyme has been reported to be an indicator of antiallergic activity.[25] Therefore, it is to be expected that pectin possesses an antiallergic potential. The same effect was described for tea extracts.[26] All tea extracts tested showed significant inhibitory effects on hyaluronidase. Results suggest that phenolic compounds such as tannins in the extracts were responsible for the inhibitory effect on hyaluronidase. Considering that the extracts showed almost the same activity regardless of the degree of fermentation of the teas, and some activity still existed after the removal of phenolic compounds, it was thought that other active components in addition to tannins were present.

Quite new procedures to neutralize allergenic effects of foods are based on treatment with a pulsed magnetic field, using a special apparatus, and by using recombinant DNA technology.[27,28]

The allergy hazard from proteins in processed foods and reduction of allergenic activity as a result of processing have been discussed. The possible increased allergenicity of new epitopes as a result of processing have been described.[29]

Finally, a search has been carried out to replace wheat, corn, and other members of the grass family, legumes, milk and milk products, eggs, nuts, and yeast by completely new foods, to which allergic individuals have no sensitivity. A large number of flours prepared from white sweet potatoes, cassava, edible aroids, yams, lotus, arrowhead, buckbean, and amaranth have been described.[30]

FOOD ALLERGY — NON-IgE-MEDIATED RESPONSE

Celiac disease, also known as celiac sprue or gluten-sensitive enteropathy, is a malabsorption syndrome that occurs in certain individuals following the ingestion of wheat, rye, barley, and sometimes, oats. Celiac disease is associated with the gliadin fraction of wheat protein and the equivalent prolamin fractions of barley, rye, and oats. A safe tolerance level cannot yet be estimated, so complete avoidance is the prudent choice, because the toxicity is not destroyed by the digestion of gliadin with pepsin and trypsin.[1]

A pure celiac-active peptide was isolated from a peptic-tryptic digest of whole gliadin. Its primary structure corresponds to residues 3 to 55 of α-gliadins. The toxicity was preserved after cleavage by chymotrypsin and the two fragment peptides (residues 3 to 24 and 25 to 55, respectively) did not significantly differ in respect to celiac activity. Another pure toxic peptide was obtained from a peptic-tryptic digest of a α-gliadin that was in fact an β-type gliadin. The amino acid composition indicated that this peptide also corresponded to the residues 3 to 24 of α-gliadins. Recently, peptides of known amino acid sequences were prepared from gliadin after cleavage with cyanogen bromide and chymotrypsin. Studies on toxicity revealed that the peptides corresponding to the residues 1 to 127, 128 to 246, 1 to 30, and 31 to 55 were toxic.[31] Even oligopeptides containing sequences Pro-Ser-Gln-Gln and Gln-Gln-Gln-Pro may be involved in the pathogenesis of celiac disease.[32,33] These results show that all peptides prepared by using enzymatic hydrolysis so far are toxic for celiac patients. An ELISA technique was developed for determination of toxic amino acids sequences in gliadins for testing of diet and/or food samples.[34]

Part B

Other Compounds (Nonimmunological Response)

In contrast to true food allergies, many of the individual adverse reactions to food do not involve the immune system. These types of body response occur through many different mechanisms. Like true food allergies, they affect only a limited number of individuals in the population. While true food allergies involve abnormal immunological responses to certain food constituents, especially proteins, nonimmunological response can occur through any one of a host of mechanisms.[1]

The three major classes of nonimmunological food intolerances are:

- Metabolic food disorders
- Idiosyncratic reactions
- Anaphylactoid reactions

Most of the nonimmunological food responses are caused by foodborne substances other than proteins.

The known metabolic food disorders involve naturally occurring substances exclusively, because they involve genetically determined deficiencies that either affect the host's ability to metabolize a food component or enhance the sensitivity of the host to some foodborne chemical via an altered metabolic pattern. An example of the former is lactose intolerance, caused by a deficiency of intestinal β-galactosidase (EC 3.2.1.23) and characterized by an inability to digest lactose. An example of the latter is favism, where a genetic deficiency in erythrocyte glucose-6-phosphate dehydrogenase (EC 1.1.1.49) causes an increased sensitivity to several hemolytic factors in fava beans.[4]

Idiosyncratic reactions to foods that affect certain individuals in the population occur through unknown mechanisms. Conceivably, a large number of different mechanisms could be involved in these idiosyncratic reactions, connected mainly with food ingredients (sulfites, aspartame, sugar, monosodium glutamate, etc.).[1]

In anaphylactoid reactions, the release of mediators from these cells occurs through yet undefined but nonimmunological mechanisms. It is presumed that some substance in the implicated food destabilizes the mast-cell membranes, causing a spontaneous release of histamine. Actually, none of these histamine-releasing substances has ever been isolated or identified in foods. The best example for anaphylactoid reaction is probably strawberry allergy. Strawberries are well known to cause adverse reactions (frequently urticaria) in some individuals. Yet strawberries contain very little protein and a strawberry allergen has never been identified, nor has any evidence been obtained for the existence of a strawberry-specific IgE.[1]

LACTOSE INTOLERANCE

Lactose malabsorption and lactose intolerance are to be distinguished from milk allergies. In normal digestive processes, lactose, a principal naturally occurring sugar in milk, is hydrolyzed into its constituent monosaccharides in the intestinal mucosa. The monosaccharides can then be absorbed and used metabolically as energy sources. In case of lactose intolerance, the key enzyme, β-galactosidase (EC 3.2.1.23), involved in this hydrolytic process is absent, or present at diminished levels.[4]

Reduced enzyme concentrations cannot be the sole cause of food intolerance because many patients report its onset in adult life and are upset by foods that they had eaten previously without effect. The bacterial flora of the gut may also have an important role.[35]

Dietary exclusion of lactose is the best way to prevent symptoms in lactose-intolerant individuals. Even complete elimination is not usually required, since lactase deficiency is seldom absolute.

A strategy for preventing symptoms in lactose malabsorbers is:

- Addition of β-galactosidase
- Use of fermented milk products
- Ultrafiltration of milk

Addition of β-galactosidase predigests some lactose, rendering the milk product more digestible for the lactase-deficient person.[36] This enzyme has been commercially produced from the yeast *Kluyveromyces lactis* or *Kluyveromyces marxianus*.[37,38] In clinical tests, infant tolerance to treated milk was excellent.[38] The disadvantage of this procedure is that it is necessary to add the enzyme to milk before ingestion, and often this changes the taste. Whether the cost of this treatment compared with simple dietary exclusion will permit its general use is unclear, but in view of the frequency of symptoms, many practitioners will be tempted to try it.

Another option is to restrict milk usage to its fermented forms, such as yogurt or some cheeses.[39] Though unpasteurized yogurt may contain lactose at percentages approaching those in milk, digestion of the yogurt is enhanced due to the inherent lactase activity in yogurt. Also, aged cheeses are very low in lactose because the lactose-rich whey is separated and removed and most of the remaining lactose is hydrolyzed during the fermentation process. On the other hand, it was reported that ingestion of other fermented or microbe-containing milk forms, such as acidophilus milk and buttermilk (or cultured milk), is more frequently associated with symptoms of lactose intolerance.[36]

Processes for manufacturing a low-lactose milk, employing ultrafiltration technology, have been described.[40] However, vitamins, minerals, and water must be added to the ultrafiltrate. A low-lactose imitation of milk can be prepared from washed curd and a small percent of edible oil or fat, together with emulsifying and/or stabilizing agent (e.g., lecithin), calcium, and sweetener (e.g., sucrose).[41]

The suppressing effect of cocoa on human lactose intolerance has been presented.[42] The addition of cocoa significantly reduced breath hydrogen level (BHL), as well as the

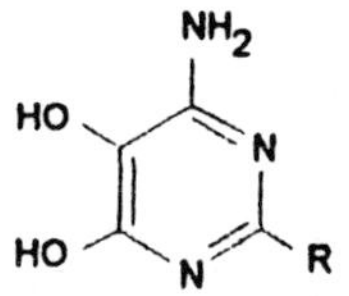

R = NH_2, divicine
R = OH, isouramil

Figure 2 Divicine and isouramil.

symptom score of both bloating and cramping. These results led to a conclusion that the suppressive effect of cocoa observed was shown by 95 and 51% of subjects with the milk and the cocoa formulas, respectively.

What can the food industry do to help the lactose-intolerant individual?[36] There are four possibilities:

1. Encourage the development of a reliable, inexpensive, home-administered test that enables the individual to pinpoint a threshold level for lactose intolerance.
2. Include on the labels of processed foods and natural-lactose foods the amount of lactose present.
3. Use reduced-lactose dairy ingredients in their processed foods.
4. Manufacture a greater variety of reduced-lactose dairy products for daily consumption.

FAVISM

The consumption of fava beans has been shown to cause favism. The causative agents are divicine and isouramil (Figure 2), which are highly reactive compounds generating free radicals and catalyzing a one-electron oxidation/reduction shuttle between reducing compounds and molecular oxygen. These compounds are produced in the gastrointestinal tract, following the hydrolysis by the microflora of the parent compounds vicine and convivine, and are absorbed by the blood. They then interact with the abundant supply of oxygen in the blood to produce superoxide radicals, which, if not neutralized by the free-radical scavenging system, cause cell damage. Therefore, several antioxidants that can protect against the toxic effects of these compounds have been tested. It was proved from direct evidence *in vivo* that free radical scavenging compounds, specifically vitamins A, C, and E and metal-chelating compounds (desferoxamine and possibly ethylenediamine tetraacetic acid [EDTA]) can protect the rat, and in many respects also humans, against divicine-induced health problems. A dosage of 250 to 500 IU of vitamin $E.kg^{-1}$ body weight provided complete protection against toxic effects of divicine.[43]

Another protective effect can be reached by soaking fava beans in water. This treatment removed approximately 80 to 90% of the original vicine and convicine content. Soaking in water for up to 35 h sometimes resulted in an unpleasant odor.[44] Similar results were obtained by steeping, blanching, and secondary steeping.[45]

REFERENCES

1. Taylor, S. L., Nordlee, J. A., and Rupnow, J. H., Food allergies and sensitivities, in *Food Toxicology, A Perspective on the Relative Risks,* Taylor, S. L. and Scanlan, R. A., Eds., Marcel Dekker, New York, 1989, chap. 10.
2. Anderson, J. A., The establishment of common language concerning adverse reactions to foods and food additives, *J. Allergy Clin. Immunol.,* 78, 140, 1986.
3. Taylor, S. L., Chemistry and detection of food allergens, in *Overview, Outstanding Symposia in Food Science and Technology,* Taylor, S. L. and Sumner, S. S., Eds., *Food Technol.,* 46, 146, 1992.
4. Taylor, S. L., Lemanske, R. F., Jr., Bush, R. K., and Busse, W. W., Food allergens: structure and immunologic properties, *Ann. Allergy,* 59, 93, 1987.
5. Otani, H., Dong, X. Y., and Hosono, A., Preparation of low-immunogenic peptide fragments from cow milk casein, *Milchwissenschaft,* 45, 217, 1990.
6. Stephan, V., Kuehr, J., Sawatzki, G., and Urbanek, R., Immunogenicity and allergenicity of an experimental cow's milk protein hydrolysate, *Z. Ernahrungswiss.,* 29, 112, 1990.
7. Hansen, S. R., Hypersensitivity — a lost or a new milk market, *North Eur. Food Dairy J.,* 55, 114, 1989.
8. Poulsen, O. M. and Hau, J., Homogenization and allergenicity of milk — some possible implications for the processing of infant formulae, *North Eur. Food Dairy J.,* 53, 239, 1987.
9. Girsh, L. S., U. S. Patent, 4,954,361, 1990.
10. Jost, R., Monti, J. C., and Pahud, J. J., Whey protein allergenicity and its reduction by technological means, *Food Technol.,* 41, 118, 1987.
11. Dannenberg, F., Zur Reaktionskinetik der Molkenproteindenaturierung und deren technologischer Bedeutung, Ph.D. thesis, *Technical University, Munich,* 1986.
12. Asselin, J., Hebert, J., and Amiot, J., Effects of *in vitro* proteolysis on the allergenicity of major whey proteins, *J. Food Sci.,* 54, 1037, 1989.
13. Asselin, J., Amiot, J., Gauthier, S., F., Mourad, W., and Hebert, J., Immunogenicity and allergenicity of whey protein hydrolysates, *J. Food Sci.,* 53, 1208, 1988.
14. de Rham, O., European Patent Appl., Societé des Produits Nestlé, EP 0 311 795 Al, 1989.
15. Chiancone, E. and Gattoni, M., Selective extraction of native beta-lactoglobulin from whey, *J. Chromatogr.,* 539, 455, 1991.
16. Akita, E. M. and Nakai, S., Lipophilization of beta-lactoglobulin: effect on allergenicity and digestibility, *J. Food Sci.,* 55, 718, 1990.
17. Burks, A. W., Butler, H., L., Brooks, J., R., Hardin, J., and Connaughton, C., Identification and comparison of differences in antigens in two commercially available soybean protein isolates, *J. Food Sci.,* 53, 1456, 1988.
18. Oste, R. E., Brandon, D. L., Bates, A. H., and Friedman, M., Effect of Maillard browning reactions in the Kunitz soybean trypsin inhibitor on its interaction with monoclonal antibodies, *J. Agric. Food Chem.,* 38, 258, 1990.
19. Doke, S., Nakamura, R., and Torii, S., Allergenicity of food proteins interacted with oxidized lipids in soybean-sensitive individuals, *Agric. Biol. Chem.,* 53, 1231, 1989.
20. Yano, M., Nakamura, R., Hayakawa, S., and Torii, S., Purification and properties of allergenic proteins in buckwheat seeds, *Agric. Biol. Chem.,* 53, 2387, 1989.
21. Watanabe, M., Yoshizawa, T., Miyakawa, J., Ikezawa, Z., Abe, K., Yanagisawa, T., and Arai, S., Quality improvement and evaluation of hypoallergenic rice grains, *J. Food Sci.,* 55, 1105, 1990.
22. Gomez, L., Martin, E., Hernandez, D., Sanchez-Monge, R., Barber, D., del Pozo, V., de Andres, B., Armentia, A., Lahoz, C., Salcedo, G., and Palomino, P., Members of the alpha-amylase inhibitors family from wheat endosperm are major allergen associated with baker's asthma, *FEBS Lett.,* 261, 85, 1990.
23. Menendez-Arias, L., Moneo, I., Dominguez, J., and Rodriguez, R., Primary structure of the major allergen of yellow mustard, *Eur. J. Biochem.,* 177, 159, 1988.
24. Kaegi, M. K. and Wuethrich, B., Falafel-burger anaphylaxis due to sesame seed allergy, *Lancet,* 338, 582, 1991.

25. Maeda, Y., Yamamoto, M., Masui, T., Sugiyama, K., Yokota, M., Okada, N., Sugiyama, K., Katayama, H., and Nakagomi, K., Hyaluronidase inhibitor in the fruit of *Citrus reticulata* Blanco, *Jpn. J. Toxicol. Environ. Health*, 37, 205, 1991.
26. Maeda, Y., Yamamoto, M., Masui, T., Sugiyama, K., Yokota, M., Nakagomi, K., Tanaka, H., Takahashi, I., Kobayashi, T., and Kobayashi, E., Inhibitory effect of tea extracts on hyaluronidase studies on antiallergic activity in tea, *J. Food Hyg. Soc. Jpn.*, 31, 233, 1990.
27. Pose, W., European Patent Appl., EP 0 266 437 Al, 1988.
28. Batt, C., A., Applying biotechnology to dairy processing, *N.Y. Food Life Sci. Q.*, 17, 30, 1987.
29. Wal, J. M., The allergy risk from technologically processed food proteins, *Med. Nutr.*, 27, 133, 1991.
30. Slimak, K. M., PCT International Patent Appl., WO 87/04599 Al, 1987.
31. Wieser, H. and Belitz, H. D., Coeliac active peptides from gliadin: large-scale preparation and characterization, *Z. Lebensm. Unters. Forsch.*, 194, 229, 1992.
32. Kocna, P., Mothes, T., Krchňák, V., and Frič, P., Relationship between gliadin peptide structure and their effect on the fetal chick duodenum, *Z. Lebensm. Unters. Forsch.*, 192, 116, 1991.
33. Hekkens, W. T. J. M. and van Twist de Graaf, M., What is gluten-free — levels and tolerance in the gluten-free diet, *Nahrung*, 34, 483, 1990.
34. Johnson, R. B., Labrooy, J. T., and Skerritt, J. H., Antibody responses reveal differences in oral tolerance to wheat and maize grain protein fractions, *Clin. Exp. Immunol.*, 79, 135, 1990.
35. Hunter, J. O., Food allergy — or enterometabolic disorder?, *Lancet*, 338, 495, 1991.
36. Houts, S. S., Lactose intolerance, *Food Technol.*, 42, 110, 1988.
37. Hussein, L., Elsayed, S., and Foda, S., Reduction of lactose in milk by purified lactase produced by *Kluyveromyces lactis*, *J. Food Protect.*, 52, 30, 1989.
38. Jodl, J. and Obermaier, O., Lactose intolerance, *Prům. Potravin.*, 39, 409, 1988.
39. Gendrel, D., Dupont, C., Richard-Lenoble, D., Gendrel, C., and Chaussain, M., Feeding lactose-intolerant children with a powdered fermented milk, *J. Pediatr. Gastr. Nutr.*, 10, 44, 1990.
40. Patel, R. S., Reuter, H., Prokopek, D., and Sachdeva, S., Manufacture of low-lactose powder using ultrafiltration technology, *Lebensm. Wiss. Technol.*, 24, 338, 1991.
41. Caldwell, M. J., Low-lactose, low-galactose imitation milk product, U.S. Patent 4,511,590, 1985.
42. Lee, C. M. and Hardy, C. M., Cocoa feeding and human lactose intolerance, *Am. J. Clin. Nutr.*, 49, 840, 1989.
43. Marquardt, R. R. and Arbid, M. S. S., Protection against the toxic effect of the favism factor (divicine) in rats by vitamins E, A and C and iron chelating agents, *J. Sci. Food Agric.* 43, 155, 1988.
44. Hussein, L., Motawei, H., Nassib, A., Khalil, S., and Marquardt, R. R., The complete elimination of vicine and convicine from the faba beans by combinations of genetic selection and processing techniques, *Qualitas Plantarum Plant Foods Hum. Nutr.*, 36, 231, 1986.
45. Terts, A., Sarosi S., and Jakab, A., Utilization of broad beans (*Vicia faba*) for food and in canned products, *Konzerv. Paprikaipar*, 4, 152, 1987.
46. Brandon, D. L., Haque, S., and Friedman, M., Interaction of monoclonal antibodies with soybean trypsin inhibitors, *J. Agric. Food Chem.*, 35, 195, 1987.

Chapter 2

Toxins

This chapter covers alkaloids, saponins, glucosinolates, cyanogens, plant phenols, lecithins, toxic amino acids, biogenic amines, marine toxins, mushroom toxins, and other toxic compounds. The part dealing with other toxic compounds includes toxic metals, mineral binding substances, nitrates, and nitrites.

In all parts of this chapter attention is focused on the changes of these compounds during processing and storage and on occurrence of these substances in raw materials and foods. The necessary information about chemistry and toxic effects is also given.

Part A

Alkaloids

Jan Velíšek and Jana Hajšlová

Alkaloids (true alkaloids, pseudoalkaloids, and protoalkaloids) discussed in this chapter are chemical constituents of higher plants that are of value or potentially of value for human nutrition. Glycoalkaloids occur in potato, tomato, and eggplant, which are grown as important vegetables. Quinolizidine alkaloids occur in lupin seeds, which are used as a food crop in South America. Purine alkaloids (stimulants of the central nervous system) are found in coffee, tea, cola beverages, cocoa, and chocolate. Quinine and alkaloids found in black pepper, red pepper, and chili represent important flavor-active ingredients. Tobacco alkaloids are an essential quality factor of commercial tobacco leaves.

No attempt has been made to cover the alkaloids that enter the food chain through livestock poisoning and those that are primarily of pharmaceutical and medicinal interest. Nor has an attempt been made to cover alkaloids accidentally ingested or taken as illicit drugs.

NICOTINE AND OTHER TOBACCO ALKALOIDS

Tobacco is one of the world's major crop plants, often considered a commodity similar to food.

CHEMISTRY

The major alkaloid of commercial tobacco, i.e., cultivars of *Nicotiana tabacum* or *N. rustica,* is nicotine [*S*-1-methyl-2-(3-pyridyl)-pyrrolidine] (Figure 1). Nicotine is always accompanied by three other major alkaloids, nornicotine [2-(3-pyridyl)-pyrrolidine], anatabine [2-(3-pyridyl)-1,2,3,6-tetrahydropyridine], and anabasine [2-(3-pyridyl)-piperidine].[1] More than 20 other minor pyridyl substances have been identified as tobacco constituents (Figure 2).[2-4]

TOXIC EFFECTS

The response of the central nervous system to nicotine is complex. At low doses, it is thought to be a stimulant of the autonomic ganglia and skeletal neuromuscular junctions.

0-8493-4623-1/95/$0.00+$.50

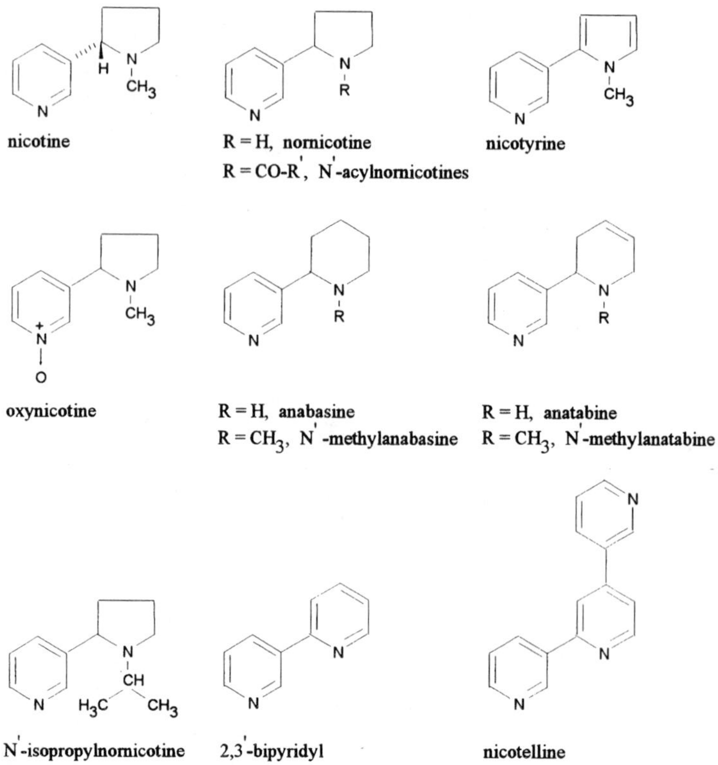

Figure 1 Structures of important tobacco alkaloids, their catabolism, and oxidation products.

Moderate doses cause increased respiratory, vasomotor, and emetic activity, while high doses result in tremors and convulsions. Nicotine may contribute to atherosclerosis by acting on lipid metabolism.[5] Animal susceptibility to the most toxic *Nicotiana* alkaloid nicotine varies between 6 to 30 $mg.kg^{-1}$. In general, *Nicotiana* alkaloids do not have equal toxicity nor the individual isomers of the same alkaloid; (+)- and (–)-nicotine have similar LD_{50} values, (–)-nornicotine is nearly as active as nicotine, (+)-nornicotine is about one-third as active as nicotine, and the (–)-anabasine LD_{50} value is 65% of that of nicotine.[6] Anabasine is a teratogenic compound, and it is speculated that anatabine could also possess teratogenic activity.[7] Acute physiologic and chronic pathologic responses of the respiratory tract to environmental tobacco smoke have been recently reviewed.[8]

OCCURRENCE

Although nicotine is most commonly associated with tobacco, it is one of the most widely distributed alkaloids, having been identified in 24 genera (12 families) of plants. Notably, it also occurs in tomato (*Licopersicum esculentum*) (page 30). The total alkaloid content of *N. tabacum* and *N. rustica* ranges from about 0.3 to 3% dry weight, depending on species in the genus, variety, plant part, environmental influences (primarily water availability, nitrogen fertility, temperature, and light), and other factors. For example, *N. tabacum* leaves containing 1.918% total alkaloids (dry weight) had 1.850% nicotine, 0.035% anatabine, 0.028% nornicotine, and 0.005% anabasine.[9] Most of the minor tabacco alkaloids are present in less than 0.005% dry weight and many are present in even lower amounts as aberrant metabolism and catabolic products.[1]

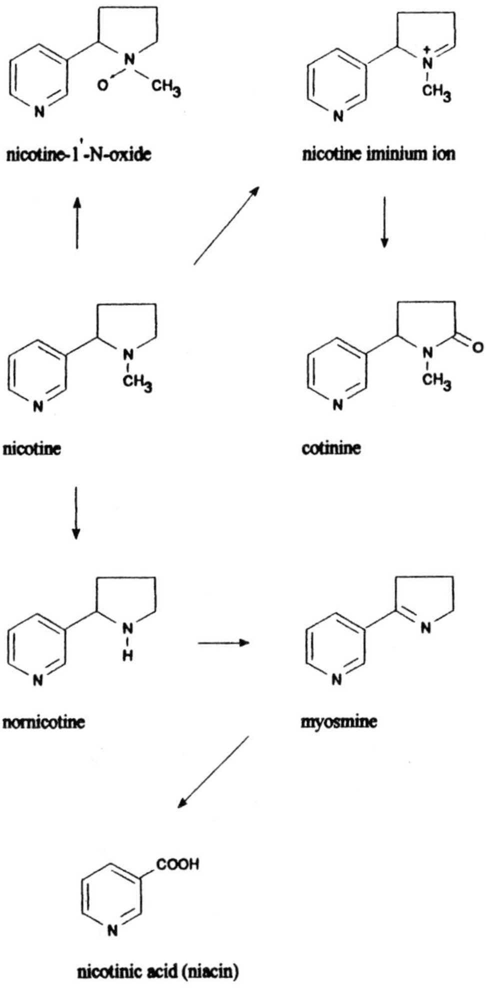

Figure 2 Major pathways of nicotine catabolism on curing.

CHANGES DURING PROCESSING AND STORAGE

The nicotine and total alkaloid content of green leaves slightly decreases during postharvest processing such as curing and drying. Sun-cured (oriental), flue-cured (Virginia), burley, air-cured, fire-cured, and other tobacco types differ in their alkaloid content. Nornicotine is produced from nicotine by transmethylation of the *N*-methyl group[10,11] and partly decomposed to nicotinic acid via myosmine (Figure 2); anabasine and anatabine probably result as catabolic products of these alkaloids.

Nicotine is mainly ingested via tobacco smoke. Tobacco legislation requires definition of the maximum amount of nicotine per cigarette and its level in the smoke of different cigarette brands. The smoke of one cigarette contains about 1 to 2 mg of nicotine, but only 0.1 to 1.0 mg in new mild cigarette brands.[12] During the burning of tobacco, nicotine is partially oxidized to cotinine and oxynicotine, the latter compound being unstable at higher temperatures and decomposing rapidly to other compounds.[13] The pyrolytic decomposition of nicotine also yields hydrogen cyanide.[14] Its content in the smoke of one cigarette varies between 0.004 to 0.270 mg (page 229). Nitrogen oxides (NO_x) produced during the burning of tobacco react with nicotine decomposition products giving rise to volatile nitrosamines (page 229). About 1.7 to 115 ng of volatile nitrosamines is produced from 1 g of tobacco.[15] The precursors of nonvolatile nitrosamines (so-called tobacco-specific nitrosamines) are mainly nornicotine, anabasine, and anatabine. Nicotine itself is a precursor of 4-(methylnitrosoamino)-1-(3-pyridyl)-1-butanone,[16-18] and nitrosonornicotine is formed during tobacco curing.[19]

QUINOLIZIDINE ALKALOIDS OF LUPINS

Since antiquity, lupins have been known as valuable grain legumes. Several species of lupins, such as *Lupinus albus*, *L. luteus*, and *L. angustifolius*, have been cultivated in Europe, Africa, and Australia, and *L. mutabilis* (tarhui or tarwi) is an important component of the diet of South American Indians. The lupin also represents one of the most interesting and valuable oilseed crops in regions of temperate climate.[20-23] Both as food and feed, the serious drawback of lupins has been their content of bitter, poisonous alkaloids occurring in both plant and seed. Other antinutritional and toxic factors reported include a very modest antitryptic activity (page 97), a saponin (page 45) content similar to that in soybeans (1.1 to 1.7%), and practically no lectin (page 95). The combined level of vicine and convicine (page 11) in lupin flour ranged from 6 to 7%.[24]

CHEMISTRY

The alkaloids of *Lupinus* species are usually bicyclic, tricyclic, and tetracyclic quinolizidines. The bicyclic alkaloids are typified by (–)-lupinine, the tricyclics by angustifoline, and the tetracyclic series by (–)-sparteine. The tetracyclic alkaloid lupanine (Figure 3), its hydroxy derivatives, and their esters with benzoic, cinnamic, angelic, and other acids occur in most lupins. Nearly 70 different compounds have been found.[20-23] For example, the major alkaloids of *L. angustifolius* cultivars are angustifoline, α-isolupanine, lupanine, and 13-hydroxylupanine (Figure 3), which account for more than 95% of the alkaloid content of this variety. Eight other minor alkaloids have been identified.[25] More than 25 alkaloids (lupanine was the major constituent) were found as components of *L. mutabilis* seeds,[26] and *L. luteus* seeds contained sparteine and lupinine as the major alkaloids.[27]

TOXIC EFFECTS

Quinolizidine alkaloids produce malaise, nausea, respiratory arrest, visual disturbances, diaphoresis, progresive weakness, or coma. The individual alkaloids vary considerably in toxicity, with lupanine and sparteine being the most toxic lupin alkaloids reported and 13-hydroxylupanine only one-tenth as toxic.[20-22] An oral dose ranging from 11 to 25 $mg.kg^{-1}$ of lupin alkaloids could result in serious consequences.[28] An average daily intake of 60 g of *L. albus* flour containing less than 0.02% alkaloid did not result in any significant changes in the main physiological indicators in blood.[29]

OCCURRENCE

The alkaloid level of lupin seeds varies depending on a number of genetic and environmental factors. In the bitter varieties of *L. angustifolius* the alkaloid content can be as high as 2 to 3%. The industry is based primarily on the sweet white seeded cultivars of *L. angustifolius*, which have less than 0.02% alkaloid. However, it has been observed that the sweet cultivars may vary in alkaloid content up to 0.2%. Climatic stress and nutritient availability may be factors that contribute to this phenomenon.[23,25]

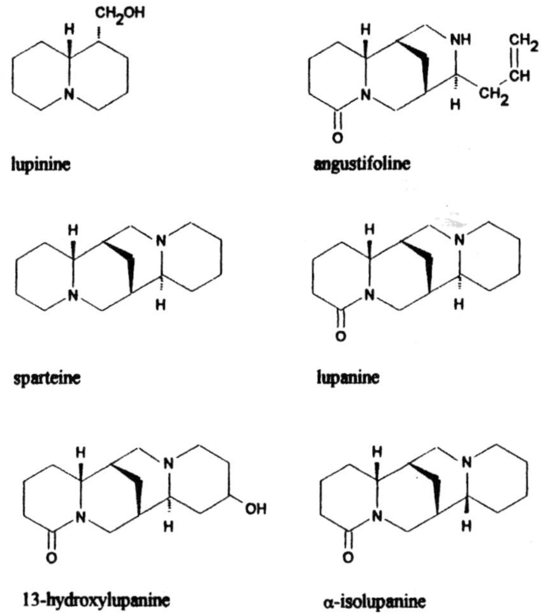

Figure 3 Major alkaloids of domesticated lupins.

CHANGES DURING PROCESSING AND STORAGE

Populations in many parts of Europe, Africa, and South America have learned through the ages to debitter lupin grains. Lupin alkaloids are water soluble; therefore the seeds can be rid of bitterness by soaking, boiling, and leaching. For example, debitter the seeds of *L. termis* by presoaking in water (1:5 v/v) for 5 h, boil for 30 min, and wash the cooked seeds with running water for 48 h almost completely removes alkaloids. Flours prepared from raw and debittered seeds had alkaloid levels of 1.52 and 0.01%, respectively.[30]

Lowering the alkaloid hazard of lupin foods is achieved by plant breeding (by selection of new cultivars of plants) and physicochemical techniques such as extraction with aqueous and organic solvents.

The oil content of lupins is low, except in the case of *L. mutabilis* (where oil content ranges up to 22 to 24% dry weight).[23] Processing lupins to oil and meal is similar to the processing of soybeans (flaking, solvent extraction of oil, and desolventizing the meal). A minor part of lupin seed alkaloids is extracted together with the oil during conventional extraction with hexane, and a major part of the alkaloids is retained in the defatted lupin flakes. Approximately 60% of alkaloids was extracted with hexane from lupin flour treated with potassium hydroxide prior to extraction.[31] Subsequently the alkaloids are removed from the oil by refining. For example, the refining, including debittering the oil by washing with diluted acids, decreased the alkaloid level from 0.14% in the raw oil to 0.0005% in the end product. The oil alkaloids were not identical with those of the seeds. In seeds, lupanine was the major alkaloid, while in the oil, 13-hydroxylupanine and *N*-methyl angustifoline were dominant.[32]

Debittering the hexane-defatted flakes or, alternatively, simultaneous extraction of oil and alkaloids from full-fat cakes or flour and/or preparing protein concentrates and isolates is a way to obtain a sweet and nontoxic product. Products with only 0.5 to 0.002% alkaloid levels have been obtained.[21,22]

Ethanol represents one of the solvents most frequently used both for debittering defatted lupin flakes and for the combined extraction of oil and alkaloids. The extraction efficiency of ethanol and its aqueous mixtures further improves by adding hydrochloric acid to the solvent. For example, hexane-defatted flakes containing 3.2% alkaloid were extracted with 80% ethanol, and protein concentrates having only 0.1 to 0.2% alkaloid were obtained.[33]

QUININE

Quinine, except for its medicinal use (as hydrochloride, hydrogen sulfate, or sulfate) as an antimalaricum and antipyreticum, is generally accepted as the standard for bitter taste (the detection threshold for quinine hydrochloride is about 10 $mg.dm^{-3}$) and is widely used as a bittering agent in beverages.

CHEMISTRY

The pure base of quinine (Figure 4) and its salts decompose on standing under the influence of acids and especially of light (photochemical reaction). Toxic quinotoxine (quinicine; Figure 4) forms on heating quinine/organic acid solutions and even during storage of pharmaceutical preparations containing quinine and organic acids such as acetylsalicylic acid.[34] The main product of the photochemical degradation in acid solutions is 9-deoxyquinine,[35] but 6-methoxyquinoline and 5-vinylquinuclidine-2-carboxaldehyde are formed in neutral solutions[36] (Figure 4).

TOXIC EFFECTS

Quinine is a strong protoplasmatic toxin inhibiting various enzymatic reactions. Its use (with respect to various secondary reactions) is regulated, and soft drink regulations require examination for quinine. The acceptable daily intake (ADI) of quinine hydrochloride for an adult is 40 mg. A dose of 200 $mg.kg^{-1}$ per day had no indications of teratogenic effects.[37]

OCCURRENCE

Quinine is the major alkaloid of the quinoline type from the bark of *Cinchona officinalis* and related trees, where it represents about 70% of the total alkaloids that occur at a level of 5 to 8%.[38] Biosynthesis of the *Cinchona* alkaloids has been studied by Battersby et al.[39]

Quinine is permitted as an additive, as a bittering agent, in carbonated beverages such as Indian or quinine tonic water and in soft drinks falling mainly in the category bitter orange or bitter lemon, which have a basis of fruit juice or comminuted fruit. Tonic water is required to contain about 60 $mg.dm^{-3}$ quinine (minimum amount), and bitter lemon beverages contain approximately 30 $mg.dm^{-3}$ quinine. The saccharin present provides a synergistic bitter taste.[40]

CHANGES DURING PROCESSING AND STORAGE

In commercial beverages exposed to full sunlight, the original quinine level of 50 $mg.dm^{-3}$ decreased to 13.5 $mg.dm^{-3}$ after 1 h, and after 3 h only traces of quinine were detected; no quinine was found after 6 h of irradiation.[41] The decrease of quinine concentrations is accompanied by the loss of the typical bitter taste and blue opalescence. Long-term storage under indirect daylight may lead to similar changes. Quinine loss in brown glass bottles was much less (47 and 21.5 $mg.dm^{-3}$ were found after 6 and 30 h of irradiation, respectively). Artificial light had almost no effect. The rate of quinine decomposition was also influenced by temperature, pH, and other factors (in nonaroma-containing beverages, the quinine concentration decreased less rapidly). The main product of the photochemical

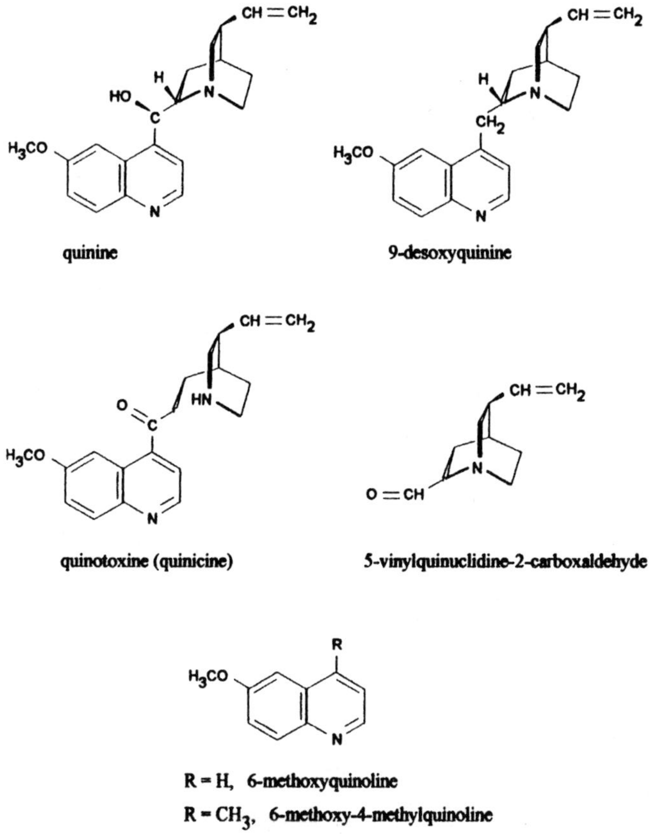

Figure 4 Structures of quinine and its decomposition products.

reaction is 6-methoxy-4-methylquinoline (Figure 4); the intermediary product of quinine decomposition was probably 9-deoxyquinine.

PIPERINE AND RELATED ALKALOIDS

Piperine is a major pungent principal, first isolated from black pepper berries (*Piper nigrum*) oleoresin, and later from other *Piper* species and other plants.

CHEMISTRY

Piperine, the piperidine amide of piperic acid or (*E,E*)-5-(1,3-benzodioxo-5-yl)-*N*-piperidinyl-2, 4-pentadienamide, is usually accompanied by three other geometric isomers (Figure 5), named chavicine, isochavicine, and isopiperine, which show little or no pungency. Several other flavor-active compounds of similar structure occur as chemical constituents of pepper berries.[42-45]

TOXIC EFFECTS

Piperine acts as a central nervous stimulant and possesses a slight antipyretic and a weak mutagenic activity. At higher levels it damages lung tissue and decreases blood pressure and respiration rate. Other related piperidine derivatives, including piperidine itself, are responsible for the irritant, antimicrobial, and insecticidal properties of *P. nigrum*.[42-45]

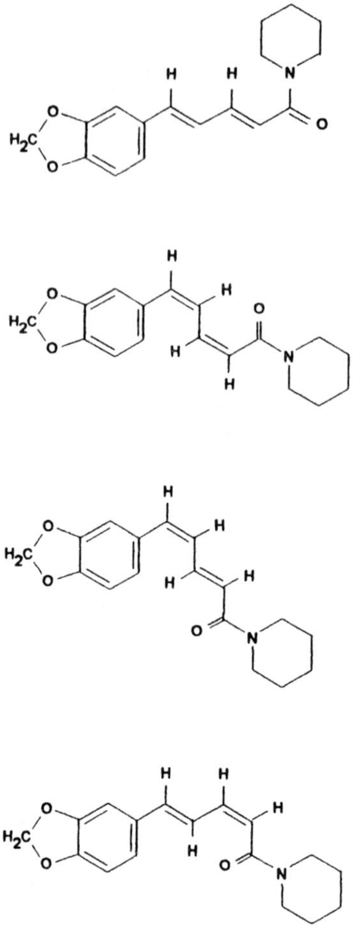

piperine

(trans, trans or E, E)

chavicine

(cis, cis or Z, Z)

isochavicine

(trans, cis or E, Z)

isopiperine

(cis, trans or Z, E)

Figure 5 Structures of piperine and its geometrical isomers.

The pharmacology of piperine, its physiological effects, and its metabolism have been recently studied in several laboratories.[46-49]

OCCURRENCE

The level of piperine in a berry of *P. nigrum* reaches a maximum just before maturity. Green pepper products prepared from the immature berries therefore have quite a high piperine content. White pepper is prepared from the ripe berries with mellow flavor, which have a lower piperine content. Since the skin is removed during processing and piperine is concentrated in the endosperm of the pepper berry, white pepper has a very high piperine content.[42]

Piperine represents 90 to 95% of the alkaloids present in black pepper. For example, Sri Lankan peppers have a very high piperine content (7 to 15%), two- to sixfold that of commercial Indian, Malaysian, and other varieties (2 to 7%).[50] The piperine content of pepper extracts is 27 to 72%.[51,52]

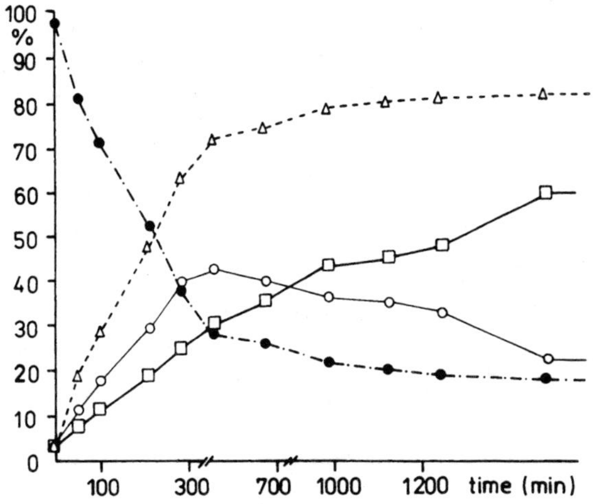

Figure 6 UV irradiation-induced isomerization of piperine dissolved in ethanol. ●, piperine; ○, chavicine; □, isochavicine and isopiperine; △, *cis* isomers together. (From Glasl, H., *Dtsch. Lebensm.-Rdsch.*, 80, 148, 1984. With permision.)

CHANGES DURING PROCESSING AND STORAGE

Piperine in solution undergoes photochemical reaction under the influence of light and ultraviolet (UV) irradiation to give a mixture of chavicine, isochavicine, and isopiperine.[53] An ethanolic solution irradiated for 10 h and then stored for 14 h in the dark contained approximately 18% piperine, 22% chavicine, and 60% isochavicine/isopiperine (Figure 6). Retention of 90% piperine was observed on exposure of piperine solutions to daylight. A dimer was obtained when a suspension of piperine was irradiated.[42] In the dark no isomerization proceeded even at a temperature of 55°C.[52] γ-Irradiation had no effect on piperine isomerization.[54] Piperine is stable during storage even after 6 months in paper bags and 10 months in aluminum foil-lined paper.[55]

Piperine gives piperic acid salts and piperidine on alkaline hydrolysis. Under slightly acidic conditions at 37°C it reacts with nitrites, forming carcinogenic nitrosamines (page 229).[56]

STEROIDAL GLYCOALKALOIDS

Steroidal glycoalkaloids (GA) are natural toxins found in plants from the *Solanaceae* family, which also includes several food crops, such as potatoes, tomatoes, and eggplants.

GLYCOALKALOIDS OF POTATOES

Chemistry

These compounds typically consist of a nonpolar, lipophilic steroidal aglycone possessing a C27 framework of cholestan with a nitrogen heterocyclic moiety and a polar water-soluble oligosaccharide portion (comprising up to five monosaccharide units) attached via glycosidic linkage.[57-62] The most important GA of tuber-bearing *Solanum* species are divided into five groups according to the structure of aglycone as given in Table 1. Although the toxic organic base was found in common potatoes in the last century, the fact that solanine is composed of two major components belonging to solanidine series α-solanine and α-chaconine (Figure 7) was revealed as late as in the middle of the 20th

Table 1 Composition of Glycoalkaloids of Tuber-Bearing *Solanum* Species

Glycoalkaloid	Sugar	Glycoside structure
Solanidine glycosides		
α-Solanine	Solatriosa	*R*–Gal < Rham, Glu
β-Solanine	Solabiose	*R*–Gal–Glu
γ-Solanine	Galactose	*R*–Gal
α-Chaconine	Chacotriose	*R*–Glu < Rham, Rham
β-Chaconine	Chacobiose	*R*–Glu–Rham
γ-Chaconine	Glucose	*R*–Glu
Dehydrocommersonine	Commertetraose	*R*–Glu < Glu, Glu
Solasodine glycosides		
Solasonine	Solatriose	*R*–Gal < Rham, Rham
Solamargine	Chacotriose	*R*–Glu < Rham, Rham
Tomatidine glycosides		
Tomatine	Lycotetrose	*R*–Gal–Glu < Glu, Xyl
Sisunine	Commertetraose	*R*–Gal–Glu < Glu, Glu
Demissidine glycosides		
Demissine	Lycotetrose	*R*–Gal–Glu < Glu, Xyl
Commersonine	Commereteraose	*R*–Gal–Glu < Glu, Glu
Leptinidine glycosides		
Leptinine I	Chacotriose	–Glu < Rham, Rham
Leptinine II	Solatriose	*R*–Gal < Rham, Glu
Acetylleptinidine glycosides		
Leptine I	Chacotriose	*R*–Glu < Rham, Rham
Leptine II	Solatriose	*R*–Gal < Rham, Glu

Note: Gal = D-galaktose, Glu = D-glukose, Xyl = D-xylose, Rham = L-rhamnose.

Adapted from Jadhav, S. J., Sharma, R. P., and Salunkhe, D. K., *CRC Crit. Rev. Toxicol.*, 5, 21, 1981.

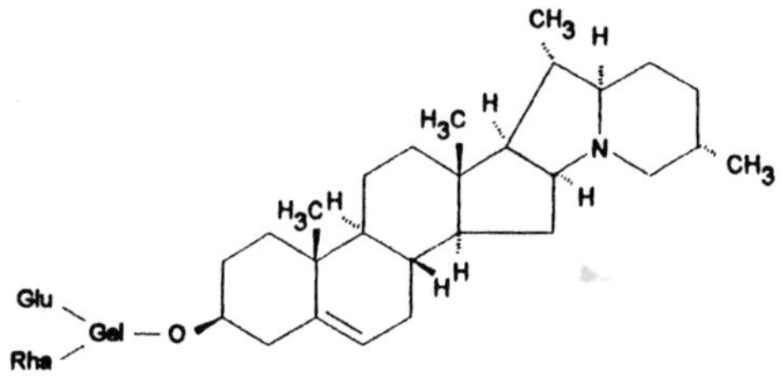

α-solanine

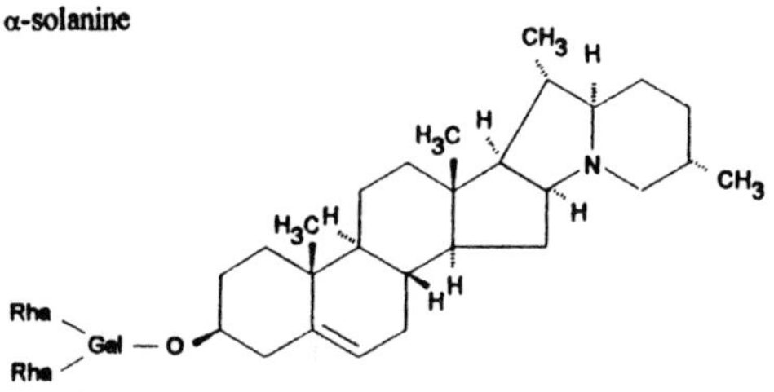

α-chaconine

Figure 7 Structures of α-solanine and α-chaconine. Glu, glucose; Gal, galactose; and Rha, rhamnose.

century. In commercial varieties these two substances represent as much as 95% of the total GA content. α-Solanine varies from 28 to 57% of solanine. Occasionally β and γ forms possessing shorter carbohydrate chains (Table 1) can be found, and free solanidine was occasionally reported to be present in bitter potatoes. Traces of other types of steroidal alkaloids such as α- and β-solamarine and/or demissidine sometimes occur in cultivated tubers.[63,64]

Toxic Effects

While many cases of GA poisoning of both livestock and domestic animals have been reported for several *Solanaceae* plants, only potato glycoalkaloids — so called solanine have been involved in recorded poisonings of humans. Typical clinical symptoms (latent period 2 to 20 h) include nausea, vomiting, diarrhea, severe stomach cramps, headache, and dizziness.[65,66]

Based on experiments with laboratory animals, solanine appears to have two toxic actions. The first of them was shown to be inhibition of blood and brain cholinesterases (EC 3.1.1.13). The other toxic effect is concerned with disruption and injury of membranes in the gastrointestinal tract and elsewhere.[67,68] Hemorrhagic and hemolytic damage results from exposure to high doses of this toxin. No carcinogenity data exist for these compounds.[69] A teratogenic effect on experimental animals was described for high doses of this compound.[70-73] A weight per day, no-observed-effect level (NOEL) has not been established. For legislative purposes the upper safety limit of 200 $mg.kg^{-1}$of whole raw (unpeeled) potato has been widely accepted. It is important to note that the dose-response curve for the effect of solanine in man is quite steep.

Occurrence

The distribution of GA within the *Solanum tuberosum* plant is very uneven with the highest concentration in parts with high metabolic activity: up to 5,000 $mg.kg^{-1}$ fresh weight of GA was found in flowers, and levels ranging from 1,950 to 4,360 $mg.kg^{-1}$ were reported for potato sprouts.[74,75] Table 2 shows a typical distribution of solanine in tubers.

Table 2 Typical Distribution of Glycoalkaloids in Potato Tuber

Part of tuber	Content of glycoalkaloids ($mg.kg^{-1}$ fresh weight)
Whole tuber	75
Skin (2–3% of tuber weight)	300–600
Peel (10–15% of tuber weight)	150–300
Peel and eye (3-mm disk)	300–500
Flesh	12–50

Adapted from Wood, F. A. and Young, D. A., *Agric. Canada Publ.* 1533, 1974. With permission.

Similar results were obtained by Kozukue et al.,[76] who determined levels of α-solanine and α-chaconine in tissue slices prepared from May Queen and Irish Cobbler potatoes. In the first cultivar, 2,907 $mg.kg^{-1}$ α-solanine (95.8% of total) and 2,580 $mg.kg^{-1}$ α-chaconine (99.8%) were contained within the first 1 mm of the outside surface; in the other cultivar these values were 2,790 $mg.kg^{-1}$ α-solanine (96.4%) and 2,580 $mg.kg^{-1}$ of α-chaconine (98.4%), respectively. The GA content significantly decreased toward the center, and only traces of toxins were found in slices taken 4 to 5 mm below the surface.

GA levels and individual GA composition are largely under genetic control. Concentrations of solanine in most commercial cultivars from around the world do not exceed levels of 200 $mg.kg^{-1}$.[77-79] However, as demonstrated later, interaction between variety and environment under some conditions including physiologic factors may lead to the accumulation of toxins.

Several wild tuber–bearing *Solanum* species, together with those cultivated in South America, are being used in breeding program to introduce desirable genes for resistance against disease, insects, and frost, and improved yield, quality, etc. This practice should be carried out with caution since unwanted properties can be transferred in this way as well (e.g., in wild tuber–bearing species 5 to 10 times higher levels of GA compared to *S. tuberosum* could be present). For example, the potato cultivar Lenape had an unusual ancestor, *Solanum chacoense,* which was used for breeding not only for improved yield, but also for attainment of a higher content of solids and lower levels of reducing sugars, as needed for the production of good french fries and having good storage quality. However, very high GA levels were detected (up to 350 $mg.kg^{-1}$ in tubers harvested in Canada and even 650 $mg.kg^{-1}$ in the U.S.), so it had to be quickly withdrawn in both countries.[80]

In addition to α-solanine and α-chaconine, other types of GA not commonly associated with commercial cultivars were also detected in various *Solanum* species, e.g., in some clones of *S. chacoense,* leptines (acetylated forms of current GA).[81] In addition to leptines, demissine or tomatine is synthesized by *S. demissum* and *S. polyadenium. Solanum demissum* and *S. acaule,* instead of solanine, contain only demissine and tomatine, respectively.[82] Solamargine and solasonine as well as α- and β-solamarine represent other unusual GA forms reported in wild tubers.[83] The latter GA, solamarines, were found in wound-healed tissues of Kennebec tubers. It was postulated that the ability to synthesize these foreign GA was inherited from an *S. demissum* ancestor. As to the recent findings, concern during breeding should also be focused on the ratio of α-chaconine and α-solanine.[84] Cultivars containing a higher portion of less toxic α-solanine ought to be preferred.

Environmental conditions such as climate, soil type, and soil moisture, as well as agricultural practices including fertilization, application of pesticides, time of harvest, etc., considerably affect the level of GA.[82] Exposure of tubers to sunlight or mechanical

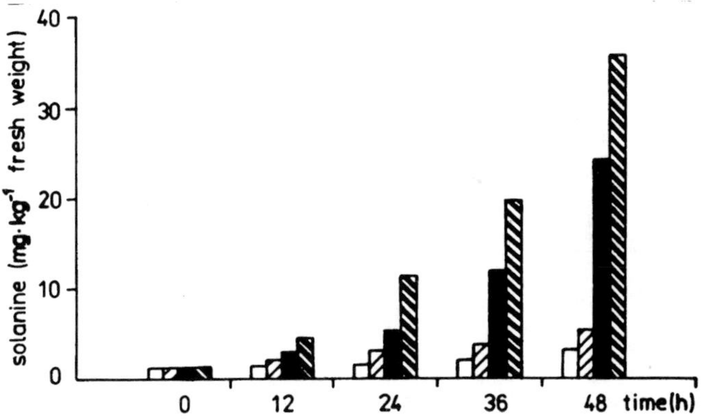

Figure 8 Effect of light exposure on solanine formation in potato slices at different temperatures. □, 0°C; ▨, 8°C; ■, 15°C; ▧, 24°C. (Adapted from Salunkhe, D. F., Wu, T. M., and Jadhav, J. S., *J. Food Sci.*, 37, 969, 1972. With permission.)

damage may also contribute to an increase in GA content. It should be emphasized that within a single variety of potato large variations in GA levels within various growing seasons can occur. Differences exist even in the levels of these toxins among tubers from individual plants. A higher GA content is typical of a cool season with a large number of overcast days.[85] In principle, small immature tubers have a higher content of GA. This is mainly due to the fact that the toxins are biosynthesized at an early stage of development and thus under unfavorable conditions, i.e., when the normal bulking and maturation process is inhibited, the GA content per unit weight is higher.

Exposure of potatoes to light results in development of green pigmentation on their surface, caused by the synthesis of chlorophyll. This so-called greening phenomenon is typically associated with elevated levels of GA. An increased content of toxins corresponds to the intensity of light and is related to the duration of exposure.[85,86] Levels of GA as high as 200 $mg.kg^{-1}$ were found[87] in tubers exposed to sunlight for 6 h with an original content of 50 $mg.kg^{-1}$. Similarly, a rapid increase of solanine during light exposure was reported in many other studies.[88-90] The amount of GA reached 450 $mg.kg^{-1}$when tubers were left in the field at low temperatures for 72 h. Tubers as well as raw potato products may be exposed to artificial light during storage and processing.[91] Stimulation of solanine formation (although not as dramatic as in the case of sunlight) may occur. The extent of this biosynthetic process depends on the character of the light: short wavelengths at the blue end of the spectrum encourage GA formation, while longer wavelengths (yellow and red) induce chlorophyll synthesis.[91-94] Figure 8 shows the effect of light exposure (18.5 lux) on GA levels in potato slices stored at different temperatures. Rapid *de novo* synthesis of solanine after an initial induction period was observed in potato tissue at higher temperatures. Some increase of GA levels occurred also in slices stored in the dark, but this process was less extensive.[95]

The formation and accumulation of abnormal metabolites in plant tissues is a well-recognized response to either mechanical injury or various diseases. This fact can be regarded as a typical phenomenon involved in a physiological defense mechanism. In general, higher levels of solanine are found in both peels and flesh of tubers injured by bruising and/or mechanical grading in the postharvest period. Inherent initial GA levels for individual varieties and breeding clones must also be considered.[96-99]

Figures 9 and 10 show the effects of various mechanical injuries of tubers stored for several days under low and ambient temperature. It is evident that higher temperatures

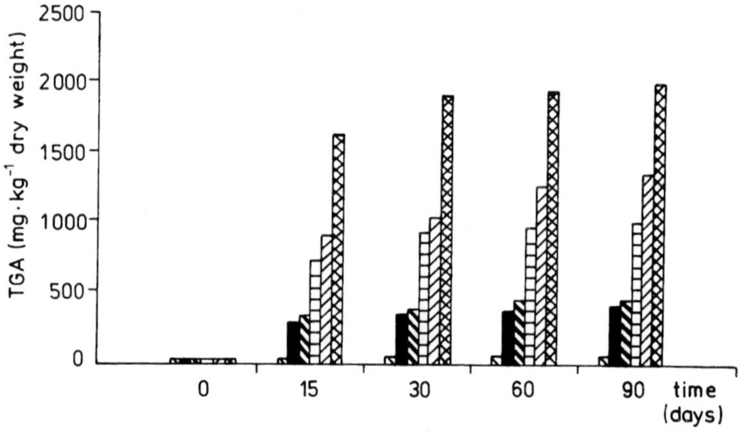

Figure 9 Effects of mechanical injuries on glycoalkaloid content of flesh during storage at 4°C. TGA, total steroidal glycoalkaloids; ▧, control; ■, brushing; ▧, hammering; ▤, dropping; ▨, puncturing; ▩, cutting. (Adapted from Salunkhe, D. F., Wu, T. M., and Jadhav, J. S., *J. Food Sci.*, 37, 969, 1972. With permission.)

stimulated more GA formation, with the highest increase occurring in both flesh and peels that have been cut (after 15 d, 77 and 88%, respectively).[100]

Changes During Processing and Storage

Because potatoes are consumed in a processed form, several investigations were conducted to obtain information about the stability of GA under conditions commonly used in practice.

As was shown earlier,[75,76] peeling removes a considerable part of GA, the final effect depending not only on the proportion of peel in relation to the weight of the intact tuber (the use of an ordinary manual household peeler results in 10 to 15% weight reduction), but also on the original GA content. It is well known that little or no GA is found in pits and in the intermediate region. According to most studies, only 4 to 40% of the original GA remains in peeled tubers, but this ratio is markedly higher if potatoes contain larger amount of GA. This was documented by Hellenas et al.,[101] who observed only a 14% decrease in GA levels in peeled Magnum Bonum potatoes, with solanine content in whole tubers 785 mg.kg^{-1}.

Many studies in the past decade have focused on potential heat-induced changes occurring in the course of household and/or industrial processing. GA stability during frying, baking, microwaving, and boiling was investigated by Bushway et al.[102] GA were stable during all these processes except frying, where a slight loss of GA was recorded. An increase of GA in fried potato chips (from 40 to 150 mg.kg^{-1} in products from peeled potatoes and from 40 to 250 mg.kg^{-1} in unpeeled potatoes) that was reported by Sizer and Maga et al.[103] can be attributed to dehydration of the raw material. The detailed study by Bushway et al.[104] was concerned with the GA content in products prepared from potato peel. This product, obtained from restaurants and retail markets, was shown to be a source of large quantities of toxins. In laboratory experiments raw peels of several commercial varieties containing 13 to 566 mg.kg^{-1} α-chaconine and 5 to 501 mg.kg^{-1} α-solanine were cooked by baking and frying. The two types of fried peels contained more α-chaconine (218.0 to 928.2 mg.kg^{-1} cooked peel) and α-solanine (109 to 721 mg.kg^{-1} cooked peel).The effects of peeling on total GA, total phenols, and sensory properties were

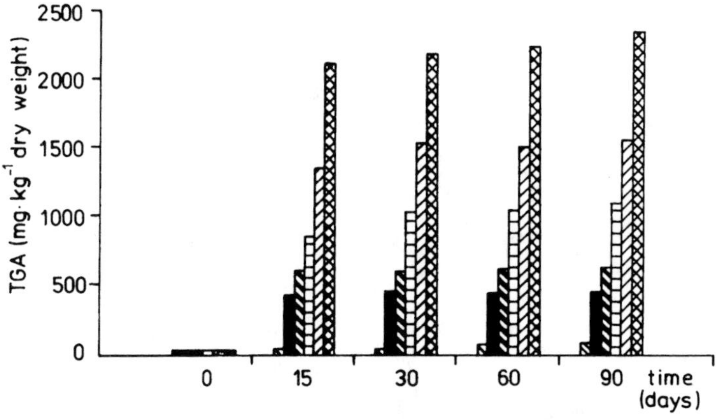

Figure 10 Effect of mechanical injuries on glycoalkaloid content of flesh during storage at 21°C. TGA, total steroidal glycoalkaloids; ▧, control; ■, brushing; ▧, hammering; ▤, dropping; ▨, puncturing; ▩, cutting. (Adapted from Salunkhe, D. F., Wu,T. M., and Jadhav, J. S., *J. Food Sci.*, 37, 969, 1972. With permission.)

studied by Mondy et al.[105,106] Three alternate ways of cooking potatoes were examined: boiling in distilled water, boiling in 16% NaCl, and steaming. The results are summarized in Table 3. In all three experiments, potatoes cooked with the peel contained considerably higher levels of solanine compared to those cooked without the surface layer. Increased levels of GA in the cortex tissue in the case of unremoved peel indicate some degree of migration into this region. However, no significant differences were recorded in the GA content in internal parts of cooked tubers. In all the cooking methods the content of GA exceeded that found in an uncooked control. This can be explained by a loss of water during such processing. The fact that boiling is ineffective as a mean of reducing the GA content was confirmed also by Japanese authors.[107] A slight decrease in toxins occurred only during microwaving in peeled potatoes cut into cubes of 5 to 10 mm^3: after 2 min 86% of original α-chaconine and 84% of α-solanine remained. When cubes of the same size were deep fried at 150°C for 5 min, the GA content did not change, but at 170°C potatoes showed a large variation in residual GA (69.7 to 98.6% for α-chaconine and 65.7 to 88.8% for α-solanine). Temperatures around 170°C were suggested as critical for decomposition of both GA. At 210°C the levels of α-chaconine were lowered after 10 min by 35%; for α-solanine this decrease was 40%. These results correspond with studies reporting decomposition of GA close to their melting points, which range from 230 to 280°C (steroidal aglycones are still stable at these temperatures).

The sensory characteristics of potato GA have been investigated quite thoroughly. Levels exceeding approximately 150 $mg.kg^{-1}$ give an unpleasant flavor to cooked potatoes. An immediate bitter taste lasting about 1 min and followed by a strong burning sensation in the throat lasting for more than 5 min is associated with eating tubers containing levels around 200 $mg.kg^{-1}$.The unpleasant taste sensation is a natural warning that the potatoes are not safe for consumption. It should be noted that salt, oil, and several other ingredients may mask the bitterness and also the hazard.[108]

The data concerning changes in solanine during storage are rather conflicting. Several studies report elevated GA levels in potatoes stored at low temperatures. As shown in Table 4 (and in accordance with several other studies), optimal storage conditions to prevent GA formation correspond to high temperatures and low air humidity.[109-112]

Table 3 Glycoalkaloid Content in Katahdin and Lemhi Potatoes Cooked With and Without Peel

	Katahdin (mg.kg^{-1})		Lemhi (mg.kg^{-1})	
	A	B	A	B
Cortex				
Uncooked	107.6	26.4	78.4	20.6
Water	123.5	34.4	88.0	20.8
Salt	130.6	34.3	88.7	21.0
Steam	130.0	34.6	92.7	21.1
Internal tissue				
Uncooked	6.9	6.9	6.2	6.2
Water	7.6	7.2	6.4	6.4
Salt	7.7	7.2	6.4	6.3
Steam	8.0	7.3	6.8	6.6

Note: A, cooked with peel; B, cooked without peel.

Adapted from Mondy, N. I. and Gosselin, B., *J. Food Sci.* 53, 3, 1988. With permission.

GLYCOALKALOIDS OF TOMATOES

Chemistry

More than 50 years ago tomatine was recognized as an allelochemical agent imparting antimicrobial properties to juice expressed from tomato plants. Since then several attempts have been made to correlate its levels with disease resistance.[113-117] α-Tomatine (Figure 11) is a steroidal glycoalkaloid consisting of an aglycone moiety tomatidine to which is attached the branched tetrasaccharide β-lycotetraose in the C3 position.

Toxic Effects

Limited data are available on the toxicity of tomatine found in immature tomatoes. Similarly to solanine, this GA possesses surfactant properties. The toxic property of tomatine is often attributed to its binding to membrane 3-β-hydroxy sterols (such as cholesterol) and consequent destabilization of the lipid bilayer.[118] More work is still required to elucidate the risk for humans resulting from exposure to tomatine.

Occurrence

α-Tomatine appears to be restricted in its taxonomic distribution to the genera *Solanum* and *Lycopersicon.*[119] While in the genus *Solanum* it is mostly accompanied by other GA. In the genus *Lycopersicon* this compound is usually the only representative of this group of substances. Occasionally, products of partial hydrolysis lacking either xylose or one glucose (called β1-, β2-, and γ-tomatine, respectively) have been isolated from certain commercial varieties and mutants of *Lycopersicon esculentum.*[120,121] With the exception of dormant seeds, tomatine can be detected in all parts of the tomato plant. Shoots are the main site where GA accumulate, with the highest level occurring in leaves in the flowers and young fruit considerable differences exist in the tomatine content. Many of these varieties appear to be attributable to such factors as the variety of plant, stage of development, time of season, and seasonal conditions. The following discussion is focused on dynamics of tomatine in tomato fruit due to its importance for human consumption.

In contrast to potatoes, GA formation in tomatoes is a temporary phenomenon and the high tomatine levels that could be hazardous for humans are associated with the early stages of development.[122,123] In an extensive study conducted by Eltayeb and Roddick,[124,125]

Table 4 Effect of Various Storage Conditions on Glycoalkaloid Content of Netted Gem Potatoes ($mg.kg^{-1}$)

Storage time (weeks)	Storage in dark at 4–8°C (cold, humid)	Storage in dark at 12–15°C (warm, dry)
1	79.3	75.0
2	56.3	79.6
3	113.0	35.2
4	137.5	57.8
5	110.9	40.1
6	154.2	87.2
Average	*108.6*	*62.6*

Adapted from Zitnak, A., Master's Thesis, University of Alberta, Edmonton, Canada, 1952. With permission.

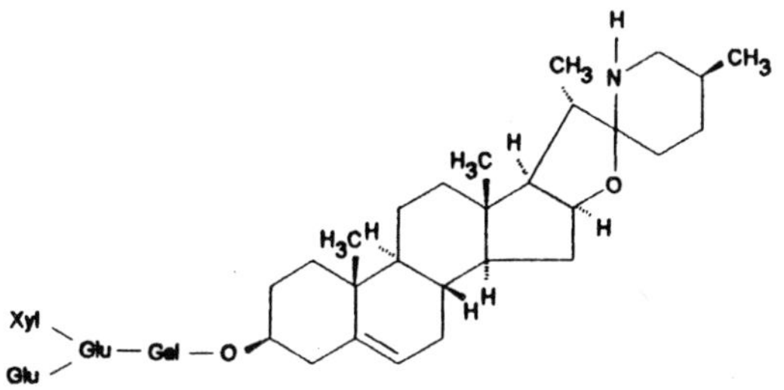

α-tomatine

Figure 11 Structure of α-tomatine. Glu, glucose; Gal, galactose; Xyl, xylose.

tomatine changes in red-fruited (Potentate Best of All, PGA), orange-fruited (Tangella, T) and yellow-fruited (Mingold Golden Sunrise, MGS) normal ripening tomato cultivars were recorded. As follows from Figure 12, no significant differences were observed between these cultivars. A rapid drop in tomatine content occurred within the first 10 d. It is noticeable that after 30 d, when the diameter of green fruits was approximately 30 mm and the average weight was 20 g, the concentrations of tomatine were very low (of order 10 $\mu g.g^{-1}$). In Figure 13 the alkaloid content is expressed on a per fruit basis. The level of tomatine gradually increased and the maximum was reached between 19 and 22 d. At this stage the diameter of fruit was 25 to 27 mm and the average weight 7 to 9 g. In terms of alkaloid per fruit, both accumulation phase and subsequent decline of α-tomatine were associated with rapid growth of green fruit. During ripening, disappearance of the toxin continued. It is noteworthy (Table 5) that the tomatine content in fruit that ripened prematurely is rather higher compared to normally ripened tomatoes.

Many authors discussed factors governing the dynamics of tomatine during development and ripening of tomatoes. It was suggested that the dilution effect (due to the weight gain) causes a decline of this alkaloid. No transport of tomatine from vegetative parts of the plant was proved by Roddic.[126] The author supposes *de novo* synthesis of this natural toxin in young fruit. As to the later tomatine disappearance, it is probable that it degrades, but more detailed information elucidating responsible processes is missing. Based on present knowledge, mitotic activity and fruit growth are the main processes contributing to tomatine disappearance, with the extent and character of this phenomena depending on the cultivar and on the development of the particular fruit.

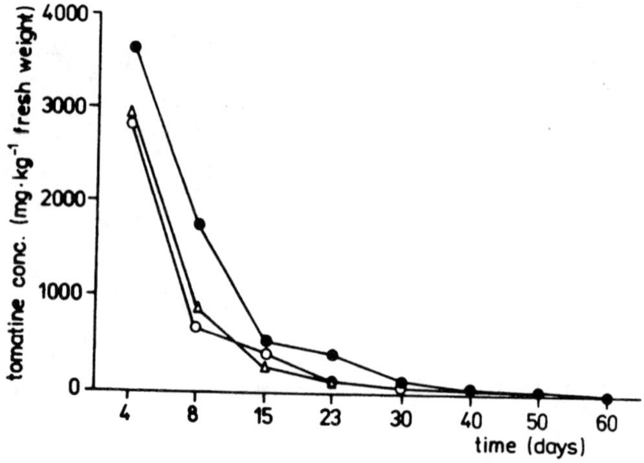

Figure 12 Changes in tomatine concentration in developing fruit of ripening tomato cultivars. ●, PBA cultivar; ○, T cultivar; △, MGS cultivar. (Adapted from Eltayeb, E. A. and Roddick, G. J., *J. Exp. Bot.*, 35, 151, 1984. With permission.)

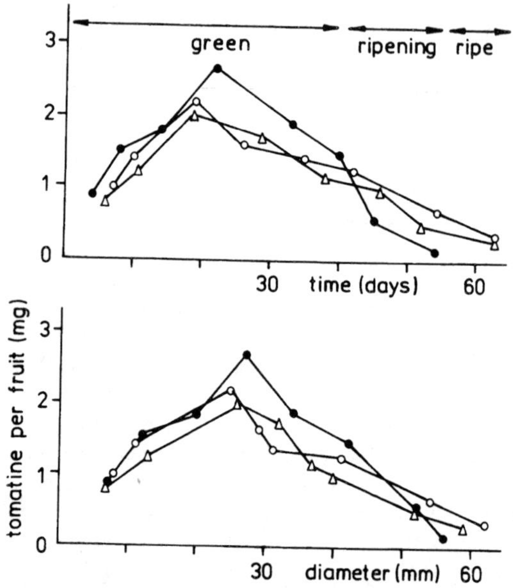

Figure 13 Changes in tomatine concentration in developing fruit of ripening tomato cultivars. ●, PBA cultivar; ○, T cultivar; △, MGS cultivar. (Adapted from Eltayeb, E. A. and Roddick, G. J., *J. Exp. Bot.* 35, 151, 1984. With permission.)

Changes During Processing and Storage

Immature green tomato fruits are occasionally used for preparation of various preserved products, especially salads, syrups, pulps, and chutney. Also, mechanized harvesting may allow the processing of a certain portion of unripe tomatoes. Kebbler et al.[127] determined tomatine levels in sweet-sour pickled fruit and in tomato chutney.

Table 5 Tomatine Content of Fruits of the Normal-Ripening Cultivar *Potentate Best of All* at Different Stages of Development

Stage of development	Diameter (mm)	Tomatine content	
		$mg.g^{-1}$ fresh weight	$mg.g^{-1}$dry weight
Small red ripe (prematurely)	28	0.011	0.25
Large red ripe (normal)	56	0.003	0.13
Large yellow to orange	54	0.004	0.19
Large green	50	0.022	0.57
Small green	27	0.300	2.67

Adapted from Eltayeb, A. E. and Roddick, J. G., *J. Exp Bot.*, 35, 151, 1984. With permission.

The observed losses are attributed mainly to a dilution effect caused by other components in the product. Peeling the fruit resulted in a slight decrease in tomatine.

Several sterilized products were prepared from unripe tomatoes by Voldřich et al.[128] The decrease of toxin in these products ranged from 8.3% (unpeeled green-yellow tomatoes with original content of tomatine 46 $mg.kg^{-1}$) to 17.3% (the same fruit, only peeled). However, due to the lack of experimental data, it is impossible to draw any general conclusions regarding all the effects of processing tomatoes.

CAPSAICIN AND RELATED ALKALOIDS

The pungent principle of different varieties of *Capsicum annuum* and *C. frutescens* fruits, often referred to as hot pepper, red pepper, or chili, consists of a mixture of capsaicinoids.

CHEMISTRY

Capsaicinoids are vanillylamides derived from C_8 to C_{11} *trans*-monoenoic and saturated branched and straight-chain fatty acids (*cis*-isomers have not been found). Capsaicin and dihydrocapsaicin together represent more than 90% of the total capsaicinoids and have been recognized as the predominant and most important pungent compounds. They are accompanied by several other minor alkaloids (Figure 14).[129-135]

TOXIC EFFECTS

Capsaicinoids show mild antioxidant properties and have been found to inhibit microbial growth. Capsaicin promotes the peristaltic reflex and increases gastric acid secretion.[136] It is partly absorbed from the gastrointestinal tract and rapidly hydrolyzed in the liver and other tissues.[137] Energy metabolism enhancement caused by increased secretion of catecholamine was observed in rats.[138] At concentrations approaching toxic levels, capsaicin showed mutagenic activity in the Ames test,[139] while in mice no mutagenicity was observed.[140] Metabolism and toxic effects of capsaicin were recently reviewed.[140-142]

OCCURRENCE

The content of capsaicinoids in *Capsicum* species varies due to varietal differences, age of plant, stage of fruit maturity, season, and growing conditions. The level of capsaicinoids in large-fruited peppers from varieties of *C. annuum* are generally low, higher amounts being found in medium-sized chilies (*C. annuum* varieties such as tabasco pepper) and the highest amounts occurring in small-sized chilies from varieties of *C. frutescens* (e.g., cayenne pepper). Most of the alkaloids are found in the pericarp, with lower amounts in the hulls and seeds. Lower levels occur at the young green stage, reaching a maximum at a stage before ripening and then dropping somewhat at the ripening stage.

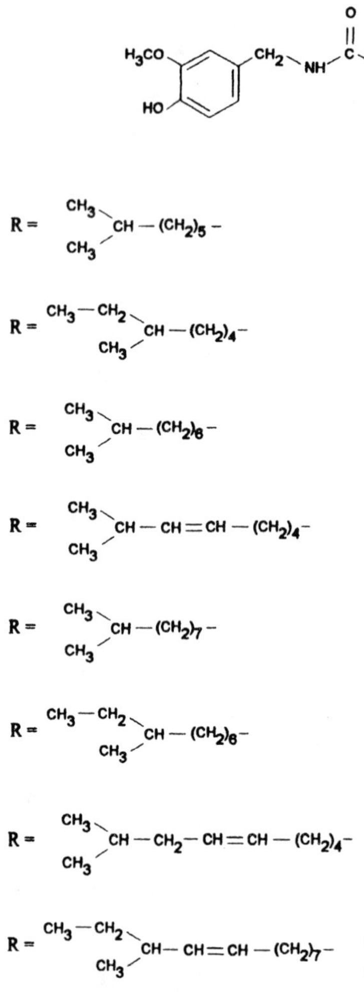

nordihydrocapsaicin (N-vanillyl-7-methyloctanamide)

nordihydrocapsaicin II (N-vanillyl-6-methyloctanamide

dihydrocapsaicin (N-vanillyl-8-methylnonanamide

capsaicin (N-vanillyl-8-methyl-6-nonenamide)

homodihydrocapsaicin (N-vanillyl-9-methyldecanamide)

homodihydrocapsaicin II (N-vanillyl-8-methyldecanamide)

homocapsaicin (N-vanillyl-9-methyl-6-decenamide)

homocapsaicin II (N-vanillyl-8-methyl-6-decenamide)

Figure 14 Structures of some capsaicinoids.

The content of capsaicinoids in paprika grown in Europe has been shown to be highly variable and on the order of about 0.01%, sometimes even as little as 0.001% or less in sweet paprika. The capsaicinoid content of various chili varieties is generally reported to range from 0.2 to 1%, and above 1% in very pungent varieties. In *C. annuum*, var. annuum, cv. Red Chili, the total capsaicinoid content, for instance, is 0.4%, with the following composition of the individual active compounds: capsaicine (49.0%), dihydrocapsaicin (43.7%), nordihydrocapsaicine (6.0%), homodihydrocapsaicine (1.0%), and homocapsaicine (0.3%).[143]

CHANGES DURING PROCESSING AND STORAGE

Pungency is the most outstanding property of capsicums, resulting from the direct effect of capsaicin and its analogs on the taste receptors in the mouth and throat. Capsaicin itself is practically devoid of odor and flavor, but it produces a burning, pungent sensation at a concentration of about 10 $mg.kg^{-1}$ that is perceptable even down to 0.1 $mg.kg^{-1}$. The pungent taste perception is enhanced by sucrose and reduced by sodium chloride,[144] while viscosity from polysaccharides retarded the perception of the mouth burn.[145]

From the culinary point of view, the pungency of *Capsicum* fruits has a unique place as it gives a characteristic hot taste to curry powders, special sauces, and a wide range of other products including meats, candy, beverages, and baked goods.

Capsaicinoids are relatively resistant to hydrolysis in aqueous solutions. Chemical hydrolysis in acid and alkali leads to vanillylamine and the corresponding fatty acid and its salt, respectively. Spontaneous hydrolysis in the enzymatically active tissue after physical disruption is an important feature as it may be employed for controlling the pungency in the culinary praxis. Sun-drying of the fruit has been found to reduce the capsaicinoid content; higher retention was obtained when fruits were air-dried in strong sunlight.[143] Capsaicinoids in red pepper millings stored in polyethylene foil, paper coated with aluminum foil or double-layered paper with an inner layer of parchment for a period of 1 year at 20 to 20°C, 0 to 2°C, and –21°C were stable throughout storage, regardless of conditions.[146] In a fermented pepper-soybean paste product (kochujang), a 20% reduction in capsaicin content was observed after 100 d of storage, while the content in a seasoned pickle containing pepper (kimchi) decreased to 82 to 83% after 12 d of pickling.[147]

Thermal processing allows capsaicinoids to spread freely throughout the fruit and brine. Blanching in boiling water and subsequent rinsing in cold water result in leaching of capsaicinoids. Peppers thermally processed without blanching contained an even higher capsaicinoid level than the fresh samples; blanched and canned peppers had a higher capsaicinoid level than the blanched ones. Freezing of peppers leads to the greatest loss of capsaicinoids (Table 6).[148,149]

Capsaicin used as a constituent of drinks containing riboflavin and ascorbic acid undergoes oxidative dimerization by the action of riboflavin/1,5-dihydroriboflavin redox system (in which riboflavin acts as a photocatalyst). *N,N′*-(3,3′-bi-4-hydroxy-5-methoxybenzyl)-di-8-methyl-non-(*E*)-6-enamide is formed as a product of this reaction (Figure 15).[150] Photochemical oxidative dimerization of capsaicin did not proceed in either the presence of ascorbic acid or in the absence of oxygen.

PURINE ALKALOIDS

Purine alkaloids occur in beverages such as coffee, tea, various herbal teas, colas, cocoa, and chocolate, as well as in many pharmaceutical drug preparations.

CHEMISTRY

Purine alkaloids are methylated derivatives of xanthine. The most abundant trimethylxanthine, caffeine, is found in about 60 genera of plants. It is accompanied by the dimethylxanthines theobromine, and theophylline, and paraxanthine, methylxanthine, heteroxanthine (Figure 16), and methyluric acids, which are, with the exception of cocoa and chocolate, the minor alkaloids.[151-153]

TOXIC EFFECTS

Caffeine is probably the most widely used drug, and there is a plethora of information, much of which is conflicting, about its physiological effects, toxicity, link to cardiovascular disease, etc. In small doses, <3 $mg.kg^{-1}$ per day, caffeine acts as a central nervous system stimulant and diuretic agent. High doses may elicit neuroendocrine effects, and very high doses may have teratogenic effects. Theobromine and theophylline are milder stimulants but stronger diuretics than caffeine. Theobromine has been shown to have teratogenic effects.[154-160]

Table 6 Effects of Processing on Capsaicinoid Levels in Jalapeno Peppers

	Content ($g.kg^{-1}$)			
Material	**CA**	**DHCA**	**NDHCA**	**Total**
Raw	7.3	6.3	1.2	14.8
Cooked (100°C, 10 min)	8.6	7.7	1.3	17.6
Blanched (100°C, 3 min) and frozen (−18°C)	4.0	3.7	0.6	8.3
Blanched (100°C, 3 min) and canned (100°C, 50 min)	4.7	4.5	0.7	9.9

Note: CA, capsaicin, DHCA, dihydrocapsaicin; NDHCA, nordihydrocapsaicin.

From Harrison, M. K. and Harris, N. D., *J. Food Sci.*, 50, 1764, 1985. With permission.

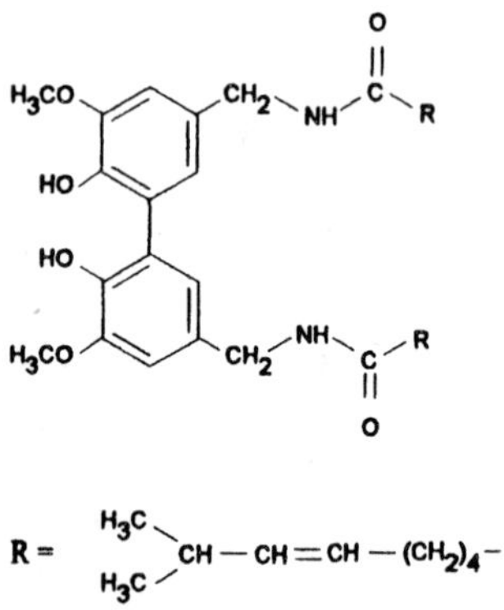

Figure 15 Structure of capsaicin dimer.

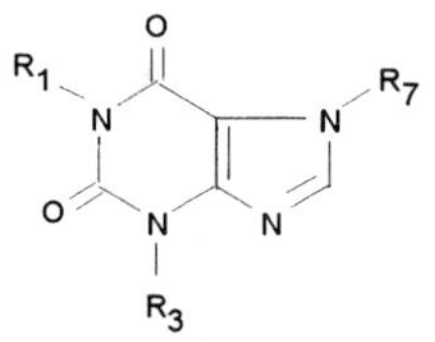

$R_1 = R_3 = R_7 = CH_3$	caffeine (1,3,7-trimethylxantine)
$R_3 = R_7 = CH_3$, $R_1 = H$	theobromine (3,7-dimethylxantine)
$R_1 = R_3 = CH_3$, $R_7 = H$	theophylline (1,3-dimethylxanthine)
$R_1 = R_7 = CH_3$, $R_3 = H$	paraxanthine (1,7-dimethylxanthine)
$R_1 = R_3 = H$, $R_7 = CH_3$	heteroxanthine (7-methylxanthine)

Figure 16 Structures of purine alkaloids.

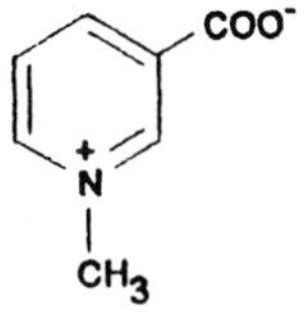

Figure 17 Structure of trigonelline.

Table 7 Alkaloid Content of Green Coffee Beans

	Percent dry weight		
Compound	**Arabica**	**Robusta**	**Liberica**
Caffeine	0.53–1.45	2.11–2.72	1.28–1.35
Theobromine	<0.005	<0.005–0.01	<0.005
Theophylline	<0.005	<0.005–0.01	0.01
Trigonelline	0.97–1.31	0.57–0.88	0.25–0.29

Reprinted from *Food Chemistry*, Vol. 26, Clifford, M. N. and Kazi, T., The influence of coffee bean maturity on the content of chlorogenic acid, caffeine and trigonelline, p. 59, Copyright 1987, with kind permission from Elsevier Science Ltd, The Boulevard, Langford Lane, Kidlington OX5 IGB, UK.

OCCURRENCE

Caffeine and its catabolic products (theobromine and theophylline) together with trigonelline (Figure 17) in green coffee beans are derived from the ripe fruit of coffee shrubs (varieties and cultivars of *Coffea arabica, C. canephora* var. *robusta,* and *C. liberica*; see Table 7). The ratio of these alkaloids is influenced by many different factors.[161,162]

CHANGES DURING PROCESSING AND STORAGE

Methylxanthines are very stable compounds and their level in individual food commodities does not change very much during processing and storage. During roasting, green coffee beans are heated to temperatures up to 200 to 250°C for 20 to 30 min. Caffeine does not change much during roasting, unlike trigonelline. Small losses of caffeine may be caused by sublimation.[163] Trigonelline is degraded to nicotinic acid (niacin) and volatile flavor-active pyridines. The trigonelline/caffeine ratio may be used as an indicator of the degree of roasting.[164] The mean caffeine content of home-prepared coffee is approximately 80 mg per cup,[165] but it can differ depending on the type of coffee. Low caffeine levels occur in decaffeinated instant coffee and coffee made from decaffeinated beans (1.7 and 1 to 6 mg/100 ml, respectively). Instant coffee contains 29 to 91 mg, percolated coffee 37 to 132 mg, and filtered coffee 93 to 127 mg caffeine per 100 ml.[154,166] Diffusion of caffeine from ground coffee is influenced by its particle size, temperature of the water, and extraction time. To obtain a more concentrated extract, an increase in temperature is more efficient than prolonged extraction time.

Tea plant leaves (*Camellia sinensis*) contain more than 2% dry weight caffeine, and theobromine content is below 0.2%. Theobromine was found only in younger leaves, and theophylline was found in zero or only trace amounts in the seedlings.[153] During the production of green tea (China tea) and the manufacture of black tea, dimethylxanthines and other purine alkaloids partly arise as products of caffeine catabolism.[167] A slight caffeine increase appears to result from the breakdown of nucleic acids.[153] A typical cup of tea provides only one-half to one-third the major tea alkaloid caffeine compared to a cup of coffee of the same size. The amount of caffeine and theobromine in the brew depends on a number of factors, including the variety, manufacture, particle size (leaf cut), and the method and time of steeping. Caffeine is extracted faster than theobromine.[168] The caffeine content of tea (loose or bags) in 1-min brews, 3-min brews, and 5-min brews averaged 8 to 28, 17 to 39, and 17 to 42 mg per 100 ml, respectively,[154] whereas decaffeinated tea brews contained 0.5 to 1.5 caffeine per 100 ml.[166]

Leaves of *Ilex paraguayensis* shrubs (maté) contain variable amounts of caffeine (the major alkaloid) and theobromine. The total alkaloid content ranges from 1.4 to 2.7% dry weight.[169] The corresponding brews contained 18 to 50 mg alkaloids per cup.

The total alkaloid content in nonroasted cocoa seeds and defatted cocoa seeds (*Theobroma cacao*) amounts to 0.7 to 3.2% and 1.4 to 4.5% dry weight, respectively; the major alkaloid theobromine occurs at a level of 0.6 to 3.1% and 1.1 to 4.2%, respectively; and caffeine concentrations are 0.02 to 0.5% and up to 2.4% dry weight, respectively.[170] Cocoa bean alkaloids do not decompose during processing. Chocolate drinks contained 26 to 44 mg theobromine and 1 to 2.5 mg caffeine per 100 ml; theobromine accounted for about 97% of the methylxanthines, and theophylline occurred at a negligible level.[166] Milk chocolate and cooking chocolate contained about 20 and 112 mg caffeine per 100 g.[154]

Present-day colas and pepper-type soft drinks derive less than 5% of their total caffeine from the cola nut (*Cola* sp.). Much of the added caffeine is obtained from other natural sources, mainly from raw coffee beans in the process of decaffeination. Unlike coffee and tea, which are brewed or steeped differently according to conditions, soft drinks are manufactured and subject to quality controls that ensure a uniform caffeine content. The caffeine content of various soft drinks ranging from about 5 to 20 mg/100 ml and 0.01 to 0.4 mg/100 ml was found in diet cola drinks.[154,166,171] Caffeine in soft drinks is quite stable during the storage period.

REFERENCES

1. Bush, L. P. and Crowe, M. W., Nicotiana alkaloids, in *Toxicants of Plant Origin, Vol. I, Alkaloids*, Cheeke, P. R., Ed., CRC Press, Boca Raton, FL, 1989, 87.
2. Matsushita, H., Tsujino, Y., Yoshida, D., Saito, A., Kisaki, T., Kato, K., and Noguchi, M., New minor alkaloids in flue-cured tobacco leaf, *Agric. Biol. Chem.*, 43, 193, 1979.
3. Miyano, M., Matsushita, H., Yasumatsu, N., and Nishida, K., *N*′-isopropylnornicotine in burley tobacco (*Nicotiana tabacum*), *Agric. Biol. Chem.*, 43, 1607, 1979.
4. Enzell, C. and Whalberg, I., Leaf composition in relation to smoking quality and aroma, *Recent Adv. Tob. Sci.*, 6, 64, 1980.
5. Martin, W. R., *Tobacco Smoking and Nicotine: A Neurobiological Approach*, Plenum Press, New York, 1987.
6. Metcalf, R. L., *Organic Insecticides, Their Chemistry and Mode of Action*, Interscience, New York, 1955.
7. Keeler, R. F. and Crowe, M. W., Anabasine, a teratogen from the *Nicotiana* genus, in *Plant Toxicology*, Seawright, A. A., Hegarty, M. P., James, L. F., and Keeler, R. F., Eds., Dominion Press, Hedges and Bell, Melbourne, Australia, 1985, 324.
8. Shephara, R. J., Respiratory irritation from environmental tobacco smoke, *Arch. Environ. Health*, 47, 123, 1992.
9. Keeler, R. F. and Crowe, M. W., Teratogenicity and toxicity of wild tree tobacco, *Nicotiana glauca* in sheep, *Cornell Vet.*, 74, 50, 1984.
10. Kisaki, T. and Tamaki, E., Phytochemical studies on the tobacco alkaloids. III. Observations on the interconversion of DL-nicotine and DL-nornicotine in excised tobacco leaves, *Arch. Biochem. Biophys.*, 94, 252, 1961.

11. Leete, E., The methylation of nornicotine to nicotine, a minor biosynthetic pathway in *Nicotiana tabacum, Beitr. Tabakforsch.*, 12, 113, 1984.
12. Chaplin, J. F., Comparison of type 32 and flue-cured tobacco cultivars produced under flue-cured culture when air- and flue-cured, *Tob. Sci.*, 19, 120, 1975.
13. Constantinescu, T., Chromatographic investigation concerning the oxidation of some β-pyridinic alkaloids in tobacco. I. Light, oxygen, temperature, peroxidase, and DPPH [2,2-diphenyl-*d*-picrylhydrazyl] effect on nicotine, cotinine, and oxynicotine, *Lucr. Cercet. Inst. Cercet. Proiect Aliment.*, 12, 67, 1973.
14. Rickert, W. S., Robinson, J. C., and Joung, J. C., Estimating the hazards of "less hazardous" cigarets. I. Tar, nicotine, carbon monoxide, acrolein, hydrogen cyanide and total aldehyde deliveries of Canadian cigarettes, *J. Toxicol. Environ. Health,* 6, 351, 1980.
15. Tso, T. C., Sims, J. L., and Johnson, D. E., Agronomic factors affecting *N*-dimethylnitrosamine content in cigarette smoke, *Beitr. Tabakforsch.*, 8, 34, 1975.
16. Hecht, S. S., Chen, C. B., Dong, M., Ornaf, R. M., Hoffmann, D., and Tso, T. C., Chemical studies on the tobacco smoke, *Beitr. Tabakforsch.*, 9, 1, 1977.
17. MacKown, C. T., Eivazi, F., Sihs, J. L., and Bush, L. P., Tobacco-specific *N*-nitrosamines: effect of burley alkaloid isolines and nitrogen fertility management, *J. Agric. Food Chem.*, 32, 1262, 1984.
18. Brunnemann, K. D., Genoble, L., and Hoffmann, D., *N*-nitrosamines in chewing tobacco: an international comparison, *J. Agric. Food Chem.*, 33, 1178, 1985.
19. Andersen, R. A., Partial characterization of condensate derived from volatiles — sublimate of homogenized leaf cured burley tobacco during storage, *J. Agric. Food Chem.*, 31, 930, 1983.
20. Leete, E., The alkaloids, in *Secondary Plant Products,* Bell, E. A. and Charlwood, B. V., Eds., Springer-Verlag, Berlin, 1980, 64.
21. Keeler, R. F., Quinolizidine alkaloids in range and grain lupins, in *Toxicants of Plant Origin, Vol. I, Alkaloids*, Cheeke, P. R., Ed., CRC Press, Boca Raton, FL, 1989, 133.
22. Petterson, D. S., Harrie, D. J., and Allen, D. G., Alkaloids, in *Toxic Substances in Crop Plants,* D'Mello, J. P. F., Duffus, C. M., and Duffus, J. H., Eds., Royal Society of Chemistry, Cambridge, U.K., 1991, 148.
23. Blaicher, F. M., Nolte, R., and Mukherjee, K. D., Lupin protein concentrate by extraction with aqueous alcohols, *J. Am. Oil Chem. Soc.*, 58, 761, 1981.
24. Aquilera, J. M. and Trier, A., The revival of the lupin, *Food Technol.*, 32 (8), 70, 1978.
25. Hatzold, T., Elmadfa, I., Gross, R., Wink, M., Hartmann, T., and Witte, L., Quinolizidine alkaloids in seeds of *Lupinus mutabilis, J. Agric. Food Chem.*, 31, 934, 1983.
26. Priddis, C. R., Capillary gas chromatography of lupin alkaloids, *J. Chromatogr.*, 261, 95, 1983.
27. Pompei, C. and Lucisano, M., Le lupin (*Lupinus albus*) comme source de proteines pour l'alimentation humaine. II. Production d'isolat par coagulation acide et par ultrafiltration-diafiltration, *Lebensm. Wiss. Technol.*, 9, 338, 1976.
28. Schmidlin-Mészáros, J., Eine Nahrungsmittelvergiftung mit Lupinenbohnen, *Trav. Chim. Alim. Hyg.*, 64, 194, 1973.
29. Gross, R., Morales, E., Gross, U., and von Baer, E., Die Lupine, ein Beitrag zur Nahrungsversorgung in den Anden. 3. Ernaerungsphysiologische Untersuchung mit dem Mehl der Suesslupine (*Lupinus albus), Z. Ernaehrung-Swiss*, 15, 391, 1976.
30. Mohamed, A. M., Youssef, M. M., Aman, M. E., and Adel-Shehata, A., Effect of debittering on chemical composition, functional properties and *in vitro* digestibility of lupine (*Lupinus termis*) flour, *Egyptian J. Food Sci.*, 15, 161, 1987.
31. Burbano, C., Muzquiz, Casinello, M., Rodenas, I., and de Cabanyes, J., Comparative study of the seeds of 2 species of lupin in the Iberian peninsula, *Lupinus luteus* L., and *L. hispanicus* Boiss et Reut., *An. Inst. Nac. Invest. Agrar. Agricola*, 28, 37, 1985.
32. Lucisano, M., Pompei, C., and Rossi, M., Oil and alkaloid removal from *Lupinus mutabilis* by extraction with hexane, *Lebensm. Wiss. Technol.*, 17, 324, 1984.
33. Hatzold, T., Gross, T. and Elmadfa, I., Production and debittering of edible oil and a protein concentrate from seeds of *Lupinus mutabilis, Fette Seifen Anstrichm.*, 84, 59, 1982.
34. Biddle, H. C., The conversion of cinchonine and quinine into their poisonous isomers, cinchotoxine and quinotoxine, and the relation of this conversion to the toxicity of the cinchona alkaloids, *J. Am. Chem. Soc.*, 34, 500, 1912.

35. Stenberg, V. I. and Travecedo, E. F., Nitrogen photochemistry. V. A new photochemical reduction of the cinchona alkaloids, quinine, quinidine, cinchonidine, and cinchonine, *J. Org. Chem.*, 35, 4131, 1970.
36. Epling, G. A. and Yoon, U. C., Photolysis of cinchona alkaloids. Photochemical degradation to 5-vinyl-quinuclidine-2-carboxaldehyde, a precursor to synthetic antimalarials, *Tetrahedron Lett.*, 29, 2471, 1977.
37. Colley, J. C., Edwards, J. A., Heywood, R., and Purser, D., Toxicity studies with quinine hydrochloride, *Toxicology*, 54, 219, 1989.
38. Goonetillake, L. A., Arambewela, L. S. R., and de Costa, R., Studies on the alkaloid contents of the bark of Cinchona found in Sri Lanka, *J. Natl. Sci. Council Sri Lanka*, 12, 141, 1984.
39. Battersby, A. R. and Parry, R. J., Biosynthesis of the Cinchona alkaloids: late stage of the pathway, *J. Chem. Soc. Chem. Commun.*, 31, 1971.
40. Egan, H., Kirk, R. S., and Sawyer, R., *Pearson's Chemical Analysis of Foods*, 8th ed., Churchill Livingstone, New York, 1981, 219.
41. Sulser, H. and Mändli, H., Photosensitivity of quinine drinks, *Mitt. Geb. Lebensmittelunters. Hyg.*, 78, 133, 1987.
42. Sumathikutty, M. A., Rajarama, K., Sankarikutty, B., Narayanan, C. S., and Mathew, M. G., Piperine, *Lebensm. Wiss. Technol.*, 14, 225, 1981.
43. Su, H. C. F. and Horvat, R., Isolation, identification, and insecticidal properties of *Piper nigrum* amides, *J. Agric. Food Chem.*, 29, 115, 1981.
44. Kollmannsberger, N., Nitz, S., and Drawert, F., Über die Aromastoffzusammensetzung von Hochdruckextrakten. I. Pfeffer (*Piper nigrum*, var. muntok), *Z. Lebensm. Unters. Forsch.*, 194, 545, 1992.
45. Semler, U. and Gross, G. G., Distribution of piperine in vegetative parts of *Piper nigrum*, *Phytochemistry*, 27, 1566, 1988.
46. Bhat, B. G. and Chandrasekhara, N., Studies on the metabolism of piperine: absorption, tissue distribution and excretion of urinary conjugates in rats, *Toxicology*, 40, 83, 1986.
47. Gauesh, B. B. and Chandrasekhara, N., Interaction of piperine with rat liver microsomes, *Toxicology*, 44, 91, 1987.
48. Gauesh, B. B., and Chandrasekhara, N., Metabolic disposition of piperine in the rat, *Toxicology*, 44, 99, 1987.
49. Muralidhara, N. K., Lack of genotoxic effects of piperine (the active principle of black pepper) in albino rats, *J. Food Safety*, 11, 39, 1990.
50. Jansz, E. R., Pathirana, I. C., and Packiyasothy, E. V., Determination of piperine in pepper (*Piper nigrum* L.), *J. Natl. Sci. Council Sri Lanka*, 11, 129, 1983.
51. Kostrzewa, E. and Karwowska, K., Characteristic of flavor and aroma of natural extracts from black pepper, *Pr. Inst. Lab. Przem. Spozyw.*, 27, 93, 1977, *Chem. Abstr.*, 9, 4793w, 1978.
52. Verzele, M., van Damme, F., Schuddinck, G., and Vyncke, P., Quantitative microscale liquid chromatography of piperine in pepper and pepper extracts, *J. Chromatogr.*, 471, 335, 1989.
53. Glasl, H., Isomerization of piperine, *Dtsch. Lebensm. Rdsch.*, 80, 148, 1984.
54. Tagaki, K., Ochiai, J., and Okuyama, T., Analysis of gamma-irradiated pepper constituents. IV. Analysis of piperine and its isomers by reverse phase HPLC and effect of gamma irradiation on racemization of piperine, *Food Irradiat.*, 23, 51, 1988.
55. Chinova, E. G., Zoloedora, S. F., Ye Reinagach, B., and Titova, V. I., Changes in essential oils during the preservation of spices, *Konserv. Ovochesush. Prom.*, 24, 31, 1969, *Chem. Abstr.*, 71, 48402a, 1969.
56. Lijinsky, W., Evelyn, C., and van de Rosalie, B., Carcinogenic nitrosamines formed by drug/nitrite interactions, *Nature*, 239, 1657, 1972.
57. Kuhn, R. and Low, I., Die Konstitution des Solanins, *Angew. Chem.*, 66, 639, 1954.
58. Kuhn, R., Low, I., and Trischmann, H., Die Konstitution des Solanines, *Chem. Ber.*, 88, 1492, 1955.
59. Kuhn, R., Low, I., and Trischmann, H., Die Konstitution des α-Chaconins, *Chem. Ber.*, 88, 1690, 1955.
60. Kuhn, R. and Low, I., Zur Konstitution der Leptine, *Chem. Ber.*, 94, 1088, 1961.
61. Prelog, V. and Jeger, O., Steroid alkaloids: the solanum group, in *The Alkaloids*, Vol. 7, Manske, R. H. F., Ed., Academic Press, New York, 1960, 343.

62. Schreiber, K., Steroid alkaloids: solanum group, in *The Alkaloids*, Vol. 10, Manske, R. H. F., Ed., Academic Press, New York, 1968, 1.
63. Lampitt, L. H., Bushill, J. H., Rooke, H. S. and Jackson, E. M., Solanine: glycoside of the potato: II. Its distribution in the potato plant, *J. Soc. Chem. Ind. (London)*, 62, 48, 1943.
64. Morris, S. C. and Pattermann, J. B., Genetic and environmental effects on levels of glycoalkaloids in cultivars of potato (*Solanum tuberosum* L.), *Food Chem.*, 18, 271, 1985.
65. Morris, S. C. and Lee, T. H., The toxicity and teratogenicity of *Solanaceae* glycoalkaloids, particularly those of the potato (*Solanum tuberosum* L.): a review, *Food Technol. Austral.*, 36, 118, 1984.
66. Mc Millan, M. and Thompson, J. C., An outbreak of suspected solanine poisoning in schoolboys: examination of criteria of solanine poisoning, *Q. J. Med.*, New Series 48, 227, 1979.
67. Roddick, J. G., Rijneberg, A. L., and Weissenberg, M., Membrane-disrupting properties of the steroidal glycoalkaloids solasonine and solamargine, *Phytochemistry*, 29, 1513, 1990.
68. Slanina, P., Solanine (glycoalkaloids in potatoes: toxicological evaluation), *Food Chem. Toxicol.*, 28, 759, 1990.
69. Friedman, M., Rayburn, J. R., and Bantle, J. A., Structural relationships and developmental toxicity of *Solanum* alkaloids in the frog embryo teratogenesis assay — *Xenopus*, *J. Agric. Food Chem.*, 40, 1617, 1992.
70. Jadhav, S. J., Sharma, R. P., and Salunkhe, D. K., Naturally occurring toxic alkaloids in foods, *Crit. Rev. Toxicol.*, 9, 21, 1981.
71. Jelínek, R., Kyzlink, V., and Blatny, C., An evaluation of the embryotoxic effects of blighted potatoes on chicken embryos, *Teratology*, 14, 355, 1975.
72. Munn, A. M., Bardon, E. S., Wilson, J. M., and Hogan, J. M., Teratogenic effects in early chicken embryos of solanine and glycoalkaloids from blighted potatoes infested with *Phytophthora infestans*, *Teratology*, 11, 73, 1975.
73. Blankemeyer, J. T., Stringer, K. B., Rayburn, J. R., Bantle, J. A., and Friedman, M., Effect of potato glycoalkaloids, α-chaconine and α-solanine, on membrane potential of frog embryos, *J. Agric. Food Chem.*, 40, 2022, 1992.
74. Wunsch, A., Glykoalkaloide in Kartoffelsorten. Verteilung innerhalb der Knolle, *Chem. Mikrobiol. Technol. Lebensm.*, 12, 69, 1989.
75. Friedman, M. and Dao, L., Distribution of glycoalkaloids in potato plants and commercial potato products, *J. Agric. Food Chem.*, 40, 419, 1992.
76. Kozukue, N. and Kozukue, E., Glycoalkaloids in potato plants and tubers, *Hortic. Sci.*, 22, 294, 1987.
77. Zitnak, A. and Johnston, G. R., Glycoalkaloid content of B5141-6 potatoes, *Am. Potato J.*, 47, 256, 1970.
78. Johns, T. and Alonso, J. G., Glycoalkaloid change during the domestication of the potato, *Solanum* section *Petota*, *Euphytica*, 50, 203, 1990.
79. Coxon, D. T., Davies, A. M., and Morgan, M. R. A., Special Report No. 7: Glycoalkaloids in potatoes, ARC Food Research Institute, Norwich, Biennial Report, 8, 1991, 1982.
80. Sinden, S. L. and Webb, R. E., Effect of variety and location on glykoalkaloids content of six potato varieties at 39 locations. *U.S. Dept. Agric. Bull.*, 1472, 30, 1974.
81. Gregory, P., Sinden, S. L., Osman, S. F., Tingey, W. M., and Chessin, D. A., Glycoalkaloids of wild, tuber-bearing *Solanum* species, *J. Agric. Food Chem.*, 29, 1212, 1981.
82. Sinden, S. L., Sanford, L. L., and Webb, R. E., Genetic and environmental control of potato glycoalkaloids, *Am. Potato J.*, 61, 141, 1984.
83. Shih, M. J. and Kuc, J., α- And β-Solamarine in Kennebec *Solanum tuberosum* leaves and aged tuber slices, *Phytochemistry*, 13, 1997, 1974.
84. Sinden, S. L. and Sanford, L. L., Origin and inheritance of solamarine glycoalkaloids in commercial potato cultivars, *Am. Potato J.*, 58, 305, 1981.
85. Maga, J. A., Potato glycoalkaloids, *Crit. Rev. Food Sci. Nutr.*, 12, 371, 1980.
86. Jadhav, S. J. and Salunkhe, D. K., Formation and control of chlorophyll and glycoalkaloids in tuber of *Solanum tuberosum* L. and evaluation of glycoalkaloid toxicity, *Adv. Food. Res.*, 21, 307, 1975.
87. Baerung, R., Influence of different rates and intensities of light on solanine content and cooking quality of potato tubers, *Eur. Potato J.*, 5, 242, 1962.

88. Salunkhe, D. K., Wu, M. T., and Jadhav S. J., Effect of light and temperature on formation of solanine in potato slices, *J. Food Sci.*, 37, 969, 1972.
89. Zitnak, A., The occurrence and distribution of free alkaloid solanidine in Netted Gem potatoes, *Can. J. Biochem. Physiol.*, 39, 1257, 1961.
90. Zitnak, A., Photoinduction of glycoalkaloids in cured potatoes, *Am. Potato J.*, 57, 415, 1981.
91. Liljemark, A. and Widoff, E., Greening and solanine development of white potatoes in fluorescent light, *Am. Potato J.*, 37, 379, 1960.
92. Conner, H. V., The effect of light on solanine synthesis in the potato tubers, *Plant Physiol.*, 12, 79, 1937.
93. Ahmed, S. S. and Muller, K., Einfluss von Lagerzeit, Licht und Temperature auf den Solanin und α-Chaconinegehalt mit und ohne Keimhemmungsmittel behandelter Kartoffeln, *Potato Res.*, 24, 93, 1981.
94. Lammerink, P., Total glycoalkaloid content of new potato cultivars, *N.Z. J. Exp. Agric.*, 13, 413, 1985.
95. Sinden, S. L., Effect of light and mechanical injury on the glycoalkaloid content of greening-resistance potato tubers, *Am. Potato J.*, 49, 368, 1972.
96. Fitzpatrick, T. J., McDermott, J. A., and Osman, S. F., Evalution of injuried commercial potato tubers, *J. Am. Soc. Hortic. Sci.*, 101, 329, 1976.
97. Ahmed, S. S. and Muller, K., Effect of wound-damages on the glycoalkaloid content in potato tubers and chips, *Lebensm. Wiss. Technol.*, 11, 144, 1978.
98. Mondy, N. I., Leja, M., and Gosselin, B., Changes in total phenolic total glycoalkaloid, and ascorbic acid content of potatoes as a result of bruising, *J. Food Sci.*, 52, 631, 1987.
99. Olsson, K., The influence of genotype on the effects of impact damage on the accumulation of glycoalkaloids in potato tubers, *Potato Res.*, 29, 1, 1986.
100. Wu, M. T. and Salunkhe, D. K., Changes in glycoalkaloid content following mechanical injuries to potato tubers, *J. Am. Soc. Hortic. Sci.*, 101, 329, 1976.
101. Hellenas, K. E., personal communication.
102. Bushway, R. J. and Ponampalam, R., α-Chaconine and α-solanine content of potato products and their stability during several modes of cooking, *J. Agric. Food Chem.*, 29, 814, 1981.
103. Sizer, C. E., Maga, J. A., and Craven, C. J., Total glycoalkaloids in potato and potato chips, *J. Agric. Food Chem.*, 28, 578, 1980.
104. Bushway, R. J., Burea, J. L., and McGann, D. F., Alfa chaconine and alfa solanine content of potato peel and potato peel products, *J. Food Sci.*, 48, 84, 1985.
105. Mondy, N. I. and Gosselin, B., Effect of peeling on total phenols, total glycoalkaloids, discoloration and flavor of cooked potatoes, *J. Food Sci.*, 53, 756, 1988.
106. Ponnampalam, R. and Mondy, N. I., Effect of cooking on the total glycoalkaloid content of potatoes, *J. Agric. Food Chem.*, 31, 493, 1983.
107. Takagi, K., Toyoda, M., Fujiyma, Z., and Saito, Z., Effect of cooking on the contents of α-solanine and α-chaconine in potatoes, *J. Food Hyg. Soc. Jpn.*, 31, 67, 1990.
108. Sinden, S. L. and Deahl, K. L., Effect of glycoalkaloids and phenolics on potato flavor, *J. Food Sci.*, 41, 520, 1976.
109. Wilson, A. M., McGann, D. F., and Buschway, R. J., Effect of growth, location and length of storage on glycoalkaloids content of road-side stand potatoes as stored by consumers, *J. Food Prot.*, 42, 495, 1979.
110. Zitnak, A., The influence of certain treatments upon solanine synthesis in potatos, Master's thesis, University of Alberta, Edmonton, 1950.
111. Linnemann, A. R., Van Es, A., and Hartmans, K. J., Changes in the content of L-ascorbic acid, glucose, fructose, sucrose, and total glycoalkaloids in potato (cv. Bintje) stored at 7, 16 and 28°C, *Potato Res.*, 28, 271, 1985.
112. Fitzpatrick, T. J., Herb, S. F., Osman, S. F., and McDermott, J. A., Potato glycoalkaloids: increase and variations of rations in aged slices over prolonged storage, *Am. Potato J.*, 54, 539, 1977.
113. Arneson, P. A. and Durbin, R. D., Studies on the mode of action of tomatine as a fungitoxic agent, *Plant Physiol.*, 13, 683, 1968.
114. Sinden, S. L., Schalk, J. M., and Stoner, A. K., Effect of daylength and maturity of tomato plants on α-tomatine content and resistence to the Colorado potato beetle, *J. Am. Soc. Hortic. Sci.*, 103, 596, 1978.
115. Barbour, J. D. and Kennedy, G. G., Role of steroidal glycoalkaloids α-tomatine-in host-plant resistence of tomato to Colorado potato beetle, *J. Chem. Ecol.*, 17, 989, 1991.

116. Steel, C. Ch. and Drysdale, R. D., Electrolyte leakage from plant and fungal tissues and disruption of liposome membranes by α-tomatine, *Phytochemistry*, 27, 1025, 1988.
117. Ford, E. J., McCance, D. J., and Drysdale, R. B., The detoxification of α-tomatine by *Fusarium oxysporum* F. sp. *Lycopersici, Phytochemistry*, 16, 545, 1977.
118. Roddick J. G., The steroidal glycoalkaloid α-tomatine, *Phytochemistry*, 19, 9, 1974.
119. Elliger, C. A., Waiss, A. C., Jr., Dutton, H. L., and Rose, M. F., α-Tomatine and resistence of tomato cultivars toward the nematode, *Meloidogyne incognita, J. Chem. Ecol.*, 14, 4, 1988.
120. Czygan, F. C. and Willuhn, G., Lipochrome und Steroidalkaloide in Tomaten, *Planta Medica*, 15, 413, 1967.
121. Duperon, R., Thiersault, M., and Duperon, P., High level of glycosylated sterols in species of *Solanum* and sterol changes during the development of the tomato, *Phytochemistry*, 23, 743, 1984.
122. Kyzlink, V., Marková, K. and Jelínek, R., Tomatine, solanine and embryotoxicity of unripe tomatoes, *Sb. Vys. Sk. Chem. Technol. Praze*, E51, 69, 1981.
123. Míková, K., Kášová, Z., and Kyzlink, V., Změny obsahu tomatinu v různě konzervovaných rajčatech, *Prům. Potravin.*, 32, 4, 1981.
124. Eltayeb, A. E. and Roddick, J. G., Changes in the alkaloid content of developing fruits of tomato (*Lycopersicon esculentum* Mill.), *J. Exp. Bot.*, 35, 252, 1984.
125. Eltayeb, A. E. and Roddick, J. G., Changes in the alkaloid content of developing fruits of tomato (*Lycopersicon esculentum* Mill.), *J. Exp. Bot.*, 35, 261, 1984.
126. Roddick, J. G., Complex formation between *Solanaceous* steroidal glycoalkaloids and free sterols *in vitro, Phytochemistry*, 18, 1467, 1979.
127. Kebler, R., Lang, H., and Ziegler, W., Einflus küchentechnischer Masnahmen auf den Solaningehalt grüner Tomatenfrüchte, *Dtsch. Lebensm. Rundsch.*, 81, 11, 1985.
128. Voldřich, M., Ondroušek, S. and Dobiáš, J., Steroidní glykoalkaloidy v čerstvých a konzervovaných rajčatech, *Potrav. Vědy*, 10, 23, 1992.
129. Bennett, D. J. and Kirby, G. W., Constitution and biosynthesis of capsaicin, *J. Chem. Soc. C*, 442, 1968.
130. Rangoonwala, R., Beitrag zur Trennung von Capsaicin, cis-Capsaicin, Pelargonsäurevanillylamid und Dihydrocapsaicin, *J. Chromatogr.*, 41, 265, 1969.
131. Rangoonwala, R. and Seitz, G., *Cis*-capsaicin. Ein Beitrag zur Synthese, Analytik und dem vermuteten Verkommen in Capsicum Fruchten, *Dtsch. Apoth. Z.*, 110, 1946, 1970.
132. Jurenitsch, J., David, M., Heresch, G., and Kubelka, M., Detection and identification of new pungent compounds in fruits of *Capsicum, Planta Med.*, 36, 61, 1979.
133. Suzuki, T., Kawada, T., and Iwai, K., Effective separation of capsaicin and its analogs by reverse-phase high performance thin layer chromatography, *J. Chromatogr.*, 191, 217, 1980.
134. Jurenitsch, J. and Leinmuller, R., Quantification of nonylic acid vanillamide and other capsaicinoids in the pungent principle of *Capsicum* fruits and preparations by gas liquid chromatography on glass capillary columns, *J. Chromatogr.*, 189, 389, 1980.
135. Jurenitsch, J. and Woginger, R., Isolation and structure of homodihydrocapsaicin II, *Sci. Pharm.*, 50, 111, 1982.
136. Limlomwongse, L., Chaitauchawong, C., and Tongyoi, S., Effect of capsaicin on gastric acid secretion and mucosal blood flow in the rat, *Am. J. Physiol.*, 245, 257, 1983.
137. Oi, Y., Kawada, T., Watanabe, T., and Iwai, K., Induction of capsaicin-hydrolyzing enzyme activity in rat liver by continuous oral administration of capsaicin, *J. Agric. Food Chem.*, 40, 467, 1992.
138. Watanabe, T., Kawada, T., and Iwai, K., Enhancement by capsaicin [pungent principle of hot red pepper] of energy metabolism in rats through secretion of catecholamine from adrenal medulla, *Agric. Biol. Chem.*, 51, 75, 1987.
139. Muralidhara, N. K., Non-mutagenicity of capsaicin in albino mice, *Food Chem. Toxicol.*, 26, 955, 1988.
140. Anon., Metabolism and toxicity of capsaicin, *Nutr. Rev.*, 44, 20, 1986.
141. Buck, S. H. and Burks, T. F., The neuropharmacology of capsaicin: review of some recent observations, *Am. Soc. Pharmacol. Exp. Ther.*, 38, 179, 1986.
142. Boujbel, A., Slim, A., and Ben Redjeb, S., Studies on mutagenic activity of hot pepper and capsaicin, *Med. Nutr.*, 27, 86, 1991.
143. Mathew, A. G., Lewis, Y. S., Kirshnamurthy, N., and Nambudiri, E. S., Capsaicin, *Flavour Ind.*, 691, 1971.
144. Sizer, F. and Harris, N., The influence of common food additives and temperature on threshold perception of capsaicin, *Chem. Senses*, 10, 279, 1985.

145. Nasrawi, C. W. and Pangborn, R. M., The influence of tastants on oral irritation by capsaicin, *J. Sensory Studies*, 3, 287, 1989.
146. Aczel, A., Application of overpressured layer chromatography in foodstuff examination, *J. High Resolut. Chromatogr. Chromatogr. Commun.*, 9, 407, 1986.
147. Chung, B. S. and Kang, K. O., The changes of capsaicin content in fresh and processed red peppers, *J. Korean Soc. Nutr.*, 14, 409, 1985.
148. Huffman, V. L., Schadle, E. R., Villalon, B., and Burns, E. E., Volatile components and pungency in fresh and processed jalapeno peppers, *J. Food Sci.*, 43, 1809, 1978.
149. Harrison, M. K. and Harris, N. D., Effects of processing treatments on recovery of capsaicin in jalapeno peppers, *J. Food Sci.*, 50, 1764, 1985.
150. Tateba, H. and Mihara, S., Photochemical oxidative dimerization of capsaicin in an aqueous solution, *Agric. Biol. Chem.*, 55, 873, 1991.
151. Clifford, M. N. and Willson, K. C., Eds., *Coffee: Botany, Biochemistry and Production of Beans and Beverage,* Croom Helm, London, 1985.
152. Clarke, R. J. and Macrae, R., Eds., *Coffee I — Chemistry*, Elsevier, London, 1985.
153. Suzuki, T., Ashihara, H., and Waller, G. R., Purine and purine alkaloid metabolism in *Camellia* and *Coffea* plants, *Phytochemistry*, 31, 2575, 1992.
154. Anon., Caffeine, *Food Technol.*, 37(4), 87, 1987.
155. Petterson, D. S., Harris, D. J., and Allen, D. G., Alkaloids, in *Toxic Substances in Crop Plants,* D'Mello, J. P. F., Duffus, C. M., and Duffus, J. H., Eds., Royal Society of Chemistry, Cambridge, 1991, 148.
156. Leonard, T. K., Watson, R. R., and Mohs, M. E., The effects of caffeine on various body systems: a review, *J. Am. Diet. Assoc.*, 87, 1048, 1987.
157. Stavric, B., Methylxanthines: toxicity to humans. II. Caffeine, *Food Chem. Toxicol.*, 26, 645, 1988.
158. Rosenkranz, H. S. and Eunever, F. K., Evaluation on the genotoxicity of theobromine and caffeine, *Food Chem. Toxicol.*, 25, 247, 1987.
159. Stavric, B., Methylxanthines: toxicity to humans. I. Theophylline, *Food Chem. Toxicol.*, 26, 541, 1988.
160. Stavric, B., Methylxanthines: toxicity to humans. III. Theobromine, paraxanthine and the combined effects of methylxanthines, *Food Chem. Toxicol.*, 26, 725, 1988.
161. Clifford, M. N. and Kazi, T., The influence of coffee bean maturity on the content of chlorogenic acid, caffeine and trigonelline, *Food Chem.*, 26, 59, 1987.
162. Suzuki, T. and Waller, G., Biosynthesis and biodegradation of caffeine, theobromine, and theophylline in *Coffea arabica* L. fruits, *J. Agric. Food Chem.*, 32, 845, 1984.
163. Puhlmann, R., Aspekte der Röstkaffeeproduktion, *Lebensmittelindustrie*, 33, 182, 1986.
164. Maier, H. G., *Kaffee*, P. Parey Verlag, Berlin, 1981.
165. Stavric, B., Klassen, R., Watkinson, B., Karpinski, K., Stapley, R., and Fried, P., Variability in caffeine consumption from coffee and tea: possible significance for epidemiological studies, *Food Chem. Toxicol.*, 26, 111, 1988.
166. Scott, N. R., Chakrabarty, J., and Marks, V., Caffeine consumptions in the United Kingdom: a retrospective survey, *Food Sci. Nutr.*, 42F, 183, 1989.
167. Suzuki, T. and Waller, G. R., Total nitrogen and purine alkaloids in the tea plant throughout the year, *J. Sci. Food Agric.*, 37, 862, 1986.
168. Price, W. E. and Spiro, M., Rates of extraction of theaflavin, caffeine and theobromine from several whole teas and sieved fractions, *J. Sci. Food Agric.*, 36, 1309, 1985.
169. Clifford, M. N. and Ramirez-Martinez, J. R., Chlorogenic acid and purine alkaloid contents of maté (*Ilex paraguayensis*) leaf, *Food Chem.*, 35, 13, 1990.
170. Paiva, M. and Janick, J., Variability of alkaloid production in *Theobroma cacao* L., *Rev. Theobroma,* 13, 249, 1983.
171. Stavric, B. and Klassen, R., Caffeine content in colas from New York State and Ontario, *J. Food Safety,* 8, 179, 1987.

Part B

Saponins

Jan Velíšek

Saponins are a group of heteroglycosides, mainly of plant origin, but also occurring in a number of marine animals. More than 100 plant families contain saponins, which generally occur as complex mixtures, varying in structure, amount, sensory properties, and physiological activities. Only a few plants containing saponins are used by humans as staple foods; some are spices, herbs, or medical plants, which are used only in trivial quantities. Saponins are chemically diverse compounds that have some common and characteristic properties, such as bitter taste, detergentlike properties, and ability to lyse erythrocytes and interact with bile acids, cholesterol, and other 3β-hydroxy steroids. Chemistry, biochemistry, toxicity, and other properties of saponins have been recently reviewed.[1-5]

CHEMISTRY

Saponins consist of an aglycone called sapogenol or sapogenin, which is either a triterpenoid or a steroid derivative linked to one or several sugar units.[2,4,5] Aglycones are generally linked to L-arabinose, D-galactose, D-glucose, D-mannose, L-rhamnose, D-xylose, and D-glucuronic acid, some of which may be acetylated. Chain length of two to five saccharide units is most frequent. The oligosaccharide chains are generally linear.

The best-known plant saponins are those present in soybeans (*Glycine max*). These so-called soyasaponins are also found in other legumes. Three different aglycones have been recognized: soyasapogenol A, soyasapogenol B, and soyasapogenol E (Figure 1). Earlier identified soyasapogenols C, D, and F seem to be artifacts.[6,7]

Soyasapogenol A is attached to two different ether-linked sugar chains at positions 3 and 22, giving rise to a variety of soyasaponins (called bisdesmosides). The sugar chain attached at position 22 of soyasapogenol A may be acetylated, and both acetylated and deacetylated group A saponins have been recognized. The former compounds (triacetyl and tetracetyl derivatives) seem to be responsible for undesirable bitter and astringent taste in soybeans. Most soybean varieties contain soyasaponins Aa and/or Ab as the major acetylated compounds. Soyasapogenol B- and soyasapogenol E-derived saponins contain a sugar attached to position 3 alone (monodesmosides). Soyasaponin Bb, also called soyasaponin I, is a common representative of the B-group saponins.[5]

Soyasaponin I has been identified also in many varieties of edible beans (*Phaseolus vulgaris*) such as navy beans and kidney beans, closely related runner beans (*P. aureus*), scarlet runner beans (*P. coccineus*), butter beans (*P. lunatus*), fava beans (*Vicia faba*), chick peas (*Cicer arietinum*), garden peas (*Pisum sativum*), and lentils (*Lens culinaris*).[8,9] It has also been found in peanuts (*Arachis hypogaea*).[7] The most abundant sapogenin of sugar and silver beets (*Beta vulgaris*) is oleanolic acid,[10] and two major spinach (*Spinacea oleracea*) sapogenols[3,11] are oleanolic acid and hederagenin (Figure 2). Quinoa grain (*Chenopodium quinoa*), consumed as a staple food in South America,[12,13] contains saponins possessing as the major aglycones phytolaccagenic acid, hederagenin, and oleanolic acid (Figure 2). The most abundant tea (*Camellia sinensis*) saponins[14] are derived from theasapogenol A to E (Figure 2). Licorice (*Glycyrrhiza glabra*) has a long history as a medical plant.[15] The root and rhizome contain large amounts of a mixture of saponins, primarily glycyrrhizin, and have an intensely sweet taste, reportedly 50 times sweeter

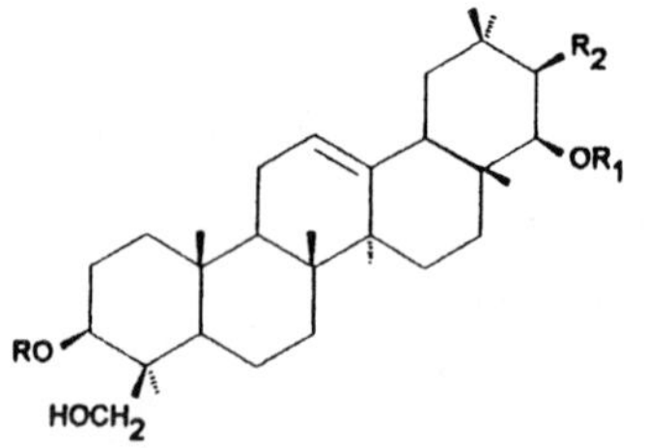

soyasapogenol A	R = R_1 = H, R_2 = OH
soyasapogenol B	R = R_1 = R_2 = H
soyasaponin Aa	R = glu-(1→2)-gal-(1→2)-gluA-(1→)- R_1 = 2,3,4-triacetyl-xyl-(1→3)-ara-, R_2 = OH
soyasaponin Ab	R = glu-(1→2)-gal-(1→2)-gluA-(1→)- R_1 = 2,3,4,6-tetracetyl-glu(1→3)-ara-, R_2 = OH
soyasaponin Bb or I	R = rha-(1→2)-gal-(1→2)-gluA-(1→)-, R_1 = R_2 = H

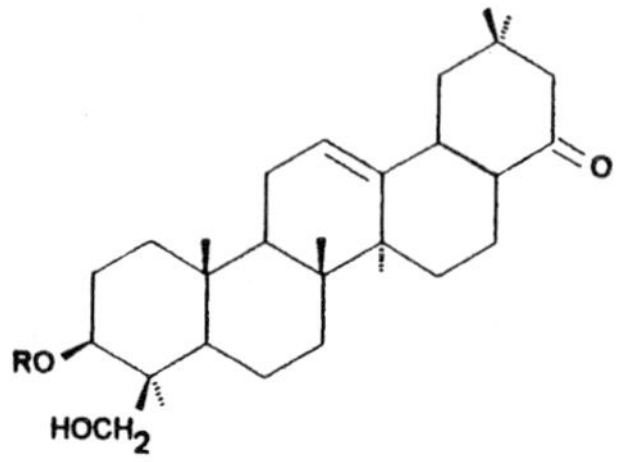

soyasapogenol E R = H

Figure 1 Structure of soyasapogenols and soyasaponins: ara, L-arabinose; gal, D-galactose; glu, D-glucose; gluA, D-glucuronic acid; rha, L-rhamnose; xyl, D-xylose.

than sucrose. The major sapogenin of licorice saponins is glycyrrhetinic acid (Figure 2). The bark of the quillaia tree (*Quillaia saponaria*) is a source of saponin used by the food industry as a foaming agent, particularly in soft drinks such as ginger beer.[4] Quillaic acid and gypsogenic acid (Figure 2) are the major aglycones.[16,17] Garlic (*Allium sativum*) saponins are based on a phytosterol sitosterol; onion (*A. cepa*) saponins contain sitosterol, oleanolic acid, and a triterpenic alcohol β-amyrin; and leek (*A. ampeloprasum*) saponins contain oleanolic acid and gitogenin.[18] Asparagus (*Asparagus officinalis*) saponins are also based on steroidal sapogenols. Typical saponins found in asparagus are officinalisnin I and II, which contain 5β-furostan-3β,22α,26-triol aglycone, and asparasaponin I and II, containing yamogenin. Sarsapogenin has been found as a minor aglycone (Figure 3).[19,20] A series of additional steroidal saponins (asparagosides) have been identified. The seeds of tomatoes contain a similar saponin.[21] Fenugreek (*Trigonella foenum-graecum*) leaves, used in India as a vegetable, and fenugreek seeds, used in the West as a spice, contain steroidal saponins called fenugrins and graecunins.[22] The major aglycone is diosgenin (Figure 3). The same aglycone is contained in saponins of yam tubers (*Dioscorea* species) used for human consumption in Southeast Asia and the Pacific region.[23,24]

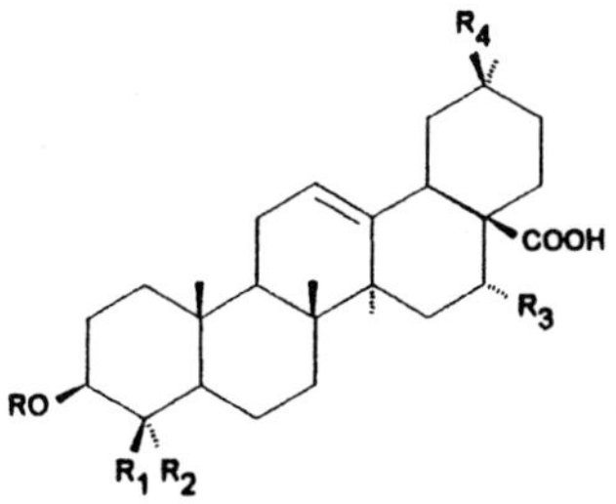

oleanolic acid	$R = R_1 = R_2 = R_3 = R_4 = H$
phytolaccagenic acid	$R = R_1 = R_3 = H$, $R_2 = CH_2OH$, $R_4 = COOCH$
gypsogenic acid	$R = R_1 = R_3 = R_4 = H$, $R_2 = CHO$
guillaic acid	$R = R_1 = R_4 = H$, $R_2 = CHO$, $R_3 = OH$
hederagenin	$R = R_1 = R_3 = R_4 = H$, $R_2 = CH_2OH$

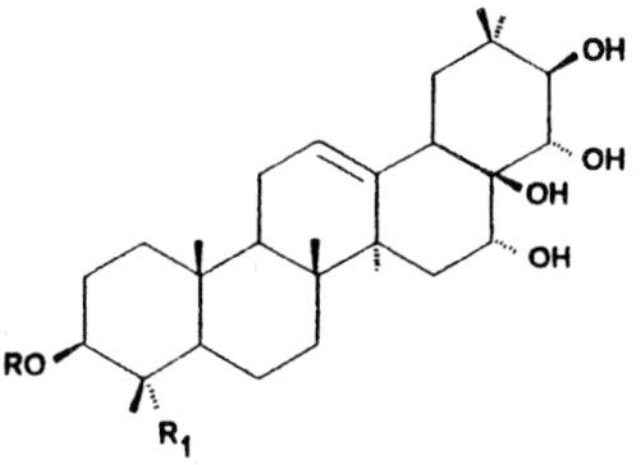

theasapogenol A	$R = H$, $R_1 = CH_2OH$
theasapogenol B	$R = H$, $R_2 = CHO$

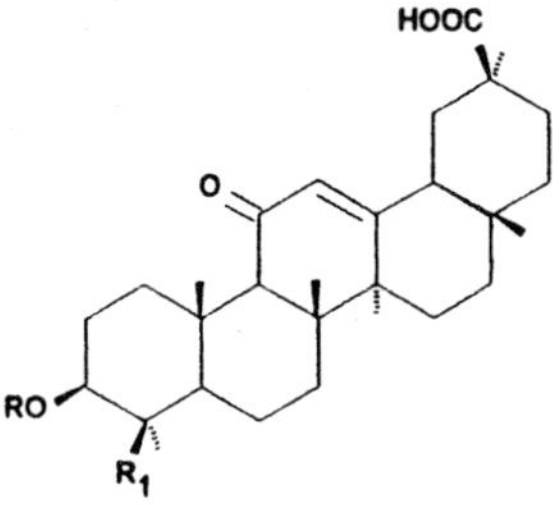

glycyrrhetinic acid	$R = H$, $R_1 = CH_3$
glycyrrhizin	R = gluA-(1 − 2)-gluA-(1 −), $R_1 = CH_3$

Figure 2 Structure of other major triterpenoid sapogenols and saponins (gluA, D-glucuronic acid).

TOXIC EFFECTS

In the past, saponins were treated as antinutritional and toxic food constituents that also influence the sensory properties of foods, such as bitterness and astringency. Some saponins are indeed toxic, but most are not. Consumed in a number of staple foods, saponins appear to have no injurious effects, and recent work has even brought to light more positive, beneficial effects of these dietary compounds.[4,5]

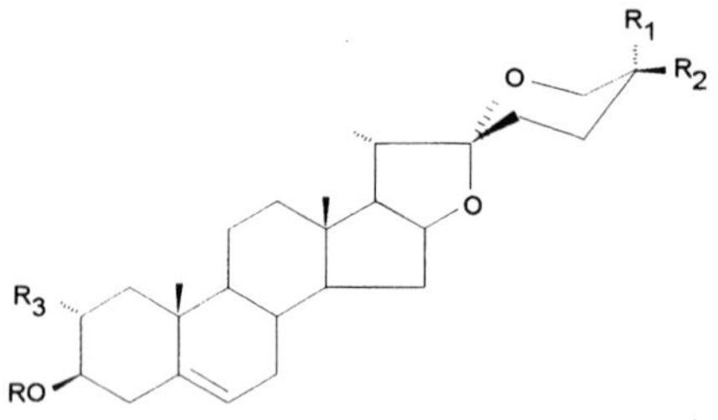

sarsapogenin	$R = R_2 = R_3 = H,\ R_1 = CH_3$
yamogenin	$R = R_1 = H,\ R_2 = CH_3,\ R_3 = OH$
diosgenin	$R = R_1 = R_2 = R_3 = H$

Figure 3 Structure of major steroid sapogenols.

Saponins are absorbed very slowly from the gastrointestinal tract of birds and mammals, but may influence the absorption and digestion of other components of the digesta and the metabolism of proteins, lipids, sugars, and minerals. Saponins are ampiphilic, strongly surface-active compounds possessing detergentlike properties. They may interact with mucosal cell membranes (causing permeability changes or loss of activity of membrane-bound enzymes) or with membrane constituents such as cholesterol and thus interfere with its absorption; they may interact with bile acids (forming micellelike aggregates) and inhibit their absorption, which is related to cholesterol metabolism, and thus become active agents in the prevention of cardiovascular diseases. For example, the alleged ability of ginseng (*Panax ginseng*), used as a medical plant to retard aging, has been attributed to the antioxidant properties of its saponins. Very high doses of toxic saponins can possibly cause intestinal irritations and lesions through which they enter the bloodstream. This can result in liver damage, hemolysis of erythrocytes, respiratory failure, convulsions, and coma. Toxic effects of saponins on cold-blooded animals (insects, fish, snails) have been known and exploited for centuries.

OCCURRENCE

Saponins are consumed in a number of staple foods and spices. Purified saponins or concentrated extracts are added to manufactured foods and drinks as foaming agents, emulsion stabilizers, or antioxidants. Glycyrrhizin has beeen used as a natural sweetening agent in confectionery, tobacco, and other products.

Saponin contents vary considerably among different plant species and varieties, depending on a number of genetic and environmental factors. Within plants, they appear to be most concentrated in the roots, rhizomes, bark, and rapidly growing shoots. Levels of saponins in some common legumes and other food plants are given in Table 1.

CHANGES DURING PROCESSING AND STORAGE

In addition to genetic, environmental, and agronomic factors, postharvest treatments, including storage, culinary, and industrial processing, affect saponin content of food plants.[3,5] Saponin solubility in water, ability to bind to other components of the plant matrix, susceptibility to partial or complete hydrolysis, and some transformation reactions may all be factors causing changes in saponin level during processing and storage in plants used for human consumption. For example, soyasaponins E are stable in the plant

Table 1 Levels of Saponins in Some Legumes and Other Food Plants

Plant	Saponin content (%)	Ref.
Soybean (*Glycine max*)	0.22–5.6	25–27
Kidney bean (*Phaseolus vulgaris*)	0.35–1.6	8,27
Runner bean (*Phaseolus aureus*)	0.34	8
Butter bean (*Phaseolus lunatus*)	0.10	8
Chick pea (*Cicer arietinum*)	0.23–6	8,27
Green pea (*Pisum sativum*)	0.11–0.18	8,27
Lentil (*Lens culinaris*)	0.11–0.51	8,27
Peanut (*Arachis hypogaea*)	0.01–1.6	8,27
Spinach (*Spinacea oleracea*)	4.7	27
Silver beet (*Beta vulgaris*)	5.8	27
Quinoa grain (*Chenopodium quinoa*)	0.14–2.3	5,13
Liquorice (*Glycyrrhiza glabra*)	2.2–15	5,15

and in crude extracts, but they are unstable in the purified form, being readily converted to the B-group soyasaponins. The glucose moiety at position 26 of steroidal saponins (such as those shown in Figure 4) may be cleaved by enzymatic or bacterial action to form spirostan derivatives. Hydrolysis to the parent compounds (aglycone and sugars), dehydration involving the β-hydroxyl, and formation of the corresponding unsaturated hydrocarbon (or dimerization to ether) is a common set of reactions of sterols.

Saponins possess undesirable bitterness and astringency in soybeans and other legumes. Bitter varieties of quinoa grain exhibit higher saponin content in comparison with semisweet and sweet varieties. Yams with high levels of saponins are bitter and often toxic. Populations in many parts of the world have learned through the ages to debitter saponin-containing foods. For example, the bitter saponins of the outer layer of quinoa grain have to be removed by washing prior to human consumption. Alternative techniques have been used, notably abrasion and decortication.[13,28] Sugar beet saponins, causing foaming of sugar juice and sugar syrups, are removed during refining of sucrose. Several procedures have been used to debitter soybeans. Mechanical removal of the outer layer of soybeans, acidic hydrolysis, fermentation,[25] and other procedures such as removal of insoluble material from the soy milk and defoaming of soy milk have been shown to reduce saponin level in traditional Japanese soybean products. Miso (fermented bean paste), natto (fermented soybeans), tonyu (soybean milk), tofu (bean curd), kori-tofu (textured bean curd), and yuba (dried bean curd) contained 0.15 to 0.44% saponin, while the full-fat soybean saponin content was 0.22 to 0.47% and that of defatted soybean was 0.67%.[5]

Cooking and canning have been claimed to have little effect on the saponin content of broad beans and navy beans (*Phaseolus vulgaris*), but soaking and canning of the hydrated beans result in significant losses.[29] The mean saponin content of raw beans was 2.06%, of soaked beans 1.08%, and of canned beans (45 min at 116°C) 0.87% (dry weight). Leaching into the soaking water and canning brine was a minor factor contributing to the decrease in the content of saponins. The major factor was hydrolysis of saponins during thermal processing. Soaking in tap water for 12 h at 30°C, 40 h of sprouting at 30°C, and ordinary cooking (15 min) of unsoaked rice beans (*Vigna umbellata*) and of green gram and black gram (*Phaseolus mungo*) caused considerable decreases in saponin content[30] (Table 2). Soaking for 12 h at 37°C, sprouting for 60 h at 25°C, ordinary cooking of presoaked seeds, and cooking for 30 min in a pressure cooker also caused significant changes[31] in the saponin content of moth beans (*Vigna aconitifolia*). For

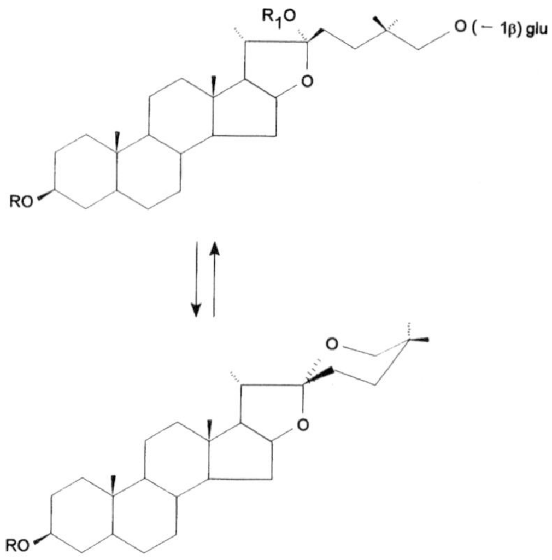

Figure 4 Interconversion of furostan-spirostan structures. (glu, D-glucose).

Table 2 Effect of Soaking, Sprouting and Cooking on the Saponin Content of Rice Beans (*Vigna umbellata*), and of Green Gram and Black Gram (*Phaseolus mungo)*

		Saponin content % (dry weight)		
Beans	**Raw**	**Soaking (12 h)**	**Sprouting (40 h)**	**Cooking (15 min)**
Rice bean[a]	2.29	2.16	1.85	1.87
Green gram	1.54	1.48	1.12	1.11
Black gram	1.68	1.55	b	1.17

[a] Average for five varieties.
[b] Not determined.

From Kaur, D. and Kapoor, A. C., *Food Chem.*, 37, 171, 1990. With permision.

example, the saponin content of seeds soaked in tap water was 2.93%, of seeds soaked in mineral salt solution 2.21%, and of sprouted seeds 0.98%. Cooking of sprouted seeds further decreased the saponin content to 0.77%; ordinary cooked presoaked seeds had a saponin level of 2.50%; pressure-cooked presoaked seeds had a saponin level of 1.75%; and pressure-cooked seeds presoaked in mineral salt solution contained 1.91% (dry weight) of saponins. The loss of saponins during soaking was attributed to the leaching into the soaking medium through simple diffusion, but the loss during cooking indicated the thermolability of saponins. Cooking was claimed[32] to have a significant effect also on the saponin content of chick peas (*Phaseolus mungo*).

Madhuca (*Madhuca butyraceae*) seeds are used as a source of oil, and the defatted flour, containing high levels of toxic saponins (about 10%), may be debittered[33] with ethanol to give a product containing 1.1% saponins.

REFERENCES

1. Oakenfull, D. G., Saponins in food: a review, *Food Chem.*, 6, 19, 1981.
2. Das, M. S. and Mahato, S. B., Triterpenoids, *Phytochemistry*, 22, 1071, 1983.
3. Price, K. R., Johnson, I. T., and Fenwick, G. R., The chemistry and biological significance of saponins in foods and feeding stuffs, *CRC Crit. Rev. Food Sci. Nutr.*, 26, 27, 1987.
4. Oakenfull, D. G. and Sidhu, G. S., Saponins, in *Toxicants of Plant Origin, Vol. II. Glycosides*, Cheeke, P. R., Ed., CRC Press, Boca Raton, Florida, 1989, 97.
5. Fenwick, G. R., Price, K. R., Tsukamoto, C., and Okubo, K., Saponins, in *Toxic Substances in Crop Plants*, D'Mello, J. P. F., Duffus, C. M., and Duffus, J. H., Eds., Royal Society of Chemistry, Cambridge, 1991, 285.
6. Kitagawa, I., Yoshikawa, M., Wang, H. K., Saito, M., Tosirusnuk, V., Fijiwara, I., and Tomita, K. I., Revised structures of soyasapogenols A, B and E, oleanene-sapogenols from soybean. Structures of soyasaponins I, II and III, *Chem. Pharm. Bull.*, 30, 2294, 1982.
7. Jurzysta, M., Arising artefacts during hydrolysis of soyasaponins, *Proc. 16th Meet. Biochem. Soc.*, Poland, 1978, 285.
8. Price, K. R., Curl, C. L., and Fenwick, G. R., The saponin content and sapogenol composition of the seed of thirteen varieties of legume, *J. Sci. Food Agric.*, 37, 1185, 1986.
9. Price, K. R. and Fenwick, G. R., Soyasaponin I, a compound possessing undesirable taste characteristics, isolated from the dried pea (*Pisum sativum*), *J. Sci. Food Agric.*, 35, 887, 1984.
10. Wagner, J. and Sternkopf, G., Chemical and physiological studies of the saponins of sugar beets, *Nahrung*, 2, 338, 1958.
11. von Tschesche, R. and Wulff, G., Triterpenes. XXVII. Saponins of spinach (*Spinacia oleracea*), *Justus Liebigs Annu. Chem.*, 726, 125, 1969.
12. Mizui, F., Kasai, R., Ohtani, K., and Tonaka, O., Saponins from brans of quinoa, *Chenopodium* Willd. I., *Chem. Pharm. Bull.*, 36, 1415, 1988.
13. Ridout, C. L., Price, K. R., DuPont, M. S., Parker, M. L., and Fenwick, G. R., Quinoa saponins — analysis and preliminary investigations into the effect of reduction by processing, *J. Sci. Food Agric.*, 54, 165, 1991.
14. von Tschesche, R., Weber, A., and Wulff, G., Über die Structur des "Theasaponins," eines Gemisches von Saponinen aus *Thea sinensis* L. mit stark antiexsuitiver Wirksamkeit, *Justus Liebigs Annu. Chem.*, 721, 209, 1969.
15. Fenwick, G. R., Lutomski, J., and Nieman, C., Liquorice, *Glycyrrhiza glabra* L. — composition, uses and analysis, *Food Chem.*, 38, 119, 1990.
16. Varshney, I. P., Beg, M. F. A., and Sankaram, A. V. B., Saponins and sapogenins from *Quillaia saponaria*, *Fitoterapia*, 56, 254, 1985.
17. Higuchi, R., Tokimitsu, Y., Fujioka, T., Komori, T., Kawasaki, T., and Oakenfull, D. G., Structure of deacylsaponin obtained from the bark of *Quillaia saponaria*, *Phytochemistry*, 26, 229, 1987.
18. Smoczkiewiczowa, M. A., Nitschke, D., and Wieladek, K., Plants of the species *Allium* (onion, garlic, leek) as sources of saponin glycosides, *Proc. Int. Congr. Commodity Science of Natural Resources*, Trieste, 1978, 407.
19. Kawano, K., Sato, H., and Sakamura, S., Isolation and structure of furostanol saponin in asparagus edible shoots, *Agric. Biol. Chem.*, 41, 1, 1977.
20. Kawano, K., Sakai, K., Sato, H., and Sakamura, S., A bitter principle of asparagus, isolation and structure of furostanol saponin in asparagus storage root, *Agric. Biol. Chem.*, 39, 1999, 1975.
21. Sato, H. and Sakamura, S., A bitter principle of tomato seeds. Isolation and structure of a new furostanol saponin, *Agric. Biol. Chem.*, 37, 225, 1973.
22. Gupta, R. K., Jain, D. C., and Thakur, R. S., Furostanol glycosides from *Trigonella foenum-graecum* seeds, *Phytochemistry*, 23, 2605, 1984.
23. Chen, A. H., Applications of the saponins of *Dioscorea*. I. Studies on the saponins of *Dioscorea* in Taiwan, *Hua Hsueh*, 43, 79, 1985.
24. Oke, O. L., Yam — a valuable source of food and drugs, *World Rev. Nutr. Diet.*, 15, 156, 1972.
25. Kitagawa, I., Yoshikawa, M., Hayashi, T., and Taniyama, T., Quantitative determination of soyasaponins in soybeans of various origins and soybean products by mean of high performance liquid chromatography, *Yakugaku Zasshi*, 104, 275, 1984.

26. Ireland, P. A. and Dziedzic, S. Z., High performance liquid chromatography on silica phase with evaporative light scattering detection, *J. Chromatogr.*, 361, 410, 1986.
27. Fenwick, D. E. and Oakenfull, D. G., Saponin content of food plants and some prepared foods, *J. Sci. Food Agric.*, 34, 186, 1983.
28. Reichert, R. D., Tatarynovitch, J. T., and Tyler, J. T., Abrasive dehulling of quinoa (*Chenopodium quinoa*) effect on saponin content as determined by an adapted hemolytic assay, *Cereal Chem.*, 63, 471, 1986.
29. Drumm, T. D., Gray, J. I., Hosfield, G. L., and Uebersax, M. A., Lipid, saccharide, protein, phenolic acid and saponin contents of four market classes of edible dry beans as influenced by soaking and canning, *J. Sci. Food Agric.*, 51, 425, 1990.
30. Kaur, D. and Kapoor, A. C., Some antinutritional factors in rice beans (*Vigna umbellata*): effects of domestic processing and cooking methods, *Food Chem.*, 37, 171, 1990.
31. Khokhar, S. and Chauhan, B. M., Antinutritional factors in moth bean (*Vigna aconitifolia*) varietal differences and effects of methods of domestic processing and cooking, *J. Food Sci.*, 51, 591, 1986.
32. Jood, S., Chanhan, B. M., and Kapoor, A. C., Saponin content of chickpea and black gram: varietal differences and effects of processing and cooking methods, *J. Sci. Food Agric.*, 37, 1121, 1986.
33. Shanmugasundaram, T. and Venkatamaran, L. V., Effect of ethanol treatment on the proteins of madhuca (*Madhuca butyraceae*) seed flour, *J. Sci. Food Agric.*, 36, 1183, 1985.

Part C
Cyanogens

Michal Voldřich

The occurrence of compounds capable of liberating hydrogen cyanide (HCN) in plants and their toxic effects have been known since antiquity, when traitorous Egyptian priests of Memphis and Thebes were poisoned with the pits of peaches.[1] The basis of the poisonous properties of cyanogenic plants was recognized about 160 years ago, when HCN was first obtained from a plant extract and when the first cyanogenic glycoside was isolated.[2,3] Since the end of the 19th century, cyanogens have maintained the interest of food chemists, due to their widespread occurrence in many important food plants and food products, and have been reviewed by several authors, e.g., Conn,[2] Davis,[3] Eyjolfsson,[4] Poulton,[5] Siegler,[6,7] Montgomery,[8,9] and Tewe and Iyayi.[10]

Generally, the ability of cyanogens to decompose, yielding free HCN (cyanogenesis) is associated with three types of compounds. The most important cyanogens are cyanogenic glycosides, which are found in several food plants. Another group with a more restricted distribution is made up of two kinds of cyanolipids, which are both derivatives of α-hydroxynitriles (cyanohydrins). The former are the gluco- or glycosides of cyanohydrins and the latter are the esters of cyanohydrins and fatty acids. Upon hydrolysis, both liberate HCN, a carbonyl component, and the sugar or fatty acid moiety, respectively. The third chemical type are the so-called pseudocyanogenic glycosides, which are glycoside derivatives of methylazoxymethanol and are not cyanogenic in the same sense, although they do release HCN when treated with alkali.

CHEMISTRY

Cyanogenic glycosides are glycosidic derivatives of 2-hydroxynitriles (cyanohydrins), with the general formula given in Figure 1.

In a majority of cyanogenic glycosides, R_1 is either an aliphatic or aromatic group and R_2 is hydrogen. Since R_1 is not the same as R_2, the carbinol atom is chiral, introducing

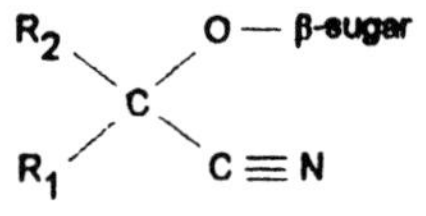

Figure 1 General formula of cyanogenic glycosides.

the possibility of epimeric pairs of glycosides. The sugar moiety, with some exceptions (amygdalin, vicianin, etc.), is D-glucose.

The most common system of glycoside classificiation is based on the known or presumed biogenetic precursors of aglycones, which include in the case of food cyanogens the amino acids L-valine, L-isoleucine, L-phenylalanine and L-tyrosine. The structures of the most important food cyanogenic glycosides are given in Figure 2. More information on chemical structure of the other cyanogens, including physical constants, spectral data, and other properties, are reviewed by the previously cited authors.[4,6]

Cyanogenic glycosides can undergo enzymatic or chemical degradation. The enzymatic hydrolysis (Figure 3) is catalyzed by two types of specific enzymes, which usually also occur in the cyanogenic tissues. With β-glucosidase (EC 3.2.1.21) the glycosidic bonds are hydrolyzed, yielding a sugar and cyanohydrin. Hydroxynitrile lyase (EC 4.1.2.10) catalyzes the subsequent cleavage of the cyanohydrin to form a carbonyl compound and HCN.[11] In almonds containing the predominant glycoside amygdalin the three specific enzymes are two β-glucosidases — amygdalin hydrolase and prunasin hydrolase — and mandelonitrile lyase, which hydrolyze amygdalin in three steps yielding glucose, benzaldehyde, and HCN.[12] The optimal pH of glucosidases ranges from 4 to 6.2 depending on the origin.

The possible path of chemical degradation of cyanogenic glycosides, under different conditions, is given in Figure 4. In dilute acid at higher temperatures the glycoside bonds can be hydrolyzed to yield sugar and cyanohydrin,[2] the reaction being acid catalyzed, while the cyanohydrin is relatively stable in acidic conditions.[13] Hydrolysis with concentrated acids can produce 2-hydroxy acids and NH_3.[14] Mild alkaline conditions [saturated $Ba(OH)_2$] typically hydrolyze the nitrile group in several glycosides without cleavage of any other bonds yielding the glycosidic acids.[2] Some glycosides (e.g., dhurrin) on the other hand, decompose to form a sugar, HCN, and a carbonyl compound under these conditions.[15] The mild alkaline conditions also facilitate epimerization of cyanogenic glycosides having electron-withdrawing groups (aromatic ring, etc.) adjacent to carbinol carbon. Amygdalin can produce a significant amount of its epimer neoamygdalin under elevated temperature at pH 7.[16]

The so-called pseudocyanogenic glycosides are glycosides of methylazoxymethanol and possess chemical properties different from cyanogenic glycosides. When treated with dilute base they liberate HCN, whereas treatment with acid or β-glucosidase liberates N_2, formaldehyde, and methanol.[6] The structure and possible pathways of pseudocyanogenic glycosides degradation are given in Figure 5.

TOXIC EFFECTS

Generally, both forms of cyanide can be expected to occur in foods, the free HCN, more or less dissociated according to the conditions in the foods, and the cyanides, stabilized in the form of original cyanogenic substances or converted to other compounds (cyanohydrins of fruit sugars, complexes with mineral ions, etc.).

The toxicity and toxic effects of HCN have been well known for a long time. The acute toxic effect of HCN is ascribed to its ability to inhibit respiration due to the inhibition of

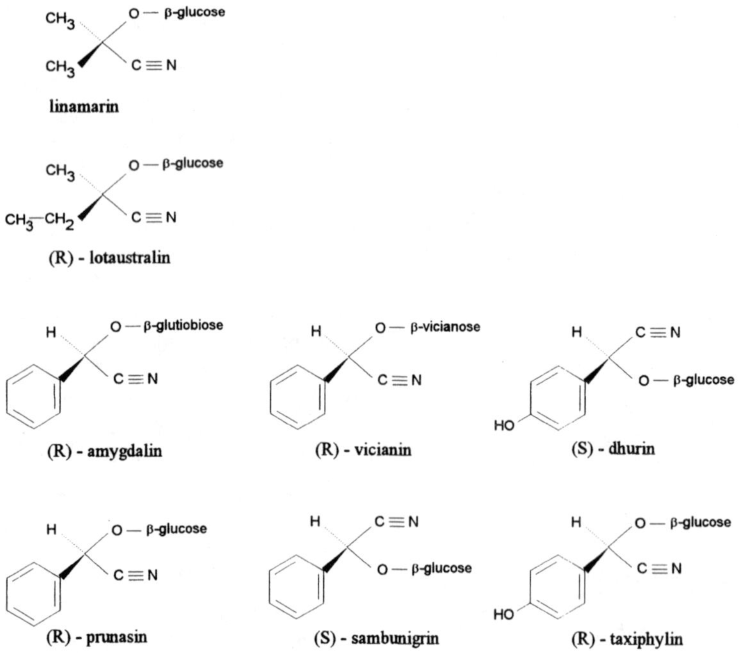

Figure 2 Structures of the most important cyanogenic glycosides.

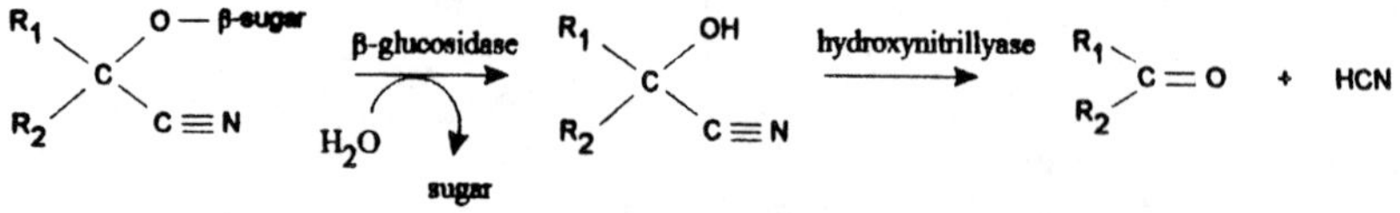

Figure 3 Enzymatic hydrolysis of cyanogenic glycosides.

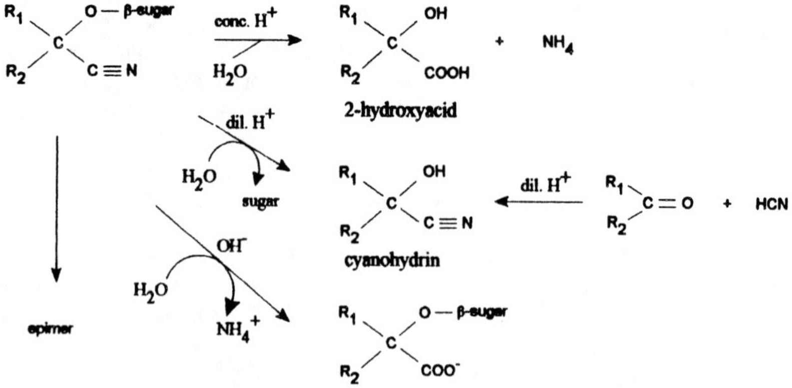

Figure 4 Chemical degradation of cyanogenic glycosides.

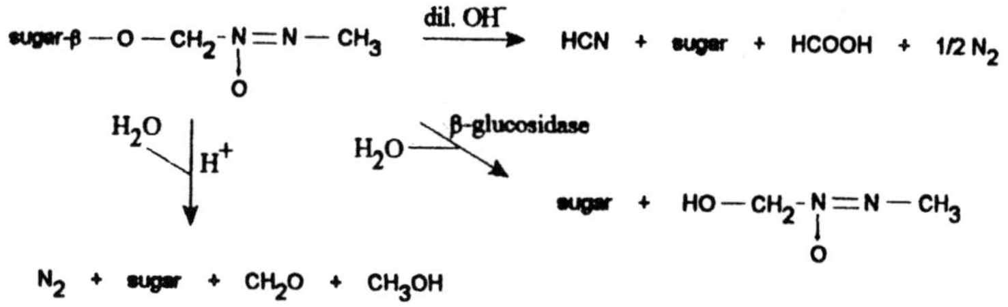

Figure 5 Degradation of pseudocyanogenic glycosides.

cytochrome oxidase (EC 1.9.3.1) in the respiratory chain. The cyanide binds with both the oxidized and reduced forms of the enzyme. Earlier opinion was that cyanide inhibition involves the copper ions of cytochromoxidase, but recent studies indicate binding with iron.[10,17] The minimum lethal dose of HCN for humans has been estimated to be in the range 0.5 to 3.5 $mg.kg^{-1}$ of body weight,[8] i.e., from 35 to 245 mg for a 70-kg adult.

Cyanides are rapidly absorbed in the intestinal system; the symptoms after intoxication with a lethal dose are peripheral numbness and light-headedness, followed by mental confusion and stupor, cyanosis, convulsions, and terminal coma. Nonlethal doses provoke similar symptoms — headache, a sensation of tightness in the throat and chest, palpitation, and muscle weakness. The intensity and duration depend on the dose and physical condition of the individual.[8,18] When nonlethal quantities of HCN are consumed, cyanide is removed by respiratory exchange or a detoxification process. But the regular intake of nonlethal doses of HCN can produce chronic cyanide intoxication. The degenerative disease known as tropical ataxic neuropathy has been shown to have an evident coherence with HCN consumed in cassava food products.[19,20]

The thiocyanates that are produced within the cyanide detoxification process are known to be a goitrogenic factor, inhibiting the intrathyroidal transfer of iodine and causing an elevation of the thyroid-stimulating hormone. The comprehensively higher occurrence of endemic goiter and cretenism has been reported in the tropical region of cassava production in Africa.[21] Furthermore, there is a higher incidence of diabetes in areas where cassava is eaten.[22] Other possible health consequences of chronic cyanide intoxication are given in the reviews of Montgomery,[8,9] Davis,[3] and Tewe and Iyai.[10] The possibility of malnutrition, especially deficiency of proteins, with particular reference to sulfur amino acids, cobalamine and thiamine, being a contributory factor to susceptibility is also suggested by all the cited authors.

When fresh cyanide plants containing intact glycosides and natural hydrolytic enzymes (or enzymes of other sources) are consumed some release of cyanide can occur in the digestive tract, but the conditions favor neither enzymatic nor chemical hydrolysis.[5] In experiments with rats orally treated, intact glucosides were excreted in urine unchanged, but an increase of thiocyanate in blood also indicated some release of cyanide.[23] The intravenous administration of cyanogens was tolerated well, and therefore it seems probable that more HCN is released by the intestinal microflora in the monogastric digestive tract than by tissues.[3]

Similar to other toxic compounds, cyanide and cyanogens have found pharmacological applications.[10] Recently, anticarcinogenic properties of the cyanogenic glucosides have also been suggested. Following the general hypothesis, the released cyanides in tissues attack the cancer cells, which are believed to be low in rhodanese (EC 2.8.1.1). The normal cells, possessing sufficient rhodanese activity, are able to detoxify cyanides.[10]

Table 1 Distribution of Some Cyanogens in Food Plants

Compound	Plant	Common name
Cyanogenic glycosides		
Linamarin	*Manihot esculenta*	Cassava
	Phaseolotus lunatus	Lima beans
Lotaustralin	*Manihot esculenta*	Cassava
	Phaseolotus lunatus	Lima beans
Dhurrin	*Sorghum* spp.	Forage sorghums
Taxiphyllin	*Bambusa* spp.	Bamboo
Amygdalin	*Prunus* spp.	Almond, peach, apricot, plum
	Malus spp.	Apple
Prunasin	*Prunus* spp.	Almond, peach, apricot, plum
	Sambucus nigra	Elderberry
	Passiflora edulis	Passion fruit
Pseudocyanogenic glycosides		
Cycasin		Cycad

In North America amygdalin and the mandelonitrile derivative of glucuronic acid are used for the treatment of cancer.[24]

OCCURRENCE

Cyanogens are widely exhibited within the plant kingdom. Although the estimated number of cyanogenic plant species is 1000 in 500 genera comprising 100 families,[2] it has been recently stated that there are only 55 direct precursors of cyanide in plants, including the pseudocyanogenic glycosides.[10] The number of isolated and characterized cyanogens gradually increases, and at present it is almost double that given in the review by Seigler in 1975.[6] Comprehensive reviews of the occurrence of cyanogenic glycosides in plants were made by Conn[2] and Poulton.[5]

Fortunately, not all cyanogenic plants are used in food production. The list of main food cyanogens and their sources is given in Table 1, and the maximum cyanogen contents in different food plants are shown in Table 2.

The most important cyanogenic plant in human nutrition is cassava (*Manihot esculenta*), also known as manioc, yucca, or tapioca, which is a major source of dietary energy for over 500 million people in tropical regions.[25] The predominant cyanogen in cassava is linamarin (also called phaseolunatin, after its other important source), which is usually found together with lotaustralin, both being synthesized from the structurally related amino acids valine and isoleucine as precursors.[30] The glycosides are present in leaves and tubers, both of which may be eaten or used for food preparation.

Linamarin also predominates in peas and beans, especially in lima or butter beans (*Phaseolus lunatus*), which are generally an important source of protein in human nutrition. It occurs in all parts of the plants throughout the entire growing period. The black varieties of lima or butter beans contain more cyanogens than others. Systematic cultivation of white varieties has greatly reduced the cyanide content (nearly 100 times), but probably no variety totally free of cyanogens could be produced.[9] Other important legumes, such as soybeans, contain only very small amounts of cyanogens, probably of nonnutritional significance.[31,32]

Table 2 Maximum Contents of Cyanogens in Food Plants

Plant	Cyanogen content expressed as HCN yield (mg.100 g^{-1} fresh weight)	Ref.
Cassava		
Young leaves	65	25
Dried root cortex	245	8
Whole root	55	8
Lima or butter bean		
Black varieties	300	8
Bamboo		
Imature stem	300	26
Tip of immature shoots	800	26
Stone fruits		
Apricot seeds	320	27
Morello cherry seeds	354	28
Pulp	1	28
Passion fruit		29
Immature	70	
Mature	10	

Grasses are another important source of cyanogens, and especially the *Sorghum* species can contain significant amounts of cyanogenic glycosides derived from tyrosine-dhurrin. This glycoside is not found in the seeds, but can account for up to 30% dry weight of immature young tissues, mainly young seedlings.[3,8] For humans, consumption of germinated seeds of sorghum could probably be dangerous, but forage species containing more than 1 g cyanogens expressed as HCN per 1 kg dry matter represent a severe risk to livestock. The arrowgrass species, in which the cyanogens are triglochinin and taxiphyllin, could also cause livestock poisoning, but taxiphyllin contained in immature bamboo shoots could also be poisonous for humans when consumed in a fresh, uncooked state or incorporated uncooked in pickles and chutney.[26]

The first isolated and characterized cyanogenic glycoside was amygdalin,[5] responsible for the toxicity of many plants of the Rosaceae family. Its well-known sources are bitter almonds and the seeds of peaches, apricots, plums, cherries, and also apples, pears, etc. Amygdalin usually occurs in seeds, while its probable precursor prunasin can be found in the pulp of immature fruits. The Rosaceae are not as dangerous as the cyanogenic plants discussed above, and instances of human poisoning arise rather through misuse, such as consumption of the bitter seeds of apricots by children[33] or preparing peach leaf tea.[34] But the processing of kernel fruits containing higher levels of cyanogen using nonstandard technologies could be a source of a regular ingestion of nonlethal doses of HCN.[28,35]

Prunasin is also the dominant cyanogen of immature passion fruits (*Passiflora edulis*), cultivated throughout the tropic and subtropic areas, where it is important in local diets and available in most markets.[36]

Sambunigrin — an epimer of prunasin — is a predominant cyanogen of *Sambucus* species, in which it occurs in all parts of the plant. It is also found in immature elderberries, in which its content decreases to zero during maturation.[2,6] As in the case of the fruit of the Rosaceae family, elderberries do not present a risk of human poisoning, but the juice of immature fruits can have an unpleasant bitter taste.[37]

The other groups of cyanogens, the cyanolipids and pseudocyanogenic glycosides, are of less nutritional importance compared with the cyanogenic glycosides. Probably the pseudocyanogenic glycoside cycasin and related compounds, occurring in the plants of the Cycadaceae family, could be of a considerable interest, because cycad seeds are used as a source of edible starch in some parts of the world.[6] But only the intact substances could have deleterious health effects, because the formation of cyanides proceeds only under alkaline conditions, and these do not occur very often during the processing of cycad seeds.

Considering the increasing number of cyanogens and sorts of plants that are used by humans, the list of cyanogenic food plants could be extended. Also, the content of HCN and cyanogens in food plants depends on the plant variety and age as well as the growing and postharvest conditions. The content of cyanogens is therefore unpredictable, and if any cyanogenic plants are processed, the risks of cyanogenesis before and within technological processing and storage of food products should be considered.

CHANGES DURING FOOD PROCESSING AND STORAGE

The cyanogen content changes even before technological processing. A number of cyanogenic fruits contain cyanogens only in their immature state,[2] but other cyanogenic plants contain significantly lower quantities of cyanogens in older tissues; e.g., the cyanogen concentration in the old (green) leaves of cassava is less than 50% of that in the young leaves of the same plant.[38] In addition to the age of plants, the content of cyanogens can be affected by fertilization, genetic and seasonal factors, and other growing conditions.[2,3,10,39] It may be supposed that cyanogenic compounds have a defensive function in plants,[1] but only the increase in dhurrin content in sorghum species caused by soil moisture stress has been described.[40]

In the intact plant tissues the glycosides and hydrolytic enzymes are spatially separated; in dark-grown sorghum seedlings and green sorghum leaves the glycosides are localized in the vacuoles of these tissues,[41,42] which do not contain glycosidases. β-Glucosidases were found in the soluble cytoplasmatic fraction.[43] Damage to cell membranes by technological processing (peeling, cutting, heating, homogenization, etc.) or during physiological changes (e.g., in overripe fruits) allows enzymes to hydrolyze glycosides to produce sugars, carbonyls, and HCN. The enzymatic hydrolysis catalyzed by endogenous enzymes — linamarase (in linamarin-containing plants), emulsine (Rosaceae), etc. — is the main factor producing HCN within the technological processing of cyanogenic plants. An acid hydrolysis of glycosides that can proceed under the higher temperatures within the processing of stone fruits[11,20] is usually terminated in production of cyanohydrine, which is stable in acidic conditions. Alkaline or neutral pH values, which can favor the cyanohydrine dissociation, do not affect the glycosidic bonds.

Another general factor affecting the HCN changes in the processing of cyanogenic plants is its volatility. HCN, with a pK_a of 9.6, is practically undissociated in plant tissues, and its low boiling point (26°C) allows it to evaporate.

People using cassava as a basic food have developed various processing techniques to decrease the cyanide content in cassava products. The traditional processing techniques comprise:

- *Sun drying.* Peeled tubers are cut and dried in the sun. The enzymatic hydrolysis of linamarin in tissues damaged by peeling and cutting could be expected (as well as the membrane permeability changes in consequence of drying) to allow the contact enzyme with substrate. But these reactions only proceed at the beginning of drying. The extent of glycoside degradation depends on cyanogen content, activity of enzymes, conditions of drying, and other factors and usually rises to a maximum of 70% of initial cyanogens.[17,44]

- *Crushing and grinding.* Homogenization of the fresh tubers allows good contact of endogenous enzymes with glycosides, depending on their condition (length of process, pH, temperature, etc.). This method, followed by a procedure eliminating evolved HCN, is very efficient in cassava detoxification.
- *Soaking by immersion in water.* The significant diminution of the cyanide content by soaking is possible only if more than 18 to 20 h is used to break the cells by osmotic pressure and to initialize the enzymatic hydrolysis.[17]
- *Fermentation.* This is the principal preparation method for popular cassava foods (farinha de mandioca, gari, tape, etc.), because it removes most of the cyanogens, and during this procedure the substances responsible for the characteristic flavor are produced. Usually, washed, peeled and grated tubers are fermented spontaneously. Within the fermentation the enzymatic hydrolysis catalyzed by endogenous plant enzymes occurs. It can also be promoted by exogenous β-glucosidases found in some of the microorganisms participating in the fermentation process.[45] Organic acids that are formed within the fermentation can favor the stabilization of HCN by reaction with carbonyl compounds present in fermented products.[3] The course of fermentation varies depending on the conditions,[45-48] leading to a decrease in the cyanogen content to about 90% of the original amount (Figure 6).[46,49]
- *Cooking.* Simple cooking in water can also reduce the cyanogen content by initiating enzymatic hydrolysis at the beginning of heating. As a result of osmotic effects and elevated temperature, the permeability of cell membranes is increased, allowing the enzymatic reactions to proceed until the enzymes are inactivated. The other detoxification effects are the extraction of cyanogens and their degradation products into surrounding water and removal of HCN in the vapor. The conditions in the plant (pH about 5) do not favor direct chemical hydrolysis of glycosides. These conclusions can be supported by the results of Essers,[50] who found, after 30 min of boiling in water, 8 and 30% of the original content of cyanogens in cassava when put in cold water and when put directly in boiling water, respectively.

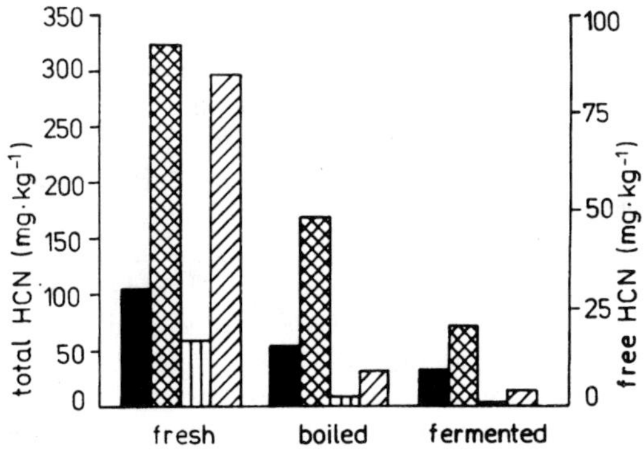

Figure 6 Total and free cyanide contents in cassava fresh, boiled (30 min), and boiled (30 min) and fermented (3 d). ■, Total HCN (minimum); ▩, total HCN (maximum); ▥, free HCN (minimum); ▨, free HCN (maximum).

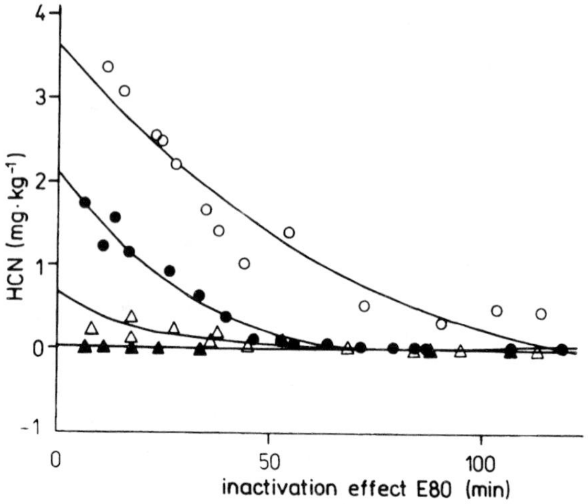

Figure 7 Dependence of HCN content in edible portion of canned stone fruit on the inactivation effect E_{80} of a heat treatment. △, Apricots; ○, plums; ●, morello cherries; ▲, peaches. (From Voldřich, M. and Kyzlink, V., *J. Food Sci.*, 57, 161, 1992. With permission.)

The stone fruits are not as important a source of cyanides as cassava products, but they could also present the possibility of regular cyanide intake in human nutrition. In contrast to cassava, which contains high quantities of cyanogens in the edible parts of the plant, stone fruits contain the majority of cyanogens in their seeds, which are not usually eaten. The processing of stone fruit should reduce the degree of glycoside degradation evolving HCN that penetrates to edible parts of fruit products. If whole wild cherries are pressed during juice production, damage to the kernels and seeds allows endogenous enzymes to hydrolyze glycosides (amygdalin, prunasin) so that the juice can contain up to 15 $mg.kg^{-1}$ HCN (depending on an initial content of glucosides in fruits), which is more than 10 times higher than when the fruits without kernels are pressed.[51,52]

The higher content of HCN can also be found in stewed (canned) stone fruits prepared from whole fruits, where the maximum reported level of HCN was 33 $mg.kg^{-1}$ of HCN in canned whole apricots in sugar solution.[53] If the cyanogen-containing fruits are processed, heat treatment — sterilization — is the main factor affecting the extent of cyanogen degradation. Similar to cassava processing, the hydrolysis is caused almost exclusively by enzymes and proceeds only at the beginning of the heating process, when the membranes are damaged and the enzymes are not inactivated. The higher the inactivation effect, the lower the HCN content of canned fruits (Figure 7).[20] The final HCN content is also affected by the course of the heat treatment. Slow heating without reaching the temperature needed to inactivate the relatively thermoresistant β-glucosidases (in addition protected by a heat isolation effect of pulp) results in higher levels of HCN in products.[54] During the storage of fruit products (juices, canned stone fruit, etc.) in the absence of enzymes, a very slow acid hydrolysis of glycosides can proceed, but the acidic conditions stabilize the cyanohydrins or catalyze their formation. The very slow increase of free HCN during long-term storage of canned morello cherries and apricots was probably caused by penetration of HCN from areas of higher concentration.[54]

Similar changes also occur during the fermentation of kernel fruits during production of stone fruit distillates, especially if the fruits with leaves and twigs are processed. At the beginning of fermentation the enzymes are in contact with substrates that produce HCN.[55]

During distillation HCN is concentrated in distillates, which can contain 0.3 to 3 $mg.kg^{-1}$ HCN.[52]

The seeds of stone fruits are also used to manufacture different products, e.g., marzipan, bitter almond oil, and macaroon paste in Europe and North America and almond jelly in Japan.[55,56] During the production of these products, kernels are crushed or soaked in water or subjected to other treatments leading to the enzymatic hydrolysis of glycosides. The evolved HCN is then usually eliminated by heating during the following steps of the manufacture.[3,55]

During the processing of other cyanogenic plants, changes similar to those described above proceed. Exceptional within the cyanogenic plants is bamboo, the predominant cyanogen of which is taxiphylin.[8] This glycoside is unusually thermolabile and decomposes during boiling,[57] thus cooking is sufficient to detoxify bamboo shoots.[8]

Cyanogenic glycosides generally have a bitter taste and with some exceptions, depending also on other factors, the degradation of glycosides results in reduction of the bitterness.[3]

Degradation products of glycosides can also undergo other reactions in foods. The acid-catalyzed formation of cyanohydrins has already been discussed. There is a hypothesis, which has not yet been confirmed, that cyanide produced by the degradation of cyanogenic glycosides could be one of the precursors of the teratogen ethyl carbamate (page 251), which was found in relatively high concentrations in the stone fruit distillates.[58,59] Benzaldehyde is the major component of stone fruit volatiles and is largely responsible for the characteristic flavor of products made from them.[54,60] Its content in wild cherries correlated positively with the hedonic sensorial quality of flavor.[54] Benzaldehyde also undergoes oxidation reactions to form benzoic acid, which can be present (depending on the glycoside content and conditions of processing) at levels of 0 to 20 $mg.kg^{-1}$ in plum and apricot juices and preserves and up to 350 $mg.kg^{-1}$ in the case of the stone fruit juice concentrates.[61]

Regardless of the extent of current knowledge, the cyanogenic glycosides will always represent risks of human poisoning. Therefore, when cyanogenic plants are processed, only techniques ensuring the lowest HCN content in products should be used. To estimate the safe dose of HCN that can be consumed without any health problems, the ADI value of Codex Alimentarius for flour treated with HCN (insecticide) (0.05 mg $HCN.kg^{-1}$ of body weight per day corresponding to 3.5 mg HCN per day for the 70-kg adult) can be used.[62]

REFERENCES

1. Hruska, A. J., Cyanogenic glucosides as defense compounds. A review of the evidence, *J. Chem. Ecol.*, 14(12), 2213, 1988.
2. Conn, E. E., Cyanogenic glycosides, in *Secondary Plant Products*, Bell, E. A. and Charlwood, B. V., Eds., Springer Verlag, New York, 1980, chap. 9.
3. Davis, R. H., Cyanogens, in *Toxic Substances in Crop Plants*, D'Mello, F. J. P., Duffus, C. M., and Duffus, J. H., Eds., Royal Society of Chemistry, Cambridge, 1991, chap. 9.
4. Eyjolfsson, R., Recent advances in the chemistry of cyanogenic glucosides, *Fortschr. Chem. Org. Naturst.*, 28, 74, 1970.
5. Poulton, J. E., Cyanogenic compounds in plants and their toxic effects, in *Handbook of Natural Toxins*, Vol. 1, Keller, R. F. and Tu, A. T., Eds., Marcel Dekker, New York, 1983.
6. Seigler, D. S., Isolation and characterization of naturally occurring cyanogenic compounds, *Phytochemistry*, 14, 9, 1975.
7. Seigler, D. S., Cyanogenic glycosides and lipids: structural types and distribution, in *Cyanide in Biology*, Vennesland, B., Conn, E. E., Knowles, C. J., Westley, J., and Wissing, F., Eds., Academic Press, London, 1981.

8. Montgomery, R. D., Cyanogens, in *Toxic Constituents of Plant Foodstuffs*, Liener, I. E., Ed., Academic Press, New York, 1969.
9. Montgomery, R. D., Cyanogens, in *Toxic Constituents of Plant Foodstuffs*, Liener, I. E., Ed., Academic Press, London, 1980.
10. Tewe, O. O. and Iyayi, E. A., Cyanogenic glycosides, in *Toxicants of Plant Origin, Vol. 1, Alkaloids,* Cheeke, P. R., Ed., CRC Press, Boca Raton, Florida, 1988.
11. Haisman, D. R. and Knight, D. J., The enzymic hydrolysis of amygdalin, *Biochem. J.*, 108, 528, 1967.
12. Haisman, D. R., Knight, D. J., and Ellis, M. J., The electrophoretic separation of the β-glucosidase of almond emulsin, *Phytochemistry*, 6, 1501, 1967.
13. Svirbely, W. J. and Roth, J. F., The effect of acid catalysis on the kinetics of cyanhydrin formation, *J. Am. Chem. Soc.*, 75, 3106, 1953.
14. Nartey, F., *Manihot esculenta* (Cassava): cyanogenesis, ultrastructure and seed germination, in *Abstracts on Cassava,* Vol. 4, Ser. 08EC-4, C.I.A.T. Publication, Columbia, 1978.
15. Mao, C. H. and Anderson, L., Partial purification and characterization of two β-glucosidases from *Sorghum* tissues, *Phytochemistry*, 6, 473, 1967.
16. Nahrstedt, A., Die Isomerisierung von Amygdalin und Homologen, *Arch. Pharm.*, 308, 903, 1975.
17. Way, J. L., Cyanide intoxication and its mechanism of antagonism, *Annu. Rev. Pharmacol. Toxicol.*, 24, 451, 1984.
18. Polson, C. J. and Tattersall, R. N., *Clinical Toxicology,* English University Press, London, 1959.
19. Osontokun, B. O., An ataxic neuropathy in Nigeria: a clinical biochemical and electrophysical study, *Brain,* 91, 215, 1968.
20. Osontokun, B. O., Cassava and cyanide metabolism in Wistar rats, *Br. J. Nutr.*, 24, 377, 1970.
21. Ekpechi, O. E., Pathogenesis of endemic goitre in Eastern Nigeria, *Br. J. Nutr.*, 21, 537, 1966.
22. McMillan, D. S. and Geevarghese, P. J., Dietary cyanide and tropical malnutrition diabetes, *Diabetes Care,* 2(2), 1979.
23. Hill, D. C., Physiological and biochemical responses of rats given potassium cyanide or linamarin, in *Cassava as Animal Feed,* Nastel, B. and Graham, M., Eds., International Development Research Centre, Ottawa, 1977.
24. Cairs, T., Froberg, J. E., Gonzales, S., Langham, W. S., Stamp, J., Howie, J. K., and Sawsek, D. T., Analytical chemistry of amygdalin, *Anal. Chem.*, 50, 317, 1978.
25. Casadei, E., Nutritional and toxicological aspects of the cassava, in *Proc. Int. Symp.,* Instituto Superiore di Sanita, Roma, Italy 14–16 March, 1987, Taylor and Francis, London, 1988.
26. Baggchi, K. N. and Gouguli, H. D., Toxicology of young shoots of common bamboos (*Bambusa arundinacea*), *Indian Med. Gaz.*, 78, 40, 1943.
27. Stoewsand, G. S., Anderson, J. L., and Lamb, R. C., Cyanide content of apricot kernels, *J. Food Sci.,* 40, 1107, 1975.
28. Voldřich, M. and Kyzlink, V., Cyanogenesis in canned stone fruits, *J. Food Sci.,* 57, 161, 1992.
29. Spencer, K. C. and Seigler, D. S., Cyanogenesis of *Pasiflora edulis*, *J. Agric. Food Chem.*, 31, 794, 1983.
30. Hahlbrock, K. and Conn, E. E., Evidence for the formation of linamarin and lotaustralin in flax seedlings by the same glucosyl transferase, *Phytochemistry,* 10, 1019, 1971.
31. Montgomery, R. D., Observation on the cyanide content and toxicity of tropical pulses, *W. Indian Med. J.,* 13, 1, 1964.
32. Honig, D. H., Hockridge, M. E., Gould, R. M., and Rackis, J. J., Determination of cyanide in soybeans and soybean products, *J. Agric. Food Chem.,* 31, 272, 1983.
33. Yatziv, A. S., Cyanide intoxication in childhood after ingesting apricot kernels, *J. Isr. Med. Assoc,* 76, 535, 1969.
34. Kingsbury, J. M., *Poisonous Plants of the United States and Canada,* Prentice-Hall, Englewood Cliffs, New Jersey, 1964.
35. Gierschner, K. and Baumann, G., Beitrage zur Analyse der Inhaltsstoffe von Fruchten und Fruchtsaften. III. Mitteilung, Bestimmung des Blausauregehaltes besonders in Sauerkirschaften und Steinen, *Z. Lebensm. Unters. Forsch.,* 139, 132, 1969.
36. Hendrick, U. P., *Sturtenant's Edible Plants of the World,* Dover, New York, 1972.
37. Kyzlink, V., *Principles of Food Preservation,* Elsevier, Amsterdam, 1990.

38. Cooke, R. D. and de la Cruz, E. M., The changes in cyanide content of cassava (*Manihot esculenta*) tissues during plant development, *J. Sci. Food Agric.*, 33, 269, 1982.
39. Kakes, P., Properties and function of the cyanogenic systems in higher plants, *Euphytica*, 48, 25, 1990.
40. Nelson, C. E., HCN content of certain sorghums under irrigation as affected by nitrogen fertilizer and soil moisture stress, *Agron. J.*, 45, 615, 1953.
41. Saunders, J. A., Conn, E. E., Lin, C. H., and Stocking, C. R., Subcellular localization of the cyanogenic glucoside of *Sorghum* by autoradiography, *Plant Physiol.*, 59, 647, 1977.
42. Saunders, J. A. and Conn, E. E., Presence of the cyanogenic glucoside dhurrin in isolated vacuoles of *Sorghum*, *Plant Physiol.*, 61, 154, 1978.
43. Butcher, H. C., Wagner, G. J., and Siegelman, H. W., Localization of acid hydrolases in protoplasts, *Plant Physiol.*, 59, 1098, 1977.
44. FAO, Roots, tubers, plantains and bananas in human nutrition, *Food and Nutrition Series, No. 24*, FAO, Rome, 1980.
45. Ikediobi, C. O. and Ohyike, E., The use of linamarase in gari production, *Process Biochem.*, July/August, 2, 1982.
46. Arihatana, M. B. and Buckle, K. A., Cassava detoxication during tape fermentation with traditional inoculum, *Int. J. Food Sci. Technol.*, 22, 41, 1987.
47. Akinrele, I. A., Fermentation of cassava, *J. Sci. Food Agric.*, 15, 589, 1964.
48. Ogunusna, A. O., Changes in some chemical constituents during the fermentation of cassava tubers (*Manihot esculenta*), *Food Chem.*, 5, 249, 1980.
49. Tinay, A. M. E., Bureng, P. L., and Yas, E. A. E., Hydrocyanic acid levels in fermented cassava, *J. Food Technol.*, 19, 197, 1984.
50. Essers, S., Development of fast detoxication methods for bitter cassava at the household level in rural North East Mosambique, in *Final Report for Ministry of Health of Mozambique*, 1986, 9.
51. Daneschwarz, M., Metodik der Bestimmung von Amygdalin in verschiedenen Fruchtpartien der Kirschen und einige Angaben über ihre Werte, *Ind. Obst. Gemüssewert.*, 61, 374, 1976.
52. Stadelman, W., Blausauregehalt von Steinobstsaften, *Flussiges Obst.*, 43, 45, 1976.
53. Pirko, P., Enstehung von Blausaure in Aprikosen Konserven wahrend der Lagerung, in *Vortag: GDCH-Fachgruppe Lebensmittelchemie und gerchtliche Chemie*, Berlin, 1967, 18–19.9.
54. Voldřich, M., Cyanogenesis within the processing of stone fruits, Ph.D. thesis, Institute of Chemical Technology, Prague, 1990.
55. Cruess, W. V., *Commercial Fruit and Vegetable Products*, McGraw-Hill, New York, 1958.
56. Kajiwara, N., Tomiyama, G., Ninomiya, T., and Hosogai, Y., Determination of amygdaline in apricot kernel and processed apricot products by HPLC, *J. Food Hyg. Soc. Jpn.*, 24(1), 42, 1983.
57. Schwarzmaier, U., Über die Cyanogenesis von *Bambusa vulgaris* and *B. guanda*, *Chem. Ber.*, 109, 3379, 1976.
58. Baumann, U. and Zimmerli, B., Entstehung von Urethan (Ethylcarbamat) in alkoholishen Getränken, *Schweiz. Z. Obst. Weinbau*, 122, 602, 1986.
59. Mildau, G., Preuss, A., Frank, W., and Heering, W., Ethylcarbamat (Urethan) in alkoholishen Getränken: Verbesserte Analyse und lichtabhangige Bildung, *Z. Lebesm. Unters. Forsch.*, 221, 147, 1971.
60. Chen, C. C., Kuo, M. C., Liu, S. E., and Wu, C. M., Volatile compounds of salted and pickled prunes (*Prunus mume*), *J. Agric. Food Chem.*, 34, 140, 1986.
61. Nagayama, T., Nishijima, M., Yasuda, K., Saito, K., Kamimura, H., Ibe, A., Ushiyama, H., Nagayama, M., and Naoi, Y., Benzoic acid in fruit and fruit products, *J. Food Hyg. Soc. Jpn.*, 24, 416, 1983.
62. Westley, J., Cyanide detoxication, in *Cyanide Compounds in Biology*, Ciba Foundation Symposium 140, Wiley, Chichester, United Kingdom, 1988.

Part D

Glucosinolates

Jan Velíšek

Glucosinolates (thioglucosides, mustard oil glucosides) occur in several families of dicotyledonous angiosperms. Most of the important plants and their seeds, which serve as vegetables, relishes, condiments, and a source of oil for humans (oilseeds) and feed for domestic animals, belong to the Brassicaceae family (cabbage, *Brassica oleracea* L. *var. capitata*; Savoy cabbage, *B. oleracea var. sabauda*; Brussels sprouts, *B. o. var. gemmifera*; cauliflower, *B. oleracea var. botrytis*; broccoli, *B. oleracea var. italica*; kohlrabi, *B. oleracea var. gongylodes*; kale, *B. oleracea var. acephala*; Chinese cabbage, *B. chinensis* L.; swede or rutabaga, *B. napus var. napobrassica*; rapeseed, *B. napus var. napus*; turnip, *B. rapa var. rapifera*; turnip rape, *B. rapa var. oleifera*; white mustard, *Sinapis alba* L.; black mustard, *B. nigra* L.; brown mustard, *B. juncea* L.; horseradish, *Armoracia rusticana* Gaert, Meyer and Scherb; radish, *Raphanus sativus* L.; watercress, *Nasturtium officinale* R. Brown; and others). Occasionally, plants belonging to other families are also consumed by humans; such as capers (Capparidaceae) and papaya seeds (Caricaceae), which are used as a substitute for pepper.[1] In recent years a number of reviews on the distribution, chemistry, biochemistry, physiological properties, and other aspects of glucosinolates in foods and feedstuffs have been published.[2-14]

CHEMISTRY

The structure of glucosinolates (Figure 1) comprises a sulfonated oxime grouping (*anti* with respect to the side chain and *syn* with respect to the thioglucosidic moiety), a sugar moiety (in almost all cases β-D-glucose and possibly glucose esterified with sinapic and other carboxylic acids), the side chain, and the cation (probably potassium; sinapine is the cation of glucosinalbin). The side chain can comprise aliphatic (straight-chain or branched, saturated or unsaturated), aromatic, or heterocyclic groupings. Common substituents include hydroxyl groups (occasionally glycosylated), terminal methylthio groups (and oxidized analogs), esters, and ketones. The side chain determines the chemical nature of glucosinolate decomposition products and, thereby, their physiological effects. Over 100 glucosinolates have now been described. The most important substances occurring in brassica vegetables and rapeseed are listed in Table 1.

BIOLOGICAL EFFECTS

Glucosinolates and their degradation products exhibit a variety of biological activities such as insecticidal, bacteriostatic, and fungistatic. Antinutritional (strumigenic) and toxic effects (hepatotoxicity, nefrotoxicity, and mutagenicity) of glucosinolates and their breakdown products in man are difficult to identify. Coupled with a low dietary iodine intake, glucosinolate breakdown products (especially thiocyanate ions and goitrin) may cause hypothyroidism, the main symptom of which is the enlargement of the thyroid gland (endemic goiter) caused by iodine deficiency. However, products of certain glucosinolates (indole glucosinolate glucobrassicin and sulfinyl glucosinolate glucoraphanin) show certain beneficial, i.e., immunomodulating and anticarcinogenic (or anti-cancer), properties.[7,15-17]

Glucosinolates and their hydrolysis products are the main factors responsible for the limited potential of rapeseed meal as a protein source for livestock and possibly in human food formulations. The most common problems associated with the feeding of rapeseed meal are goitrogenicity,

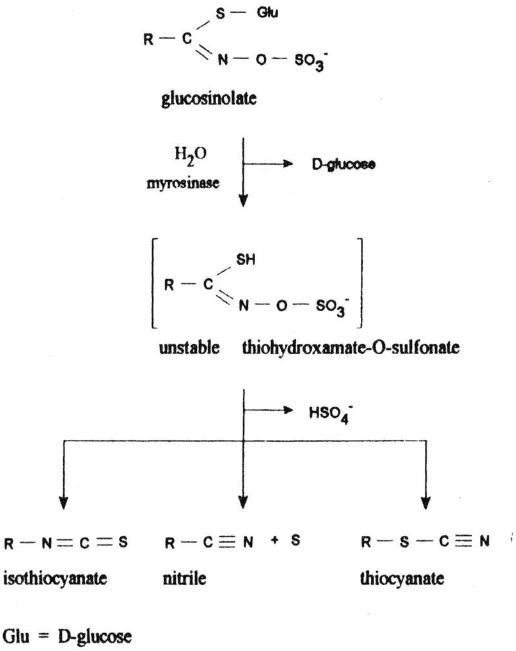

Figure 1 Enzymatic decomposition of glucosinolates.

liver hemorrhage, reduced palatability effecting low growth rates in animals, egg taint in hens, and an off-flavor imparted to milk. Adverse effects due to the occurrence of glucosinolates in feed arising from the use of rapeseed have been well documented.[2,4,13,18]

The levels of glucosinolates have been reduced by breeding in summer and winter rapeseed varieties (the summer varieties are generally lower in glucosinolate content than the winter ones) from 100 to 150 $\mu mol.g^{-1}$ seed to 20 to 30 $\mu mol.g^{-1}$ seed. Double zero varieties containing less than 35 $\mu mol.g^{-1}$ glucosinolates and less than 3% erucic acid in their oils are being widely grown in Europe and Canada.

Methods suggested for the detoxification of rapeseed meal involve the destruction of glucosinolates by heat,[19] extrusion,[20] chemicals, or their extraction with water or aqueous solvents.[21-23] Most of these processes proved to be expensive and have resulted in high protein losses or reduced protein quality.

The levels of the main glucosinolate degradation products, such as isothiocyanates and nitriles, found in rapeseed oil during its production are listed in Table 2.

OCCURRENCE

Glucosinolates are not confined to any particular part of the plant, being found in seeds, leaves, stems, and roots. Higher concentrations are found in the growing plant and its seeds. The level in brassica vegetables ordinarily ranges from about 100 to 4000 $mg.kg^{-1}$ fresh weight in the vegetative parts of plants, whereas in seeds up to about 60,000 $mg.kg^{-1}$ may be found.[2]

Usually more than one glucosinolate is found, but in some cases (for example, glucocapparin in capers, glucotropaeolin in cress and papaya seeds, and glucosinalbin in white mustard) the species contain essentially only a single glucosinolate. In the *Brassica* species, 10 to 20 individual glucosinolates are usually present, but only a few predominate.

Table 1 Structure, Common Names, And Occurrence Of Glucosinolates

R[a]		Common name	Occurence[b]
I	Methyl	Glucocapparin	CA
II	2-Propenyl (allyl)	Sinigrin	BM, BS, CB, CF, HR, MB, SC, SW
III	Isopropyl (1-methylethyl)	Glucoputranjivin	BS, SW
IV	3-Butenyl	Gluconapin	BR, BS, BS, CB, CC, CF, MB, RS, SC, SW, TU
V	2-Butyl (1-methylpropyl)	Glucocochlearin	SW, TU
VI	4-Pentenyl	Glucobrassicanapin	CB, CB, CC, MB, RS, SW, TU
VII	2(R)-Hydroxy-3-butenyl	Progoitrin	BR, BS, CB, CC, CF, RS, SC, SW, TU
VIII	2(S)-Hydroxy-3-butenyl	Epiprogoitrin	CR
IX	2-Hydroxy-4-pentenyl	Gluconapoleiferin	BR, BS, CC, CF, RS, SW, TU
X	3-Methylthiopropyl	Glucoibervirin	CB, CF, SW
XI	4-Methylthio-3-butenyl	—	RA
XII	4-Methylthiobutyl	Glucoerucin	BR, CB, CF, SW, TU
XIII	5-Methylthiopentyl	Glucoberteroin	SW, TU
XIV	3-Methylsulfinylpropyl	Glucoiberin	BR, BS, CB, CF, SC
XV	4-Methylsulfinyl-3-butenyl	Glucoraphenin	RA
XVI	4-Methylsulfinylbutyl	Glucoraphanin	BR, CB, CC, CF, RA, SC
XVII	5-Methylsulfinylpentyl	Glucoallysin	CB, CC, SW
XVIII	3-Methylsulfonylpropyl	Glucocheirolin	BS, SW
XIX	4-Methylsulfonylbutyl	Glucoerysolin	CB
XX	Benzyl	Glucotropaeolin	CB, CS
XXI	4-Hydroxybenzyl	Sinalbin (glucosinalbin)	BS, WM
XXII	2-Phenylethyl	Gluconasturtiin	BR, CB, CC, CF, HR, SW, TU
XXIII	2-Hydroxy-2-phenylethyl	Glucobarbarin	—
XXIV	3-Indolylmethyl	Glucobrassicin	BR, BS, CB, CC, CF, RA, RS, SC, SW, TU
XXV	1-Methoxy-3-indolylmethyl	Neoglucobrassicin	BR, BS, CB, CC, CF, RS, SC, SW, TU
XXVI	4-Methoxy-3-indolylmethyl	4-Methoxyglucobrassicin	BR, BS, CB, CC, CF, SC, SW, TU
XXVII	4-Hydroxy-3-indolylmethyl	4-Hydroxyglucobrassicin	BR, BS, CB, CC, CF, RS, SW

[a] See Figure 1.

[b] BM, black mustard; BR, broccoli; BS, Brussels sprouts; CA, capers; CB, cabbage; CC, Chinese cabbage; CF, cauliflower; CR, crambe; CS, cress; HR, horseradish; MB, brown mustard; RA, radish; RS, rapeseed; SC, Savoy cabbage; SW, swede; TU, turnip; WM, white mustard.

Table 2 Changes in Rapeseed Oil Isothiocyanates and Nitriles During Processing

	Amount ($mg.kg^{-1}$)			
	Pressed oil		Extracted oil	
Oil	Isothiocyanates	Nitriles	Isothiocyanates	Nitriles
Crude	0.1–1.0	8.0–10.0	9.0–25.0	90.0–110.0
Neutralized and bleached	0.0–0.1	0.6	12.0	70.0
Refined (deodorized)	0.0	4.0–18.0	0.0	4.0–18.0

From Velíšek, J., Davídek, J., Michová, J., and Pokorný, J., *J. Chromatogr.*, 502, 167, 1990. With permission.

The glucosinolate pattern varies considerably within different parts of the plant during its development. The same glucosinolates usually occur in a particular subspecies, but large variations in the absolute amounts of glucosinolates are found within different varieties and cultivars belonging to the same species. The absolute amount of glucosinolates is further subject to a wide range of other agronomic and environmental interferences.

CHANGES DURING PROCESSING AND STORAGE

Glucosinolates in enzymatically active plant tissues are hydrolyzed by the enzyme termed myrosinase (thioglucosidase or thioglucoside glucohydrolase, EC 3.2.3.1), present in all glucosinolate-containing plants. The myrosinase occurs in a number of isoenzymic forms, showing activity over a wide pH range and stablility at temperatures up to 60°C, with an optimum temperature of approximately 50°C. Myrosinase activity was not lost even when cabbage or Brussels sprouts were dried overnight at 50°C.[24] Cooking cauliflower in water for 10 min led to an approximately 20% decrease of myrosinase activity.[25]

Most cruciferous crops for human consumption are processed by pulping, cutting, chopping, blanching, cooking, freezing, pickling, and fermenting. Processes causing disruption of cells result in some glucosinolate autolysis by myrosinase. To various degrees, enzymatic hydrolysis continues during storage, cooking, and fermentation of brassica vegetables.

Enzymatic degradation of glucosinolates starts with the release of glucose and labile aglucones, which give rise to bisulfate, isothiocyanate (by a Lossen-type rearrangement), or nitrile and elemental sulfur (Figure 1). Organic thiocyanates have also been found as products of enzymatic hydrolysis of several glucosinolates, and benzylthiocyanate is one of the major products arising from glucotropaeolin.

The nature of the breakdown products is affected by the parent glucosinolate structure, pH, and the presence of certain cofactors. Most glucosides can be divided into three groups according to the products of their hydrolysis. Glucosinolates having an alkyl or alkenyl side chain yield in almost neutral media (at pH 5 to 7) primarily the relatively stable isothiocyanates (mustard oils). Those possessing a β-hydroxyl substituent in the alkyl or alkenyl side chain (e.g., progoitrin, its isomer epiprogoitrin, gluconapoleiferin, and glucobarbarin) form unstable β-hydroxy isothiocyanates, which spontaneously cyclize to oxazolidinethiones (Figure 2). Glucosinolates having an indole nucleus (glucobrassicins), sometimes treated as alkaloids (page 15), hydrolyze to unstable isothiocyanates, which (if indeed formed) decompose to the more stable 3-hydroxymethylindoles, also called 3-indolemethanols (Figure 3). For example, glucobrassicin possesses the corresponding 3-indolemethanol and thiocyanate (rhodanide) ion.[12,14] The former product reacts nonenzymatically with L-ascorbic acid to yield ascorbigen (acorbigen A), which, in vegetables rich with ascorbic acid, represents the major indole-containing product of glucobrassicin transformation.[15] In acidic media (of pH below 7), ascorbigen releases ascorbic acid, and addition of 3-indolemethanol cation to another molecule of ascorbigen yields ascorbigen dimer and ascorbigen trimer. In the same media, 3-indolemethanol releases formaldehyde and forms di- and polyindolemethanes.[12,14,26] Other glucobrassicins give analogous products, the proportion of which varies with the reactivity of the indole ring as affected by substitution.

In more acidic conditions (at pH around 3) all glucosinolates produce increasing amounts of nitriles. Significant amounts of nitriles also arise during autolysis of cruciferous plants, even when the pH would be expected to favor isothiocyanate formation. It seems that under acidic conditions Fe(II) ions depress myrosinase-induced isothiocyanate formation, facilitating desulfurization of the aglucone to the nitrile, but they have little

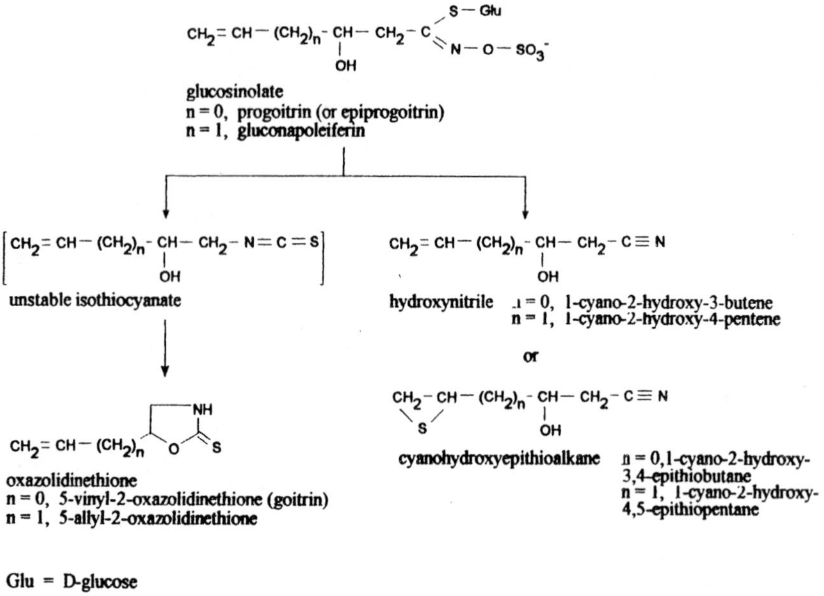

Figure 2 Enzymatic decomposition of progoitrin and gluconapoleiferin.

effect at neutral pH. In combination with thiols, Fe(II) ions inhibit isothiocyanate formation even in neutral media.[27,28]

Another cofactor, termed epithiospecifier protein[29] (by itself devoid of myrosinase activity), is necessary for a myrosinase-induced formation of diastereoisomeric (*threo* and *erythro*) forms of epithionitriles (cyanoepithioalkanes) from glucosinolates bearing unsaturated aliphatic side chain; 1-cyano-2,3-epithiopropane arises from sinigrin, 1-cyano-3,4-epithiobutane from gluconapin, 1-cyano-4,5-epi-thiopentane from glucobrassicanapin, 1-cyano-2-hydroxy-3,4-epithiobutane from progoitrin, and 1-cyano-2-hydroxy-4,5-epithiopentane from gluconapoleiferin (Figure 2).

Glucosinolates are also relatively easily decomposed chemically. In strong acids, the decomposition products of glucosinolates are the corresponding carboxylic acids, glucose, hydroxylammonium ions, and hydrogen sulfate ions. In alkaline media, glucosinolates having an active hydrogen at the first carbon atom (e.g., sinigrin and glucotropaeolin) yield 2-amino acids and thioglucose in a reaction involving a Neber-type rearrangement.[30] In mild alkaline media, a reducing sugar 1-deoxy-1-(3-indolyl)-α-L-sorbopyranose is formed from ascorbigen via decarboxylation and isomerization.[31] The same compound seems to be present in blood serum after administration of ascorbigen to animals.[15]

In aqueous solutions containing Hg(II), Ag(I), or probably some other metal ions, glucosinolates capable of forming insoluble sulfides split off glucose, and the resulting metal derivative of aglucone rearranges to isothiocyanate or nitrile, depending on the solution pH. Glucosinolates can be reduced to primary amines using Raney nickel catalysis in aqueous solutions at room temperature.[32] The same amines are formed from isothiocyanates upon hydrolysis. Glucosinolates are also thermally decomposed to products identical with those obtained conventionally on enzymatic hydrolysis, i.e., mainly isothiocyanates and nitriles.[33] In general, nitriles are produced as major products. Glucosinolates possessing a β-hydroxy group yield atypical products. For example, 3-hydroxy-4-pentenethionamide[34] and 5-vinyloxazolidinone[29] arose from progoitrin in solutions of pH 8 to 12 in the presence of Fe(II) ions (Figure 4), but goitrin has not been

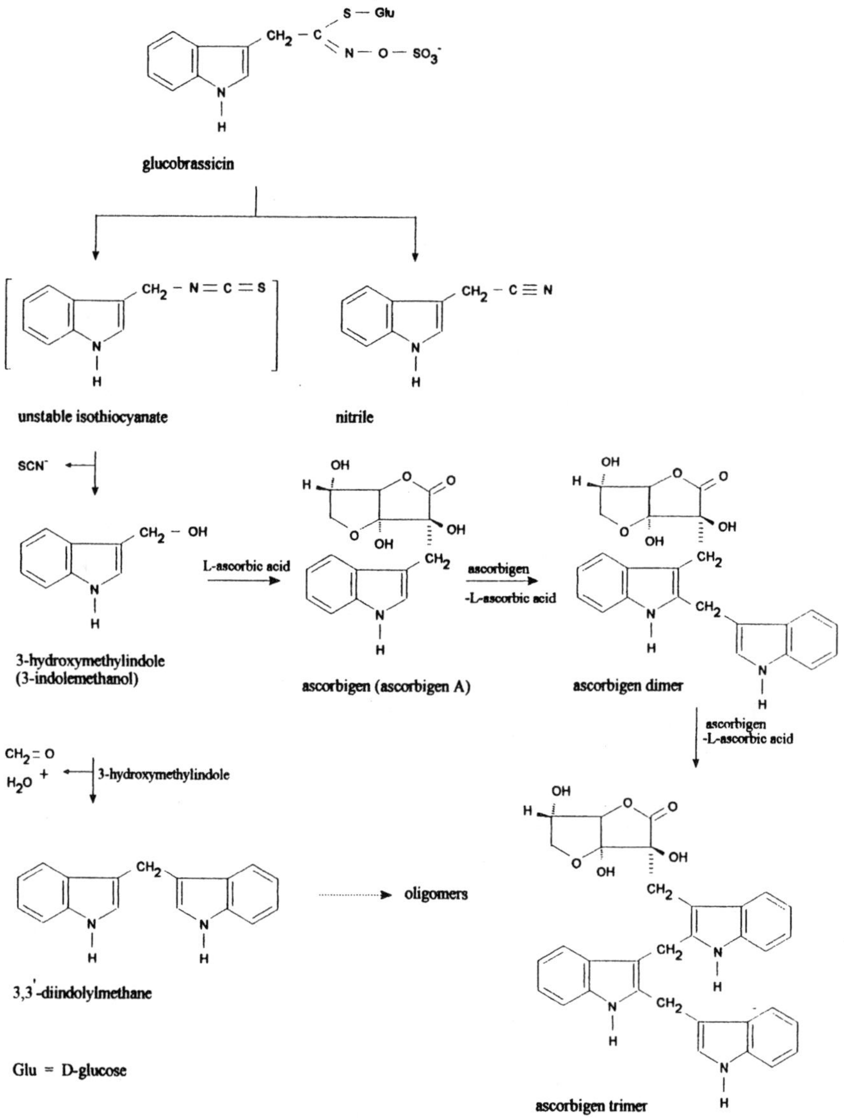

Figure 3 Enzymatic decomposition of glucobrassicins.

identified (sinigrin in the presence of ferrous ions gave rise to 3-butenethionamide).[35] The effect of ferrous ions was not produced by other metal ions.[34] Goitrin is easily nitrosated by nitrite yielding mutagenic *N*-nitroso-5-vinyl-2-oxazolidinethione with a loss of sulfur.[36] The chemical breakdown of glucobrassicin is summarized in Figure 5.

Autolysis of fresh cabbage heads and Brussels sprouts prepared by pulping with water at a pH of 5.6 to 6.3, gave a preponderance of nitriles instead of the related isothiocyanates and goitrin.[24] The total amounts of nitriles in the autolyzed products were 28 to 95 mg.kg^{-1} for cabbage and 110 mg.kg^{-1} for Brussels sprouts. In addition to 1-cyano-2-hydroxy-3-butene and the two forms of 1-cyano-2-hydroxy-3,4-epithiobutane from breakdown of progoitrin, other nitriles identified were 1-cyano-2,3-epithiopropane, 1-cyano-3,4-

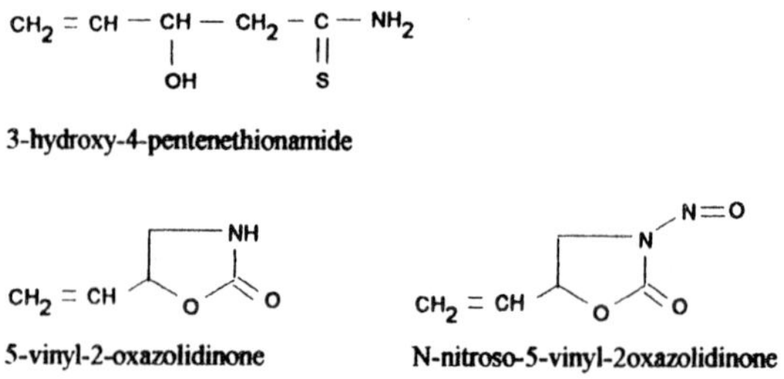

Figure 4 Chemical degradation products of progoitrin.

epithiobutane, 1-cyano-3-methyl-thiopropane, 1-cyano-3-methylsulfinylpropane, 1-cyano-4-methylthiobutane, 1-cyano-4-methylsulfinylbutane, 1-cyano-2-phenylethane, and 1-cyano-3-methylsulfinylpropane from the breakdown of glucoiberin, one of the major glucosinolates of the majority of cabbage varieties. Isothiocyanates and goitrin were obtained when the same cabbage was air-dried prior to autolysis. Browning of shredded cabbage was suppressed by the addition of allylisothiocyanate.[37] A cabbage homogenate contained ascorbigen as the major glucobrassicin breakdown product (about 24 to 55 $mg.kg^{-1}$ fresh weight), ascorbigen dimer as a minor component (about 1 $mg.kg^{-1}$), and trace amounts of ascorbigen trimer.[15] Homogenizing Savoy cabbage resulted in total degradation of glucosinolates; 3-indolemethanol, 3-indoleacetonitrile, 3,3′-diindolylmethane, and ascorbigen were found as glucobrassicin breakdown products.[14] Ascorbigen and 3-indolemethanol were the major products, comprising 75 and 20% of the theoretical yield, respectively. In homogenized Brussels sprouts, the initial level of 3-indolemethanol (30 $mg.kg^{-1}$ fresh weight) decreased to about 5 $mg.kg^{-1}$ within 24 h, perhaps due to the formation of ascorbigen.[25]

Blanching and cooking result in glucosinolate loss by leaching. The total and individual glucosinolate contents of fresh and boiled brassica vegetables are given in Table 3. Cooking caused a decrease in glucosinolate level in vegetables by an average of 36%, the loss being greatest in swede-turnip (48%) and Brussels sprouts (45%) cooked for 5 min and being least in cauliflower (31%) and cabbage (28%) cooked for 10 min. Average losses of the individual glucosinolates ranged from 34% (sinigrin) to 59% (neoglucobrassicin).[16] For example, cabbage steam-blanched or blanched in boiling water resulted in a 30 and 50% reduction of isothiocyanate-forming glucosinolates and indole glucosinolates, respectively.[9] About one-half to two-thirds of the original amount of glucosinolates remained unchanged during boiling. Volatile isothiocyanates, such as allyl isothiocyanate, completely disappeared. Goitrin and 3-methylsulfinylpropyl isothiocyanate were partly decomposed upon boiling, while inorganic thiocyanate remained in the boiled vegetable. In cooked cabbage and Savoy cabbage glucobrassicin-derived products (i.e., 3-indolemethanol, 3-indoleacetonitrile, and 3,3′-diindolylmethane) were low. Ascorbigen levels increased about 2.5-fold, with 380 and 970 $mg.kg^{-1}$ dry weight being present in cooked cabbage and Savoy cabbage, respectively. In cooked Brussels sprouts, no goitrin or thiocyanate ions were detectable.[38]

Freezing seems to have a pronounced effect on the glucosinolate content in brassica vegetables. The average level of thiocyanate ions in fresh Brussels sprouts was almost double that in frozen material. Oxazolidinethione levels of the frozen material reached only one-third those of the fresh one.[39]

Freeze-drying or air-drying results in lower losses of glucosinolates.[40] Hydrolysis of glucosinolates occurred even in dried cabbage and Brussels sprouts homogenized with water.[24] In contrast to the autolysis of fresh material, where the major products were nitriles, autolysis of the dried vegetables yielded mainly isothiocyanates and goitrin. The

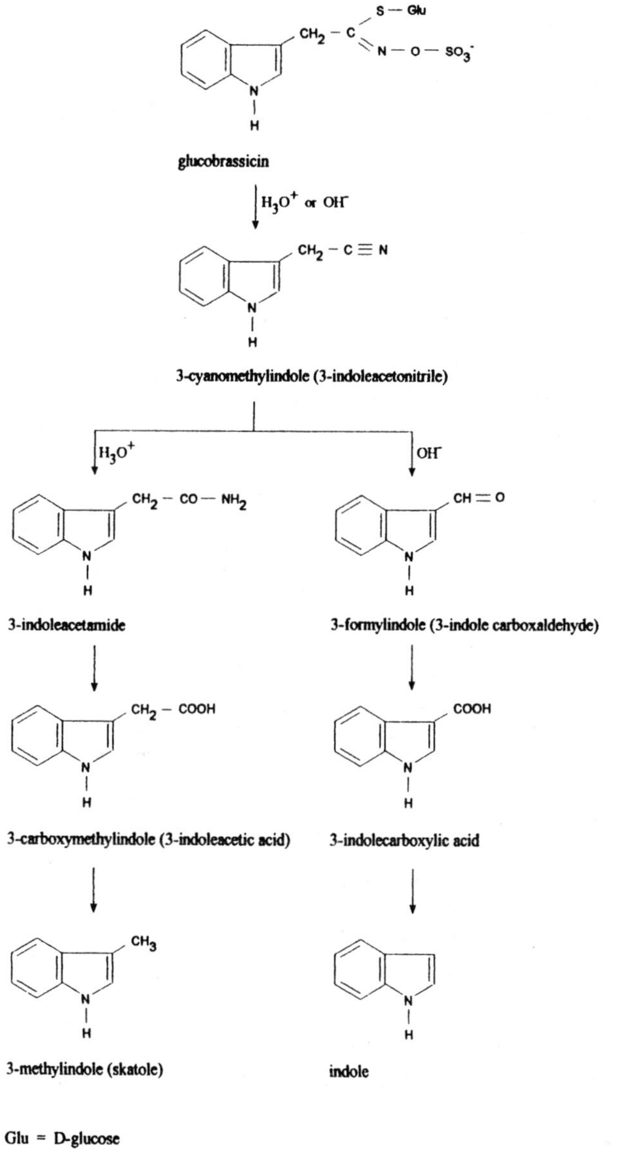

Figure 5 Chemical degradation of glucobrassicins.

contents of the latter compound were 8 to 32 $mg.kg^{-1}$ in cabbage and 61 $mg.kg^{-1}$ in Brussels sprouts (calculated on a fresh weight basis).

Pickled japanese nozawana (turnip) had a characteristic pungent flavor due to 3-butenyl, 4-pentenyl, 4-methylthiobutyl, and 2-phenylethyl isothiocyanates.[41]

Fermentation of cabbage to produce sauerkraut results in total breakdown of the glucosinolates during the first 2 weeks of fermentation.[42] The degradation products were thiocyanate ions, isothiocyanates, goitrin, and the nitriles 1-cyano-3-methylsulfinylpropane (from glucoiberin) and 1-cyano-2,3-epithiopropane (from sinigrin). In the final sauerkraut,

Table 3 Content of Glucosinolates in Some Fresh and Cooked Brassica Vegetables

	Total glucosinolates (mg.kg^{-1} fresh weight)		Individual glucosinolates (mg.kg^{-1} fresh weight)										
Vegetable	**Range**	**Mean**	**II**[a]	**IV**	**VI**	**VII**	**IX**	**XII**	**XIII**	**XIV**	**XXII**	**XXIV**	**XXV**
Cabbage													
Fresh	360–2,754	1,089	263	18	—	38	—	—	—	450	—	295	25
Cooked	315–1,651	786	202	13	—	27	—	—	—	300	—	174	11
Cauliflower													
Fresh	138–2,083	620	142	7	—	23	—	—	—	173	—	227	48
Cooked	94–1,111	420	100	3	—	14	—	—	—	122	—	151	30
Brussels sprouts													
Fresh	1,455–3,939	2,260	445	252	—	478	—	—	—	353	—	624	110
Cooked	597–2,542	1,237	264	148	—	299	—	—	—	195	—	298	33
Swede-turnip													
Fresh	392–1,657	560	—	42	37	371	42	46	71	—	97	48	96
Cooked	205–944	291	—	24	26	206	23	23	39	—	58	23	38

[a] See Table 1.

From Sones, K., Heaney, R. K., and Fenwick, G. R., *J. Sci. Food Agric.*, 35, 712, 1984. With permission.

the thiocyanate ion levels were 9 to 17 mg.kg^{-1} and those for 1-cyano-3-methylsulfinylpropane were 16 to 25 mg.kg^{-1} (about 50% of theoretical values obtainable from glucoiberin). Losses may be attributed to drainage of the juice or heat decomposition during canning or cooking. Isothiocyanates, 1-cyano-2,3-thiopropane, and goitrin were not detectable throughout fermentation. In fermentation carried out at 19°C, no intact glucosinolates were detectable after 3 d, at 15°C after 4 d, at 10°C after 6 d, and at 5°C after 8 d.[43] Allyl isothiocyanate was detected in the headspace of some sauerkraut packages. Irradiation with ionizing rays prior to fermentation accelerated degradation of glucosinolates, but the degradation rate could not be further increased by inoculation with lactic acid bacteria. Sauerkraut contained ascorbigen as the major glucobrassicin breakdown product (about 31 to 52 mg.kg^{-1} fresh weight) together with smaller quantities of ascorbigen dimer (1 to 3 mg.kg^{-1}), ascorbigen trimer (1 to 3 mg.kg^{-1}), 3-indolemethanol (2 to 3 mg.kg^{-1}), and indoleacetonitrile (1 to 5 mg.kg^{-1}).[15]

Glucosinolate degradation products are often associated with pungent, cabbagy, garlicky, acrid, biting, and bitter flavors of cruciferous vegetables, relishes, and condiments. They are the major contributors to the desirable flavor of radish, horseradish, mustard, and watercress, while the flavor of leaf vegetables is more complex. Generally, at low concentrations, isothiocyanates have a pleasant appetite-stimulating flavor, whereas nitriles have a garlic-like flavor. Off-odors associated with overcooked and rehydrated vegetables and the bitterness of some brassica vegetables can be attributed to glucosinolate degradation products formed either by enzymatic or chemical reactions. All factors that affect the glucosinolate content of the plant, together with the degree of tissue disruption, processing, and culinary conditions, affect flavor of cruciferous vegetable and condiment products.

Glucosinolates and their breakdown products at a maximum level of up to about 50 mg per person per day are regular chemical constituents of the human diet, mainly derived from brassica vegetables and to a smaller extent from condiments. Trace amounts can be derived from refined (deodorized) rapeseed oils. They can also pass into the food chain indirectly through animals feeding on cruciferous plants.[2,4,13,18]

REFERENCES

1. Chan, H. T. and Tang, C.-S., The chemistry and biochemistry of papaya, in *Tropical Foods*, Vol. I, Inglett, G. E. and Charlambous, G., Eds., Academic Press, New York, 1979, 144.
2. Fenwick, G. R., Heaney, R. K., and Mawson, R., Glucosinolates, in *Toxicants of Plant Origin*, Vol. II, Cheeke, P. R., Ed., CRC Press, Boca Raton, FL, 1991, 1.
3. Fenwick, G. R., Heaney, R. K., and Mullin, W. J., Glucosinolates and their breakdown products in food and food plants, *CRC Crit. Rev. Food Sci. Nutr.*, 18, 123, 1983.
4. Heaney, R. K. and Fenwick, G. R., Identifying toxins and their effects: glucosinolates, in *Natural Toxicants in Food, Progress and Prospects*, Watson, D. H., Ed., Ellis Horwood, Chichester, England, 1987, 76.
5. VanEtten, C. H. and Tookey, H. L., Glucosinolates, in *Handbook of Naturally Occurring Food Toxicants*, Recheigl, M., Jr., Ed., CRC Press, Boca Raton, FL, 1983, 15.
6. Tookey, H. L., VanEtten, C. H., and Daxenbichler, M. E., Glucosinolates, in *Toxic Constituents of Food Crops*, 2nd ed., Liener, I., Ed., Academic Press, New York, 1980, 103.
7. Beier, R. C., Natural pesticides and bioactive components in foods, in *Reviews of Environmental Contamination and Toxicology*, Ware, G. W., Ed., Springer Verlag, New York, 1990, 48.
8. Duncan, A. J., Glucosinolates, in *Toxic Substances* of *Crop Plants*, D'Mello, J. P. F., Duffus, C. M., and Duffus, J. H., Eds., Royal Society of Chemistry, Cambridge, 1991, 126.
9. de Vos, R. H. and Blijleven, W. G. H., The effect of processing conditions on glucosinolates in cruciferous vegetables, *Z. Lebensm. Unters. Forsch.*, 187, 525, 1988.
10. Underhill, E. W., Glucosinolates, in *Secondary Plant Products*, Bell, E. A. and Charlwood, B.V., Eds., Springer Verlag, Berlin, 1980, 493.
11. Dietz, H. M. and Harris, R. V., Novel and rapid methods of glucosinolate analysis with particular reference to their application to 00-rapeseed, in *Food Control*, 1990, 84.
12. McDanell, R., McLean, A. E. M., Hanley, A. B., Heaney, R. K., and Fenwick, G. R., Chemical and biological properties of indole glucosinolates (glucobrassicins): a review, *Food Chem. Toxicol.*, 26, 59, 1988.
13. Fenwick, G. R. and Curtis, R. F., Rapeseed meal in poultry diets: a review, *Anim. Feed Sci. Technol.*, 5, 255, 1980.
15. Alexandrova, L. G., Korolev, A. M., and Preobrazhenskaya, M. N., Study of natural ascorbigen and related compounds by HPLC, *Food Chem.*, 45, 61, 1992.
16. National Research Council, Inhibitors of carcinogenesis, in *Diet, Nutrition and Cancer*, National Academy Press, Washington, D.C., 1982, 358.
17. Zhang, Y., Talalay, P. Cho, Ch.-G., and Posner, G. H., A major inducer of anticarcinogenic protective enzymes from broccoli: isolation and elucidation of structure, *Proc. Natl. Acad. Sci. U.S.A.*, 89, 2399, 1992.
18. Walker, N. J. and Gray, I. K., The glucosinolate of land cress (*Coronopus didymus*) and its enzymic degradation products as precursors of off-flavor in milk — a review, *J. Agric. Food Chem.*, 18, 346, 1970.
19. Rutkowski, A., Effect of processing on the chemical composition of rapeseed meal, *International Conference on the Science, Technology and Marketing of Rapeseed and Rapeseed Products, St. Adele, Quebec, 1970*, Rapeseed Association of Canada, Quebec, 1970, 496.
20. Fenwick, G. R., Spinks, E. A., Wilkinson, A. P., Heaney, R. K., and Legoy, M. A., Effect of processing on the antinutrient content of rapeseed, *J. Sci. Food Agric.*, 37, 735, 1986.
21. Kirk, L. D., Mustakas, G. C., Griffin, E. L., and Boath, A. N., Crambe seed processing: decomposition of glucosinolates (thioglucosides) with chemical additives, *J. Am. Oil Chem. Soc.*, 48, 845, 1971.
22. Shahidi, F., Naczk, M., Hall, D., and Synowiecki, J., Insensitivity of the amino acids of canola and rapeseed to methanol-ammonia extraction and commercial processing, *Food Chem.*, 44, 283, 1992.
23. Sosuski, F., Soliman, F. S., and Bhatty, R. S., Diffusion extraction of glucosinolates from rapeseed, *Can. Inst. Food Sci. Technol. J.*, 5, 101, 1972.
24. Daxenbichler, M. E., VanEtten, C. H., and Spencer, G. F., Glucosinolates and derived products in cruciferous vegetables. Identification of organic nitriles from cabbage, *J. Agric. Food Chem.*, 25, 121, 1977.
25. Bradfield, C. A. and Bjeldanes, L. F., High-performance liquid chromatographic analysis of anticarcinogenic indoles in *Brassica oleracea*, *J. Agric. Food Chem.*, 35, 46, 1987.

26. Spande, T. F., Hydroxyindoles, indole alcohols, and indolethiols, in *Indoles*, 2nd ed., Houlihan, W. J., Ed., Wiley Interscience, New York, 1979, 1.
27. Uda, Y., Kurata, T., and Arakawa, N., Effects of pH and ferrous ion on the degradation of glucosinolates by myrosinase, *Agric. Biol. Chem.*, 50, 2735, 1986.
28. Uda, Y., Kurata, T., and Arakawa, N., Effects of thiol compounds on the formation of nitriles from glucosinolates, *Agric. Biol. Chem.*, 50, 2741, 1986.
29. Petroski, R. J. and Kwolek, W. F., Interactions of a fungal thioglucoside glucohydrolase and cruciferous plant epithiospecifier protein to form 1-cyanoepithioalkanes: implications of an allosteric mechanism, *Phytochemistry*, 24, 213, 1985.
30. Friis, P., Larsen, P. O., and Olsen, C. E., Base catalysed degradation of glucosinolates, *J. Chem. Soc. Perkin Trans.*, 1, 661, 1977.
31. Plikhtyak, I. L., Yartseva, I. V., Kluev, N. A., and Preobrazhenskaya, M. N., Transformation of ascorbigen and its derivatives into substituted 1-deoxy-1-(indol-3-yl)-α-L-sorbopyranoses, *Khim. Geterocykl. Soedin.*, 5, 607, 1989.
32. Olsen, C. E. and Sorensen, H., Recent advances in the analysis of glucosinolates, *J. Am. Oil Chem. Soc.*, 58, 857, 1981.
33. Mac Leod, A. J., Panesar, S. S., and Gil, V., Thermal degradation of glucosinolates, *Phytochemistry*, 20, 977, 1981.
34. Austin, F. L., Gent, C. A., and Wolff, I. A., Degradation of natural thioglucosides with ferrous salts, *J. Agric. Food Chem.*, 16, 752, 1968.
35. Youngs, C. G. and Perlin, A. S., Fe(II)-catalysed decomposition of sinigrin and related thioglycosides, *Can. J. Chem.*, 45, 1801, 1967.
36. Lüthy, J., Carden, B., Bachmann, M., Friedrich, V., and Schlatter, C., Identifizierung und Mutagenität des Reaktionsproduktes von Goitrin und Nitrit, *Mitt. Geb. Lebensmittelunters. Hyg.*, 75, 101, 1984.
37. Nagata, M., Yano, M., and Saijo, R., Inhibitory mechanism of allylisothiocyanate on browning of shredded cabbage, *Nippon Shokuhin Kogyo Gakkaishi*, 39, 322, 1992.
38. McMillan, M., Spinks, E. A., and Fenwick, G. R., Preliminary observations on the effect of dietary Brussels sprouts on thyroid function, *Hum. Toxicol.*, 5, 15, 1986.
39. Mullin, W. J. and Sahasrabudhe, M. R., An estimate of the average daily intake of glucosinolates via cruciferous vegetables, *Nutr. Rep. Int.*, 18, 273, 1978.
40. Kojima, M., Hamada, H., and Toshimitsu, N., Changes in isothiocyanates of *Wasabia japonica* roots by drying, *Nippon Shokuhin Kogyo Gakkaishi*, 32, 886, 1985.
41. Uda, Y., Suzuki, K., and Maeda, Y., Off-flavor constituents generated in pickled nozawana (*Brassica campestris* L. *var. rapifera*) leaves during early pickling process, *Nippon Shokuhin Kogyo Gakkaishi*, 39, 200, 1992.
42. Daxenbichler, M. E., VanEtten, C. H., and Williams, P. H., Glucosinolate products in commercial sauerkraut, *J. Agric. Food Chem.*, 28, 809, 1980.
43. Gail-Eller, R. and Gierschner, K., Zum Gehalt und Verhalten der Glucosinolate in Weiskohl und Sauerkraut, *Dtsch. Lebensm. Rundsch.*, 80, 341, 1984.
44. Sones, K., Heaney, R. K., and Fenwick, G. R., An estimate of the daily intake of glucosinolates from cruciferous vegetables in the UK, *J. Sci. Food Agric.*, 35, 712, 1984.
45. Daxenbichler, M. E. and VanEtten, C. H., Glucosinolates and derived products in cruciferous vegetables: gas liquid chromatographic determination of the aglucon derivatives from cabbage, *J. Ass. Offic. Anal. Chem.*, 60, 950, 1977.
46. Heaney, R. K. and Fenwick, G. R., The analysis of glucosinolates in Brassica species using gas chromatography. Direct determination of the thiocyanate ion precursors, glucobrassicin and neoglucobrassicin, *J. Sci. Food Agric.*, 31, 593, 1980.
47. Mossoba, M. M., Shaw, G. J., Andrzejewski, D., Sphon, J. A., and Page, S. W., Application of gas chromatography (matrix isolation) Fourier transform infrared spectrometry to the identification of glucosinolates from Brassica vegetables, *J. Agric. Food Chem.*, 37, 367, 1989.
48. Lewis, J. A. and Fenwick, G. R., Glucosinolate content of brassica vegetables-Chinese cabbages Pe-tsai (Brassica pekinensis) and Pak-choi (Brassica chinensis), *J. Sci. Food Agric.*, 45, 379, 1988.
49. Lewis, J. A., Fenwick, G. R., and Gray, A. R., Glucosinolates in Brassica vegetables: green-curded cauliflowers (Brassica oleracea L. botrytis group) and purple-headed broccoli (B. oleracea L. italica group), *Lebensm. Wiss. Technol.*, 24, 361, 1991.
50. Carlson, D. G., Daxenbichler, M. E., VanEtten, C. H., Hill, C. B., and Williams, P. H., Glucosinolates in radish cultivars, *J. Amer. Soc. Hortic. Sci.*, 110, 634, 1985.

Part E

Plant Phenols

Jana Dostálová and Jan Pokorný

Phenolic compounds are among the most numerous and widely distributed classes of natural components in materials of plant origin.[1] Despite the wide occurrence of phenolic substances, their content in food products is mostly very low. They occur only in traces in animal products. Their toxicity and their biological importance are generally only moderate,[1] so they are not a focus of attention among food scientists.

CHEMISTRY

The number of various phenolic substances occurring in food materials is enormous, so it is possible to mention here only a few examples of the most important classes of compounds. Phenolic substances (in the narrow sense) contain only one hydroxyl group, whose hydrogen atom may be substituted. Substances that contain two or three hydroxyl groups in the molecule are called polyphenols. Essentially, they are not polymers of phenols, so the name is incorrect from the terminological standpoint, but they are traditionally so called.

Phenolic substances are easily oxidized into polyphenolic derivatives under conditions of food preparation or storage. The oxidation may be enzymatic, catalyzed by various oxygenases, or chemically by molecular oxygen, usually under the catalytic effect of heavy metal ions (Figure 1). This latter reaction is mostly a free radical reaction. The polyphenolic compounds produced by these reactions are usually derivatives of pyrocatechol or pyrogallol. They are derived less frequently from resorcinol,[2] though some phenolic substances from cereal grains belong to this group.

Carboxylic derivatives of phenols or polyphenols are important constituents of many foods of plant origin.[3] They belong either to the benzoic acid or to the cinnamic acid series. The cinnamic acid moiety, containing an allylic group, may have either a (*Z*) or an (*E*) configuration. Their hydroxyl groups are frequently substituted by a methoxy or an acyl group.

Esters of caffeic acid (3,4-dihydroxycinnamic acid) with quinic acid are called chlorogenic acids,[4] the most important representative being 3-caffeoylquinic acid. Some esters of this group contain two caffeoyl groups bound to one molecule of quinic acid; e.g., cynarin is a 1,5-disubstituted derivative of quinic acid. Other acids of the cinnamic acid series may be bound as esters as well, such as ferulic or sinapic acids. Rosmarinic acid,[5] an ester of caffeic and hydroxydihydrocaffeic acid, is present in rosmarine and is an active natural antioxidant. Gallic acid is often bound in the form of digallic acid.

Phenolic acids of both of these series form esters with sugars. More often, sugars are bound as glycosides; e.g., linocaffein is a glucoside of caffeic acid.

Both hydroxybenzoic and hydroxycinnamic acids, also form esters with higher aliphatic alcohols, glycols, or glycerol. These esters have good antioxidant activities in edible oils, such as esters isolated from oat extracts. Esters of sinapic acid or related acids with choline are called sinapin,[6] which is present in Brassicaceae, such as mustard or rapeseed. They have an objectionable strong bitter taste. Similar esters are formed even with flavonoids, mainly gallates and digallates.

Alcohols corresponding to the above hydroxycarboxylic acids occur in plant materials as well, such as coniferyl and sinapyl alcohols, respectively. The respective aldehydes are very common as well, such as vanillin.

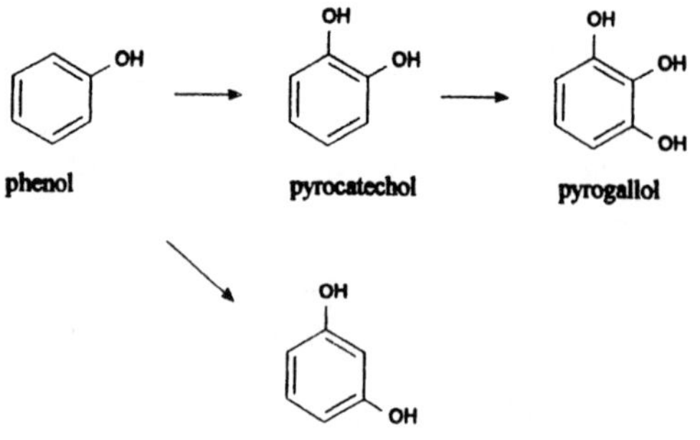

resorcinol

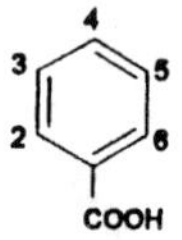

benzoic acid

2-hydroxy = salicylic
3,4-dihydroxy = o-pyrocatechuic
2,5-dihydroxy = gentisic
3,4,5-trihydroxy = gallic
3-methoxy, 4-hydroxy = vanillic
3,5-dimethoxy, 4-hydroxy = syringic

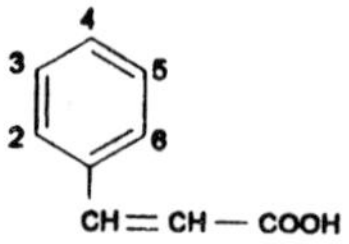

cinnamic acid

2-hydroxy = o-coumaric
3-hydroxy = m-coumaric
4-hydroxy = p-coumaric
3,4-dihydroxy = caffeic
3-methoxy, 4-hydroxy = ferulic
3-hydroxy, 4-methoxy = isoferulic
3,5-dimethoxy, 4-hydroxy = sinapic

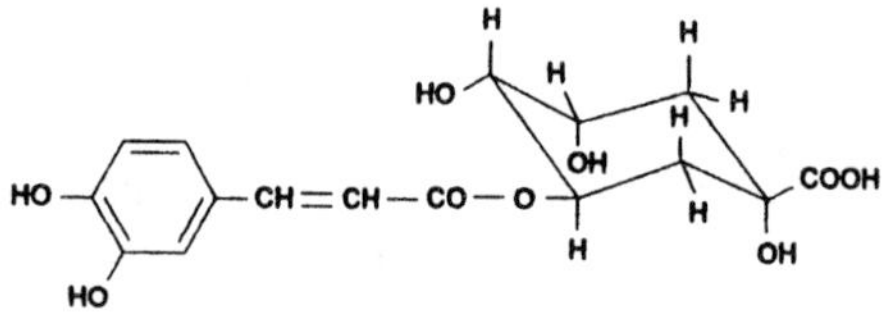

chlorogenic acid

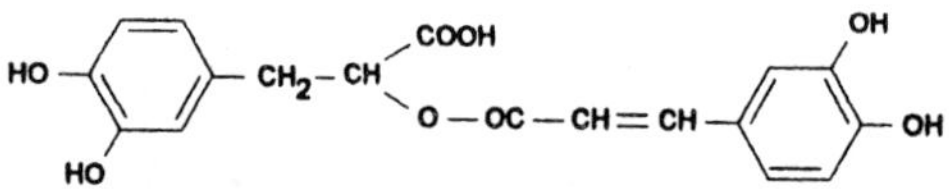

rosemarinic acid

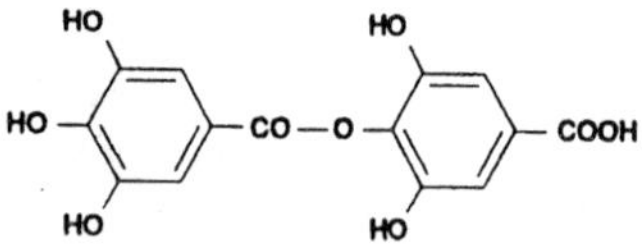

digallic acid

Figure 1 Phenolic substances derived from benzoic or cinnamic acids.

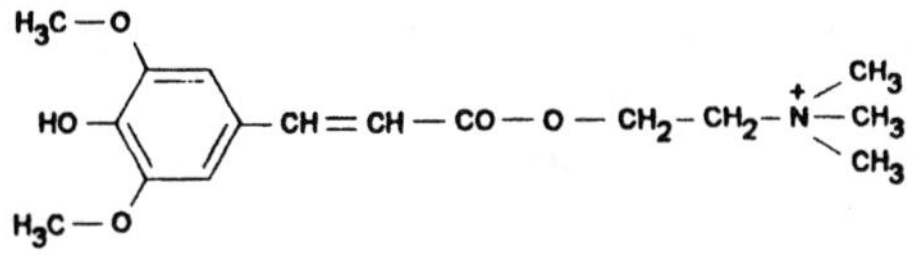

sinapin

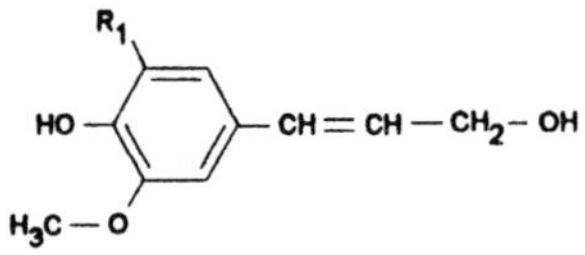

R_1 = H coniferyl alcohol
R_1 = $O-CH_3$ sinapic alcohol

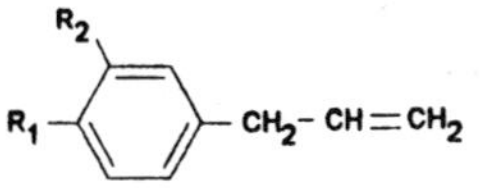

R_1 = $O-CH_3$, R_2 = H estragole
R_1 = $O-CH_3$, R_2 = $O-CH_3$ methyleugenol

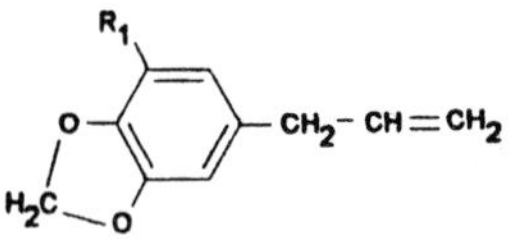

R_1 = H safrole
R_1 = $O-CH_3$ myristicin

Figure 1 (continued)

The products of decarboxylation of cinnamic acid series are decomposed with the formation of propenyl benzene. They are intense flavor compounds. The chemical structures of the above-mentioned compounds are given in Figure l.

A special large group of phenolic substances consists of two substituted benzene rings connected with a chain of 3-substituted carbon atom[7] (the 3-6-3 type compounds).They are derivatives of flavan or its respective unsaturated compound, flaven. Hydroxylic derivatives of flavan are flavanols or flavandiols. The respective oxo-derivatives are flavanones or flavanonols. Oxo-derivatives of flaven are called flavones and flavonols. They form flavylium salts in acidic medium. Isomeric derivatives exist as well, for instance, isoflavones. Another isomer of flavone is aurone, containing a five-member ring. The middle ring is cleaved in chalkones, which consist of two-benzene rings connected with a 3-carbon aliphatic chain.

Both benzene rings in all the above derivatives are mainly substituted with hydroxyl groups. For example, catechin is a tetrahydroxylic derivative, and the respective gallocatechin contains an additional hydroxyl group. A typical trihydroxyl derivative of flavanones is naringenin. Anthocyanidins[8] are the most important natural derivatives of flavylium salts, such as cyanidin or the respective pyrogallol derivative, delphinidine. All the above derivatives frequently (mainly) occur as mono- or diglycosides or may be present as esters, e.g., gallates. The chemical structures of flavan and flaven derivatives are given in Figure 2.

Hydroxylated cinnamic acids easily form lactones (mainly γ–lactones). Various lactones[9] naturally occur in some foods. The simplest compound of this kind is coumarin, and its hydroxy derivative is umbelliferone. Still higher substituted coumarins are scopoletin and aesculetin. Their isomers are isocoumarins. Coumarins may contain another condensed heterocycle, such as a pyran ring or a furan ring in the molecule. Ellagic acid is a diketone of digallic acid.The chemical structures of coumarin derivatives are given in Figure 3.

TOXIC EFFECTS

Only a few phenolic compounds occurring in nature are potent toxins, at least in concentrations consumed. Some phenolics cause serious toxic effects in livestock, but the risks for humans from phenolic substances present in normal food consumed under usual circumstances seem negligible. In a few instances, a toxic effect was observed as a result of abnormal consumption of phenols in plant materials or consumption of abnormal diets.[10]

Data on the toxicity of phenolic compounds are rather controversial. A few phenols have been found to be carcinogenic, while in other cases or under other experimental conditions, anticarcinogenic activity was observed. This contradiction may be partially explained as follows. The primary mechanism of the anticarcinogenic effect is the reaction of polyphenols with free radicals *in vivo* (Figure 4). Free polyphenol radicals produced in this way are relatively stable, and not sufficiently active to initiate cancer, in contrast to peroxy (ROO·) or hydroxyl (HO·) radicals. They are slowly deactivated by various recombination reactions (Figure 5).

In addition to the above very rapid reaction (Figure 4), a slow, free-radical-producing back reaction may occur as well, which is negligible under normal concentrations of phenolic substances. If the concentration of phenols increases, the reaction (Figure 4) cannot increase because of limited availability of free radicals. The back reaction, however, is dependent only on the concentration of phenols, so that at extremely high concentrations the back reaction may even prevail and the antioxidant becomes a prooxidant (Figure 6). The reports on the carcinogenic effect of polyphenolic compounds may be derived from the above inversion of the antioxidant activity under high experimental concentrations of polyphenolics in the test.

The most potent carcinogens among phenolic substances are aflatoxins,[11] which, however, cannot be truly considered as natural components of food (page 171). Among other phenolics, a few substances are carcinogenic or otherwise toxic, such as safrole or coumarin. Unrealistic doses were necessary in most cases to produce a significant carcinogenic effect. Common flavonols are bacterial mutagens. People have used plants containing phenolics since ancient times because of their antiviral, antimicrobial, antipyretic, diuretic, and many other properties.[12] The toxicity and possible therapeutic effect can overlap, and in most cases, the resulting activity depends on the doses. For example, dicoumarol causes bleeding in cattle and is used as rat poison, but on the other hand, dicoumarol and its derivatives are useful drugs, preventing unwanted clotting in cases of a threat of embolism or stroke. Gossypol[13] (Figure 7) is used in China as a male contraconception agent, but may cause liver damage at higher concentrations.

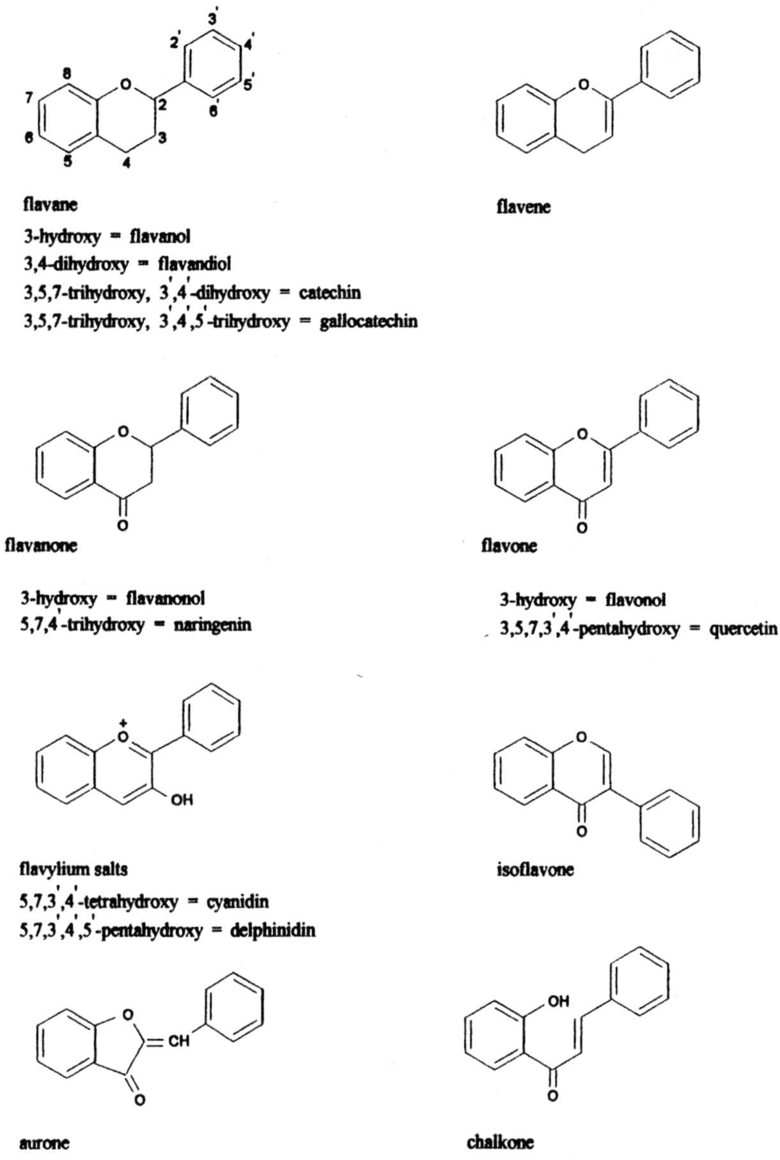

Figure 2 Flavan and flaven derivatives.

Some phenolic substances are not carcinogenic but may have cocarcinogenic activity, such as catechol in cigarette smoke condensate or chlorogenic acid in coffee. Chlorogenic acid catalyzes the formation of *N*-nitrosamines from nitrates and secondary amines. In other studies, gallic acid and its derivatives were found to be inhibitors of nitrosation at gastric pH values.[11]

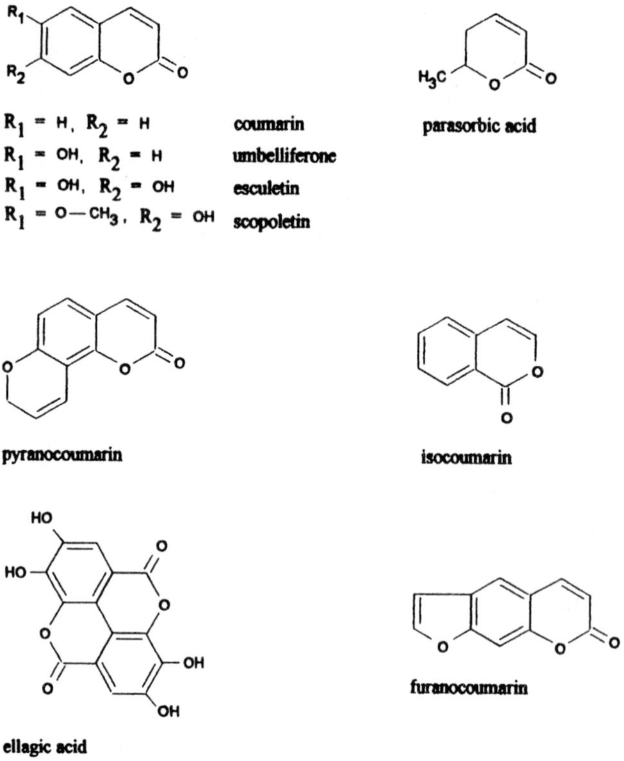

Figure 3 Coumarin and its derivatives.

$$\mathrm{Ph{-}H} + \mathrm{ROO}\cdot \longrightarrow \mathrm{Ph}\cdot + \mathrm{ROOH}$$

Ph—H = polyphenol

Ph· = polyphenol free radical

Figure 4 Reaction of polyphenolic substances with free peroxy radicals.

$$\mathrm{Ph}\cdot + \mathrm{ROO}\cdot \longrightarrow \mathrm{Ph{-}OOR}$$

or

$$\mathrm{Ph}\cdot + \mathrm{Ph}\cdot \longrightarrow \mathrm{Ph{-}Ph}$$

Figure 5 Termination reactions of free phenolic radicals.

Some examples of the direct toxic effect of phenolic substances are summarized in Table 1. Coumarins, the more toxic isocoumarins, pyranocoumarins, and furanocoumarins belong to the group of the most potent toxins in this group of compounds.

The antinutritional activity of phenolic substances is more important than the direct toxicity. This is summarized in Table 2. Polyphenols are oxidized into quinones under the catalytic activity of polyphenol oxidases (EC 1.14.18.1, EC 1.10.3.2). Quinones react

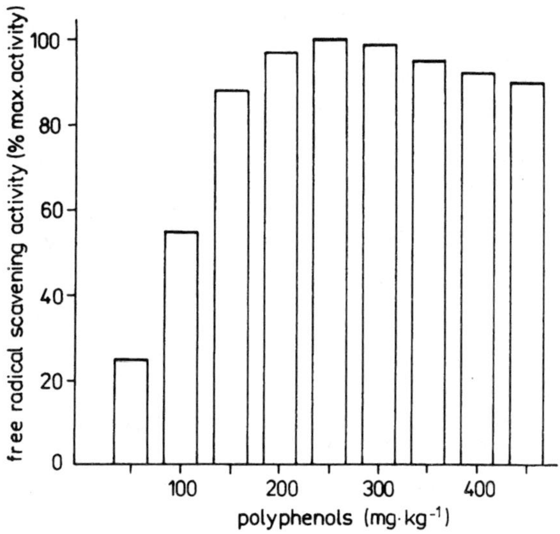

Figure 6 Effect of concentration on the free-radical scavenging activity of polyphenolic compounds.

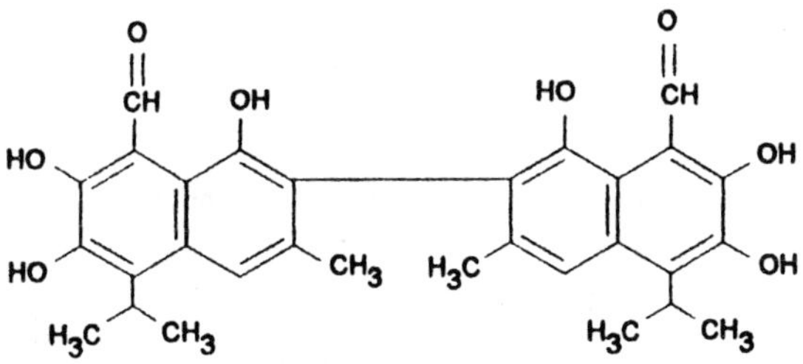

Figure 7 Gossypol.

with lysine and methionine bound in proteins with formation of complexes that are not cleaved by digestive enzymes. The protein digestibilities of 55.4 and 85.1% were reported for high-phenolic and low-phenolic materials, respectively.[14] Multiple hydrogen bonds, which are not cleaved by digestive enzymes, are formed between condensed tannins and food proteins (page 192). They are similar to complexes formed during the tanning of hides, and they prevent the digestion of the protein moiety.

Some phenolic substances reduce the sensory value of foodstuffs, if present in higher amounts. Typical examples are apples, pears, various other fruits and vegetables, red wine, and tea. Phenolic substances in these foodstuffs cause excessive astringency[15] or bitterness (sinapin and various other polyphenols, for instance, in herbs). The color acceptance is decreased by enzymatic browning. Some phenolic substances have an irritant effect on mucosa of the oral cavity or of other parts of the digestive system.

OCCURRENCE

Phenolic substances are found in nearly all plant products, but their amount is usually very low. With some exceptions, amounts do not exceed 1 to 2%, but they are mostly much

Table 1 Samples of Direct Toxicity of Some Phenolic Compounds

Compounds investigated	Toxic effect
Coumarins, isocoumarins, pyranocoumarins, furanocoumarins, aflatoxins, parasorbic acid, some flavonoids	Direct carcinogenity
Catechols or some flavonoids	Cocarcinogenity
Furanocoumarins	Smasmolytic and vasodilating activity
Furanocoumarins	Skin sensitizers to sunlight
Coumarin, gossypol	Hepatotoxicity
Phloridzin	Glycosuria
Some flavonoids	Mutagenicity

Table 2 Antinutritional Activities of Phenolic Substances

Chemical reaction	Antinutritional effect
Enzymic browning	Decrease of biological value, formation of unavailable lysine and methionine
Tannin-protein interactions	Decrease of protein digestibility, inhibition of digestive enzymes
Interaction with carbohydrates	Decrease of starch digestibility
Interaction with mineral components	Inhibition of iron absorption, precipitation of some mineral components into unavailable salts or complexes
Formation of complexes with thiamine	Antithiamine effect

lower. Food products of animal origin do not contain phenolics, except for smoked foods. The average total daily intake of phenolics in the human diet may thus approach 1 g.[16]

There is much data available on the content of phenolics in plant products, but they are difficult to compare because of different methods used for their evaluation and various factors affecting their content in the material. Some examples of their content in typical food products are given in Table 3. The highest content is found in green tea and in other similar herbal materials, which are, however, not consumed much. Cereal brans and some oilseeds and vegetables are also rich in phenolics.

The content of coumarins is evident from Table 4. Coumarins are widely distributed in natural flavorings such as Tonka or Tonkin beans (ripe seeds of *Coumarenna odorata* [Dutch Tonka] or *C. oppositifolia* [English Tonka], Leguminosae). They are also present in essential oils. Scopoletin and aesculetin were found in carrots, celery, and other vegetables.

Many toxic furanocoumarins (psoralens) are natural constituents of hundreds of plant species, including the family Umbelliferae, such as parsnip, celery, and parsley, and also in citrus fruits, figs, etc. Common concentrations are of the order of 1 $mg.kg.^{-1}$ Several factors affect the content of phenolics in plant species, such as variety (cultivars), plant part, age, stage of ripening, climatic conditions, and stress conditions (drought, irradiation, insects, molds, etc.). Because of the astringent taste of tannins and other phenolics, plants are usually improved by selection to have the minimum phenolic content.

Colored plant parts are often high in phenolics; for instance, white common beans *(Phaseolus vulgaris* L.) are lower in phenolics than black, red, or bronze cultivars.[28] Rapeseed with a dark skin is higher in phenol compounds than are yellow seeds, which

Table 3 Content of Phenolics in Some Food Materials

Food material	Compound	Content (%)	Ref.
Sorghum	Polyphenols (as catechin)	0.01–7.45	17
Finger millet	Condensed tannins (as catechin)	0.04–3.47	14
Wheat flour	Phenolic acids (free and bound)	0.0105–0.0134	18
Maize	Tannin	0.00–0.01	19
Soybeans	Phenolic acids	0.00119–0.00355	20
Soybean flour	Phenolic acids	0.0234	21
Chick peas	Tannins	0.51–0.85	22
Cow peas	Tannins	0.46–0.76	22
Mung bean	Tannins	1.32–1.55	22
Fruits (apples, pears)			
Peel	Flavonoids	0.02	23
Pulp	Flavonoids	0.0002–0.001	23
Vegetables	Flavonoids	0.0002–0.4000	23
Paprika	Flavonols	0.0033–0.0205	23
Spice plants	Flavonoids	0.007–0.2	23
Tea leaves, green	Catechins	20	18
Tea leaves, fermented	Catechins	3	18
Cocoa beans	Catechins	3	18
	Leucoanthocyanidins	2.5	18
Coffee beans	Chlorogenic acid	6–8	18
Roasted	Chlorogenic acid	4–5	18

are more suitable to the production of edible proteins. Bean and pea varieties with white flowers have substantially lower phenolic content than varieties with colored flowers. The occurrence of furanocoumarins in flax seeds of *Angelica archangelica* was 35 times higher than in tangial seeds.[29]

Changes in the content of phenolics observed during the maturation of fruits are due to the polymerization of polyphenols. These processes are accompanied by loss of solubility and reactivity of phenolics with proteins, and thus by loss of astringency.[30] During the maturation of sorghum, the content of phenolics increases to become constant or decreases again in later stages.[31] In tea leaves, the tannin content increases with the increasing age of the leaf.

The formation of flavonols and flavones depends on the irradiation intensity; therefore, they are concentrated in outer tissues, such as outer leaves of onion bulbs.[7] Various stress-inducing factors, such as ultraviolet (UV) light, cold temperature, mechanical damage, exposure to acidic fogs, and application of pesticides, have been shown to increase the content of furanocoumarins in celery.[26] The γ–irradiation dose of 2 kGy induced accumulation of coumarins in citrus flavedo.[32]

The effect of microorganisms on the synthesis of furanocoumarins is very important. For example, the total contents of furanocoumarins in the whole healthy parsnip root, peel of healthy roots, and diseased area of roots were 97, 300, and 2460 $mg.kg^{-1}$, respectively.[33] In celery infected by *Sclerotonia sclerotiorum*, the content of furanocoumarins rose from 1.84 $mg.kg^{-1}$ to 43.82 $mg.kg^{-1}$, with occasional samples reaching 95.52 $mg.kg^{-1}$.[34] Furanocoumarins also accumulate during long-term storage (over 6 months at 4°C and 95% relative humidity) in celeriac (*Apium graveolens* cv. Monarch), uncoated or coated with various polysaccharides. The increase was much higher in the peel portion than in the edible portion of the tuber.[35] Parsnip roots infected with a strain of *Fusarium sporotrichinoides* accumulated high levels of fungitoxic furanocoumarins, mainly

Table 4 Content of Coumarins and Their Derivatives in Some Food Materials

Material	Compound	Content (%)	Ref.
Lime oils	Coumarin	7	24
Orange oils	Coumarin	0.5	24
Calabrian bergamot oil	Bergamottin	1.02–2.272	25
	5-Geranyloxy-7-methoxycoumarin	0.08–0.22	25
	Citropten	0.14–0.35	25
	Bergapten	0.10–0.32	25
Dutch and English Tonka	Coumarin	1–3	18
Vegetables	Scopoletin, aesculetin	1[a]	10
Celery petioles	Furanocoumarin	0.34–1.84[b]	26
Celery leaves	Furanocoumarin	2.95–15.85[b]	26
Apricots	Scopoletin	0.03–0.07[c]	27
	Aesculetin	0.02–0.05[c]	27
Apples	Aesculetin	0.20–0.45[c]	27

[a] $mg.kg^{-1}$; [b] $\mu g.kg^{-1}$; [c] $mg.dm^{-3}$.

xanthotoxin and angelicin.[36] Roots and petiole tissues of celery and celeriac accessions were shown to contain linear furanocoumarins. Amounts were very low (less than 5 $mg.kg^{-1}$) in young celery and celeriac roots after 7 weeks of incubation, but levels as high as 50 $mg.kg^{-1}$ were found in severely rotted celery root and crown tissues of mature plants. Petioles of young mature plants contained higher amounts of linear furanocoumarins than roots.[37] Bioproducts (products of ecological agriculture) are produced under higher stress conditions than products of modern agriculture; however, literature on the content of phenolics in bioproducts is very scarce. The phenolic compounds, which are induced in plants by stress conditions, particularly disease, may be assumed to rise as well. Phenolic derivatives should protect plants against birds, insects, and microorganisms. Therefore, the content of phenolic substances is probably higher in bioproducts than in products of modern, sophisticated agriculture.

CHANGES DURING PROCESSING AND STORAGE

Various chemical and enzyme-catalyzed reactions of phenolic compounds proceed during food processing and storage (Table 5).

The most important reaction of phenolic substances is a complex series of oxidation reactions, which are mostly catalyzed by oxygenases. The first step is the oxidation of phenolic substances into the respective polyphenolic derivatives. The reaction is mainly catalyzed by various enzymes,[38] such as peroxidases (EC 1.11.1.7) and catalases (EC 1.11.1.6), and usually proceeds via the Fenton reaction[39] (Figure 8). The free-radical character of this reaction explains the inhibitory effect of some polyphenols, such as nordihydroguaiaretic acid.

The further oxidations of polyphenols of the pyrocatechol or pyrogallol type into the respective quinones are reactions widely occurring in various foods of plant origin. The reaction is catalyzed by polyphenol oxygenases (EC 1.10.3.2)[40] and results in formation of the respective quinones (Figure 9). Resorcinol derivatives cannot react in this way, as they do not form any corresponding quinones on their oxidation.

Quinones are very reactive compounds. They are involved in many subsequent reactions, the most important being their reaction with various amino or thiol derivatives[41] (Figure 10). Both free amino acids and amino acids bound in proteins, such as lysine or cysteine, react with quinones with the formation of substituted quinones. Reactions of

Table 5 Main Reactions of Phenols and Polyphenols Under Conditions of Food Processing and Storage

Type of reaction	Products formed
Oxidation of phenols	Polyphenols
Oxidation of polyphenols	Quinones, followed by enzymic browning reactions
Esterification of phenolic acids and hydrolysis of phenolic esters	Esters or acids
Methoxylation of phenols and the reverse reaction	Methoxy derivatives or free hydroxylic derivatives
Hydrolysis of heteroglycosides into polyphenols and sugars	Polyphenolic aglycones or heteroglycosides
Formation of hydrogen bonds with proteins	Insoluble tannin-protein complexes
Polymerization	Dimers and polymeric pigments

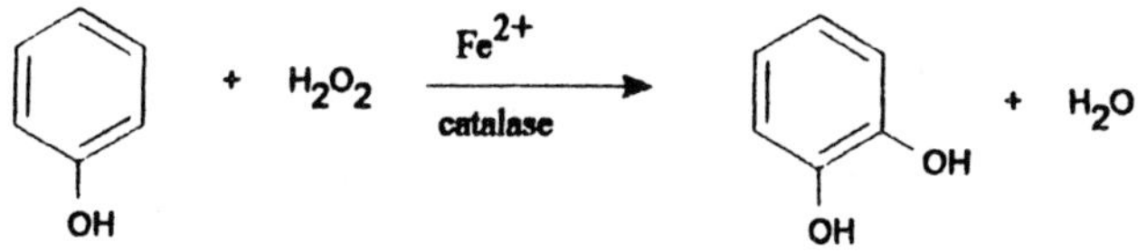

Figure 8 Oxidation of phenols into pyrocatechol derivatives.

3,4-dihydroxyphenylalanine (dopa) are the best known mechanism of this type, studied in detail. The final resulting products are deep-brown-colored polymers, called melanins. They impart a brown discoloration to many food materials, such as apples, potatoes, pears, bananas, figs, cocoa beans, or olives. The reaction is called enzymatic browning,[42] even when only the first stage (formation of quinones) is enzyme catalyzed.

The enzymatic browning affects both the nutritional and the sensory values of foods in different ways, mainly by binding essential amino acids into unavailable polymers and by changing the appearance and the flavor of foods. Therefore, it is generally considered undesirable. During food processing, the enzymatic browning is inhibited in various ways. The most important method is the blanching process.[40] Another method is the inhibition of subsequent reactions of quinones by treatment with sulfites[43,44] or by simply changing the pH value, as the reaction is much slower in acidic medium.

Enzymatic browning should be differentiated from the nonenzymatic browning or Maillard reaction, which involves the formation of brown macromolecular substances (called melanoidins) by interactions of reducing sugars with amino acids. Polyphenols do not directly participate in nonenzymatic browning, but they may stimulate nonenzymatic browning in the following way.

Quinones are oxidizing agents that react with α-amino acids. They are oxidized into aldehydes, with cleavage of carbon dioxide and ammonia (Figure 11). The reaction is usually more complicated, as aldehydes may react with ammonia, and the mechanism depends on both partners — amino acids and quinones. It is called the Strecker degradation.[45] Aldehydes and amines produced in this way are precursors of nonenzymatic browning reactions.

Another reaction of quinones is their polymerization (Figure 11). Polymers are yellow, red, or brown, and thus contribute to enzymatic browning of food materials. A typical example of dimerization is the conversion of green tea catechins into quinones,[46] and their

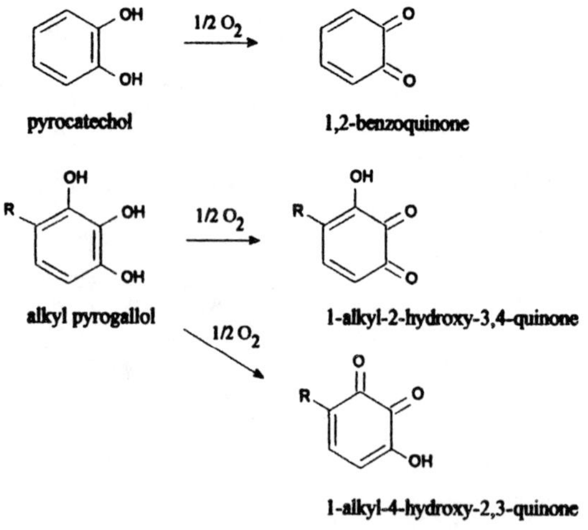

Figure 9 Oxidation of pyrocatechol and pyrogallol derivatives into quinones.

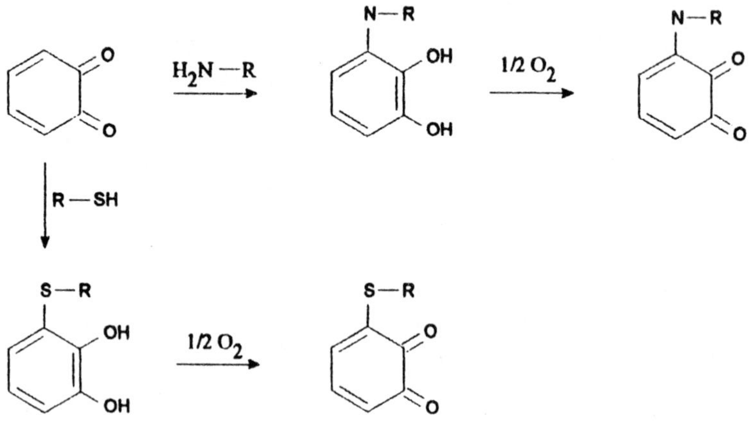

Figure 10 Reactions of quinones with amines or sulfur derivatives.

further dimerization into a yellow pigment, theaflavin (Figure 12) and a red pigment, thearubigin (Figure 12). They are typical pigments of black (fermented) tea. Gallocatechins, their gallates and digallates, form analogous pigments. The polymerization of quinones is usually a favorable reaction, suppressing the astringency of the original material, such as green tea infusions. Browning, accompanying the reaction, does favorably influence the appearance in some cases, e.g., in tea, cocoa, figs, or olives.

The discoloration of foods in the presence of phenolics may be due to another group of reactions, the formation of colored complexes with polyvalent metals, mainly with bivalent ions of iron.Trivalent iron may be transformed into bivalent iron by oxidation of a polyphenol molecule into a quinone. The production of traditional ink is based on this reaction. Violet complexes are produced by reaction of quercetin or catechin with ferrous ions.[47] Iron is not stable in these complexes; it is further oxidized into ferric ions, which form orange- or brown-colored complexes.

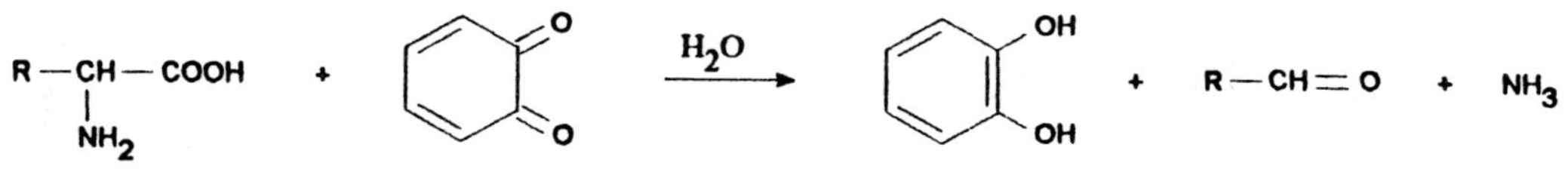

Figure 11 Strecker degradation of α-amino acids with quinones.

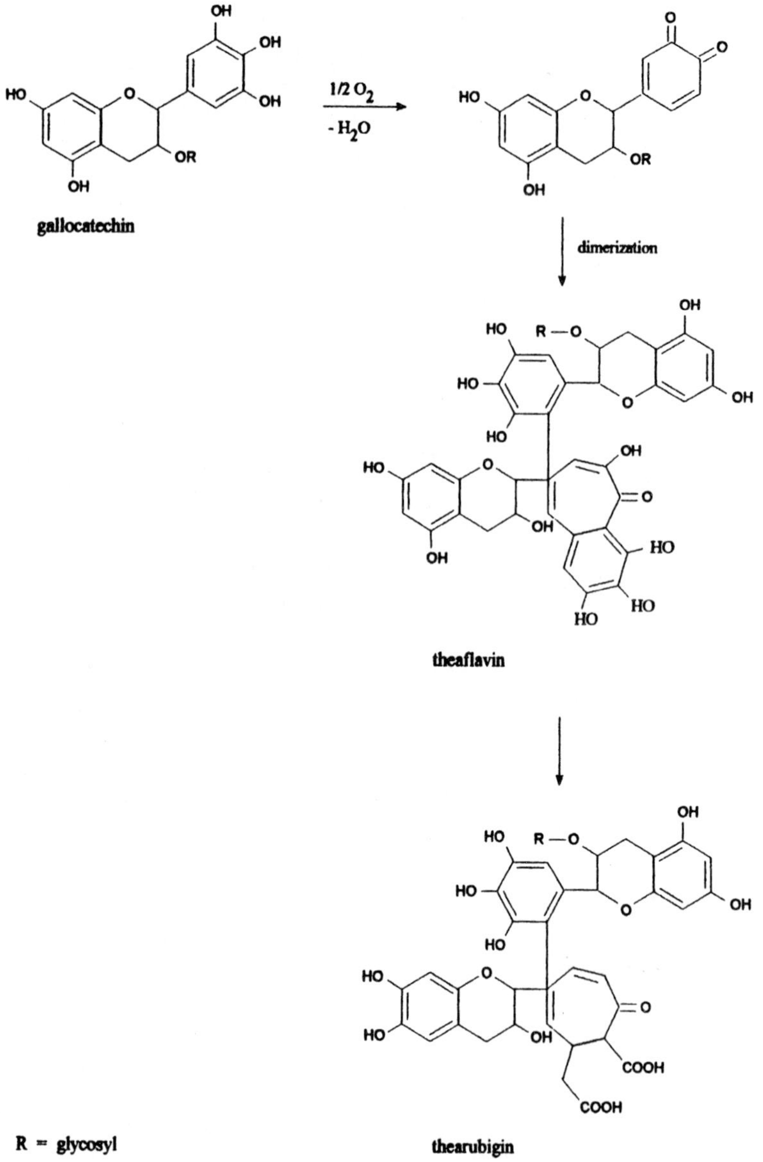

Figure 12 Formation of theaflavin and thearubigin.

Different reactions may occur during the storage of food materials, if enzymes have not been deactivated. For example, polyphenols may be converted into the respective methoxy derivatives (Figure 13), they may be esterified with quinic, tartaric,[48] caffeic, or other acids (Figure 14), or the existing esters may be enzymatically hydrolyzed.

Polyphenols are mainly bound as glycosides or diglycosides in fruits and similar food materials. Glycosides may be cleaved by hydrolases into free phenols and sugars, and of course, the reverse reaction is possible as well (Figure 15). The sensory character is often

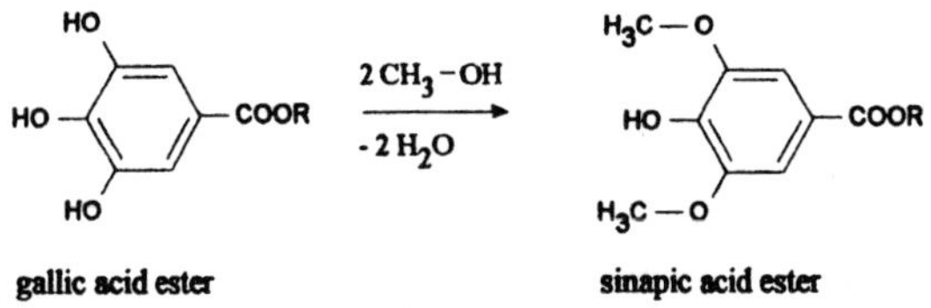

Figure 13 Formation of methoxy derivatives from polyphenols.

affected by these reactions. The bitterness of polyphenols in citrus fruits depends on the formation and hydrolysis of these heteroglycosides.[49]

In addition to chemical reactions, multiple physical bonds may be formed between hydroxyl groups of polyphenols and amine or peptide groups of proteins. Insoluble complexes produced[50] in those processes are attacked by proteolytic enzymes only partially and with difficulty,[51] and therefore the nutritional value of food is impaired by these reactions.[52] The sensory value is affected as well. The astringency decreases, but on the other hand, the texture may deteriorate somewhat.

Phenolic substances are usually removed from foodstuffs if their content is particularly high, since they reduce the sensory value or decrease the nutritional value of feedstuffs for monogastric animals.

Polyphenolic substances are removed from cereals, legumes, and oilseed meals using various methods, such as extraction, dehulling, soaking, thermal processing, germination, fermentation, treatment with different chemicals, especially with alkali, or by combination of these processes.

Various solvents are used for extraction of phenolics from food or feed materials. Most processes are based on extraction with methanol or ethanol, their mixtures with water and with alkali, and in some instances with hydrochloric acid. Another effective process is the removal of phenolics by soaking cereals or legumes, followed by heating to denaturate proteins. The effect of soaking is pH dependent. Reichert and Youngs[53] recommended soaking millet seeds in dilute hydrochloric acid or citric acid. The color of millet grains is thus markedly reduced. Other acids have a similar effect, such as lactic acid in sour milk and in similar acidic solutions. In contrast, Chavan et al.[54] used 0.05 *M* solution of sodium hydroxide for removing tannins from high-tannin sorghum. The soaking is often followed

Table 6 Detoxification of Food and Feed Materials by Extraction of Phenolic Compounds

Extracted material	Extracted compounds	Solvent system used	Removal of phenolics (%)
Millet	Polyphenols	Methanol	65
Alfalfa meal juice	Polyphenols	2-Propanol	65
Sunflower meal	Polyphenols	Acetone-water-acid	65
Sunflower meal	Polyphenols	50% Acetone, 40% Ethanol, 40% Methanol	95–98
Rapeseed meal	Tannins	Methanol	16
Rapeseed meal	Tannins	95% Methanol	36
Defatted sunflower meal	Polyphenols	Acidic butanol	99.9
Canola meal	Phenolics	0.2 *M* Ammonia in ethanol	82
Canola meal	Phenolics	Methanol-ammonia-water-hexane	73.4
Grapeseed meal	Polyphenols	Acidified methanol	61.2–70.5
Grapeseed meal	Polyphenols	95% Methanol and 5% or 10% ammonia	41–75

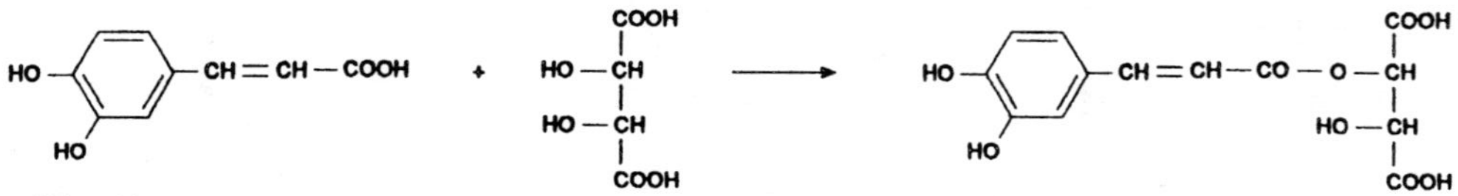

caffeic acid   tartaric acid   caffeyltartaric acid

Figure 14 Esterification of polyphenols with tartaric acid.

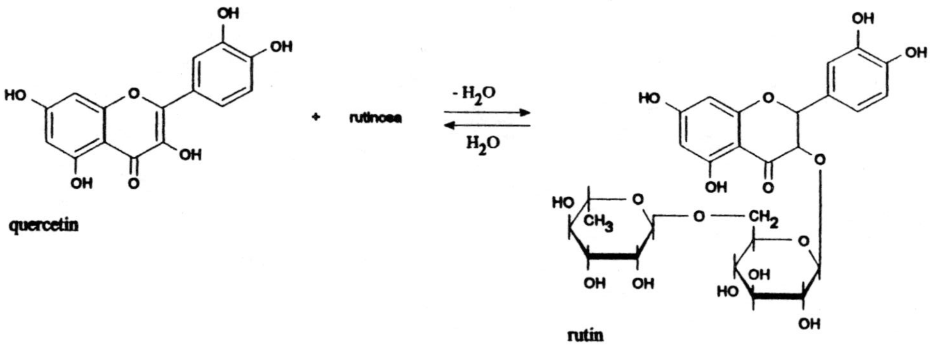

Figure 15 Hydrolysis of polyphenolglycosides.

by heating. The efficiency of tannin reduction in sorghum depends on the time of incubation, temperature, and concentration of alkali. For a given time and temperature, it was found that as alkali concentration was increased, tannin extracted was also increased up to 80%. At a given temperature and alkali concentration, time caused an increase of tannin extraction up to 80%, while high temperature reduced the time needed.[55]

The content of tannins in fruit juices may be influenced by technology. Juice treated by hot pressing and proteolytic enzymes contained more tannins than cold-pressed juice.[56]

The tannin content also decreases during germination, such as in fermented fava bean flour. It decreased after 7 d of germination by 29.7%, but the tannin content in hulls did not change.[57] Observations on the tannin degradation by germination are controversial. Obizoba and Atii[58] reported substantial reduction of tannins during the fermentation of sorghum seed (Guinersia), but according to Kheterpaul and Chaubaṅ,[59] the polyphenol content in flour from pearl millet (*Pennisetum tryptoideum* Rid.) fermented at 30°C increased from 761 to 860 mg.100 g^{-1}. Tannins in grain sorghum and millet are located in pericarp and testa. The antinutritional activity can be improved by removing pericarp and testa by pearling. The polyphenolic pigments were reduced to 66.9 to 71.3% in grains dehulled and soaked in 0.2 *N* HCl.[60] According to Reichert,[61] the concentrations of C-glycosylflavones and alkali-labile ferulic acid markedly decreased after dehulling the millet grain. After nearly 50% of the kernel was removed with the laboratory pearler the concentrations of both C-glycosylflavones and alkali-labile ferulic acid in dehulled grains were about 20% of the concentrations in the whole grains. Tannins can be reduced by dehulling rapeseed as well. Hull removal reduced tannin content of raw brown beans (*Phaseolus vulgaris* L.) by a factor of about 4.5.[62] The *in vitro* protein digestibility could be increased by 69.1% after dehulling the grain.[14] Decorticated millet grain contained far less phenolic acids than whole kernels, approaching those in whole wheat.[63] Whole grains of proso millet contained 0.055 to 0.178% tannins (expressed in catechin equivalents). After decortication, grain contained only trace amounts (0.023 to 0.034%) of polyphenols.[64]

The changes of phenolics of apple, pear, and white grape juices with processing and storage are summarized in the review by Spanos and Wrolstad.[65]

Very little data exist on the detoxication of food by removal of coumarins. Five coumarins present in grapefruit juice can be removed by more than one-half by centrifugation.[66] Another successful method[67] is the removal of coumarin and flavonoids from orange and grapefruit juices by treatment with β-cyclodextrin polymer. In filtered navel orange juice limonin was reduced from 8 to 4 ppm. Similar treatment of grapefruit juice reduced limonin from 3 to1 ppm. Naringin content in aqueous solutions decreased from 436 to 161 ppm and in filtered grapefruit juice from 432 to 207 ppm. Coumarins were removed from mechanically treated citrus oil by winterizing.[68]

As is evident, the literature on the toxicity and antinutritional activity of phenolics is far from complete, and available information is often controversial. Surprisingly, data on various coumarin derivatives are very scarce despite their relatively high toxicity and carcinogenity. The probable reason is their low content in the diet due to low consumption of coumarin-containing foods. With the development of vegetarian diets and bioproducts from ecological agriculture, the need for more information becomes urgent.

REFERENCES

1. Griffiths, D. W., Condensed tannins, in *Toxic Substances in Crop Plants,* D'Mello, J. P. F., Duffs, C. M., and Duffus, J. H., Eds., Royal Society of Chemistry, Cambridge, 1991, 180.
2. Hengtrakul, P., Lorenz, K., and Mathias, M., Alkylresorcinols in U.S. and Canadian wheats and flours, *Cereal Chem.,* 67, 413, 1990.
3. Herrmann, K., Hydroxyzimtsauren und Hydroxybenzoesauren enthaltende Nahrstoffe in Pflanzen, in *Fortschritte der Chemie Organischer Naturstoffe,* Vol. 35, Herz, W., Grischbach, H., and Kirby, G. W., Eds., Springer, Wien, Germany, 1978, 73.
4. Herrmann, K., Caffeic and chlorogenic acid, *Pharmazie,* 11, 433, 1956.
5. Wu, J. W., Lee, M. H., Ho, C. T., and Chang, S. S., Elucidation of the chemical structures of natural antioxidants isolated from rosemary, *J. Am. Oil Chem. Soc.,* 59, 339, 1982.
6. Zadernowski, R. and Kozlowska, H., Phenolic acids in soybean and rapeseed flours, *Lebens. Wiss. Technol.,* 16, 110, 1983.
7. Herrmann, K., Flavonols and flavones in food plants: a review, *J. Food Technol.,* 11, 433, 1976.
8. Mazza, G. and Miniati, E., *Anthocyanins in Fruits, Vegetables, and Grains,* CRC Press, Boca Raton, Florida, 1992.
9. Murray, R. D. H., Méndez, G., and Brown, S., *The Natural Coumarins: Occurrence, Chemistry and Biochemistry,* Wiley, Chichester, England, 1982.
10. Davídek, J., Velíšek, J. and Pokorný, J., *Chemical Changes during Food Processing,* Elsevier, Amsterdam, 1990, chap. 6.
11. Singleton, W. L., Naturally occurring foods toxicants: phenolic substances of plant origin common in foods, *Adv. Food Res.,* 27, 149, 1988.
12. Strube, M., Dragstes, L. O., and Larsen, J. C., *Antimutagenic and Antitumourigenic Effects of Plant Phenols,* National Food Agency of Denmark, Soborg, 1992, chap. 2.
13. Chang, C. C. and Segal, S. J., Assesment of toxicity and antifertility efficacy of gossypol in male rats, in *Gossypol,* Segal, New York, 1985, 45.
14. Ramachandra, G., Virupuska, T. K., and Shadaksharaswany, M., Comparison of the protein fractions of finger millet, *Phytochemistry,* 17, 1487, 1978.
15. Lee, C. B. and Lawless, H. T., Time-course of astringent sensations, *Chem. Senses,* 16, 225, 1991.
16. Brown, J. P., A review of the genetic effects of naturally occurring flavonoids, anthraquinones and related compounds, *Mutat. Res.,* 75, 243, 1980.
17. Earp, C. F., Akingbala, J. O., Ring, S. H., and Rooney, L. W., Evaluation of several methods to determine tannins in sorghum with varying kernel characteristics, *Cereal Chem.,* 58, 234, 1981.
18. Davídek, J., Janíček, G., and Pokorný, J., *Chemie Potravin,* SNTL, Praha, 1983, 250.
19. Lorenz, K. J. and Kulp, K., *Handbook of Cereal Science and Technology,* Marcel Dekker, New York, 1991, 265.
20. Ramakrisna, B. M. V., Mital, B. K., Gupta, K. C., and Sand, K. C., Determination of phenolic acids in different soybean varieties by reversed phase HPLC, *J. Food Sci. Technol. India,* 26, 154, 1989.
21. Shahidi, F. and Naczk, M., An overview of the phenolics of canola and rapeseed: chemical, sensory and nutritional significance, *J. Am. Oil Chem. Soc.,* 69, 917, 1992.
22. Khan, M. A., Jacobsen, I., and Eggum, B. O., Nutritive value of some improved varieties of legumes, *J. Agric. Food Chem.,* 40, 1501, 1992.
23. Kopec, K. and Minárová, E., Bioflavonoidy v zelenině, *Rostlinná výroba,* 31, 889, 1985.
24. Stanley, W. L. and Jurd, L., Citrus coumarins, *J. Agric. Food Chem.,* 19, 1106, 1981.
25. Mondelo, L., Stagno-d'Alcontres, I., del Duce, R., and Crispo, F., On the genuineness of citrus essential oils. XL. The composition of the coumarins and psoralens of Calabrian bergamot essential oil (*Citrus bergamia* Risso), *Flavor Fragrance J.,* 8, 17, 1993.
26. Trumble, J. T., Millar, J. G., Ott, D. E., and Carson, W. C., Seasonal patterns and pesticidal effects on the phototoxic linear furanocoumarins in celery, *Apium graveolens* L., *J. Agric. Food Chem.,* 40, 1501, 1992.
27. de Simon, B. F., Perez-Ilzarbe, J., Hernandez, T., Gomez-Cordoves, C., and Estrella, I., Importance of phenolic compounds for the characterisation of fruit juices, *J. Agric. Food Chem.,* 40, 1531, 1992.

28. Bressani, R. and Elias, L. G., The nutritional role of polyphenols in beans, in *Proc. Symp. Polyphenols in Cereals and Legumes*, IFT, St. Louis, Missouri, 1979, 61.
29. Zobel, A. M. and Brown, S.A., Furanocoumarin concentrations in fruit and seeds of *Angelica archangelica, Environ. Exp. Bot.*, 31, 447, 1991.
30. Goldstein, J. L. and Swain, T., Changes in tannins in ripening fruits, *Phytochemistry*, 2, 371, 1963.
31. Bullard, R. W. and Elias, D. J., Sorghum polyphenols and bird resistance, in *Proc. Symp. Polyphenols in Cereals and Legumes*, IFT, St. Louis, Missouri, 1979, 43.
32. Dubery, I. A., Elicitation of enhanced phenylpropanoid metabolism in citrus flavedo by gamma-radiation, *Phytochemistry*, 31, 2659, 1992.
33. Ceska, O., Chaudhary, S., Warrington, P., Poulton, G., and Ashwood-Smith, M., Naturally-occurring crystals of photocarcinogenic furocoumarins on the surface of parsnip roots sold as food, *Experientia*, 42, 1302, 1986.
34. Chaudhary, S. K., Ceska, O., Warrington, P. J., and Ashwood-Smith, M. J., Increased furocoumarin content of celery during storage, *J. Agric. Food Chem.*, 33, 1153, 1985.
35. Roeber, M., Pydde, E., and Knorr, D., Storage time dependent accumulation of furocoumarins in polysaccharide gel coated celery tubers, *Lebensm. Wiss. Technol.*, 24, 466, 1991.
36. Desjardins, A. E., Spencer, G. F., Plattner, R. D., and Beremand, M. N., Furanocoumarin phytoalexins, trichothecene toxins, and infection of *Pastinaca sativa* by *Fusarium sporotrichioides, Phytopathology*, 79, 170, 1989.
37. Heath-Pagliuso, S., Matlin, S. A., Fang, N., Thompson, R. H., and Rappaport, L., Stimulation of furanocoumarin accumulation in celery and celeriac tissues, *Phytochemistry*, 31, 2683, 1992.
38. Robinson, D. S., Peroxidases and catalases in foods, in *Oxidative Enzymes in Foods*, Robinson, D. S. and Eskin, N. A. M., Eds., Elsevier, London, 1991, chap. 1.
39. Al-Hayek, N. and Dore, M., Oxidation of organic compounds by Fenton´s reagent: possibilities and limits, *Environ. Technol. Lett.*, 6, 87, 1985.
40. Zawistowski, J., Biladeris, C. G., and Eskin, N. A. M., Polyphenol oxidases, in *Oxidative Enzymes in Foods*, Robinson, D. S. and Eskin, N. A. M., Eds., Elsevier, London, 1991, chap. 7.
41. Finley, K. T., The addition and substitution chemistry of quinones, in *The Chemistry of the Quinoid Compounds*, Vol. 2, Patai, S., Ed., John Wiley & Sons, London, 1974, 877.
42. Guenter, M., Enzymatic browning of foods. Quantitative relationships between browning and food constituents, *Z. Lebensm. Unters. Forsch.*, 76, 454, 1983.
43. Janowitz-Klapp, A. H., Richard, F. C., Goupy, P. M., and Nicolas, J. J., Kinetic studies on apple polyphenol oxidase, *J. Agric. Food Chem.*, 38, 1437, 1990.
44. Paschoalina, J., Fereira, V. L. P., and Letao, M. F. de F., Prevention of browning of palm heart during retorting, *Colot. Inst. Technol. Alim.*, 20, 51, 1990.
45. Schonberg, A. and Moubascher, R., The Strecker degradation of α-amino acids, *Chem. Rev.*, 50, 261, 1952.
46. Bokuchava, M. A. and Skobelava, M., Chemistry and biochemistry of tea and tea manufacture, *Adv. Food Res.*, 17, 25, 1969.
47. Okunev, A. S. and Pokrovskaya, M. V., Formation of chlorogenic acid/iron complexes, *Izv. Vyssh. Ucheb. Zaved. Pishch. Tekhnol.*, 5, 101, 1987.
48. Tadera, K., Suzuki, Y., Kawai, F., and Mitsuda, H., Studies on a new *p*-coumaryl derivative isolated from spinach leaves. II., *Agric. Biol. Chem. (Tokyo)*, 34, 517, 1970.
49. Belitz, H. D. and Wieser, H., Bitter compounds: occurrence and structure-activity relationship, *Food Rev. Int.*, 1, 271, 1985.
50. Sekyia, J., Kajiwara, T., Monma, T., and Hatanaka, A., Interaction of the tea catechins with proteins: formation of protein precipitate, *Agric. Biol. Chem. (Tokyo)*, 48, 1963, 1984.
51. Mori, Y. and Mitani, A., Effect of the browning system of catechol and polyphenol oxidase on proteolytic enzyme, *Kaseigaku Zasshi*, 28, 259, 1977.
52. Kumar, P. and Singh, M., Tannins: their adverse role in ruminant nutrition, *J. Agric. Food Chem.*, 32, 447, 1984.
53. Reichert, R. D. and Youngs, C. G., Bleaching effect of acid in pearl millet, *Cereal Chem.*, 56, 287, 1979.

54. Chavan, J. K., Kadam, S. S., Ghonsikar, C. P., and Salunkhe, D. K., Removal of tannins and improvement of *in vitro* protein digestibility of sorghum seeds by soaking in alkali, *J. Food Sci.*, 44, 1319, 1979.
55. Babiker, E. E. and El-Tinay, A. H., Effect of alkali on tannin content and *in vitro* protein digestibility of sorghum cultivars, *Food Chem.*, 45, 55, 1992.
56. Sandhu, G. S., Bawa, A. S., and Bains, G. S., Studies on the effect of variety, processing and storage on the quality of grape juices, *Indian Food Packer,* 42, 36, 1988.
57. Savelkoul, F. H. M. G., Boer, H., Tamminga, S., Schepers, A. J., and Elburg, L., *In vitro* enzymatic hydrolysis of protein and protein pattern change of soya and fava beans during germination, *Plant Food Hum. Nutr.*, 42, 275, 1992.
58. Obizoba, I. C. and Atii, J. V., Effect of soaking, sprouting, fermentation and cooking on nutrient composition and some anti-nutritional factors of sorghum (*Guinessia*) seeds, *Plant Food Hum. Nutr.*, 41, 203, 1991.
59. Kheterpaul, N. and Chauhan, B. M., Effect of natural fermentation on phytate and polyphenolic content and *in vitro* digestibility of starch and protein of pearl millet *(Pennisetum typhoideum), J. Sci. Food Agric.*, 55, 189, 1991.
60. Pawar, V. D. and Parlikar, G. S., Reducing the polyphenols and phytate and improving the protein quality of pearl millet by dehulling and soaking, *J. Food Sci. Technol. India,* 27, 140, 1990.
61. Reichert, R. D., The pH sensitive pigments in pearl millet, *Cereal Chem.*, 56, 291, 1979.
62. Loewgren, M., The effect of hull on the protein quality of brown beans (*Phaseolus vulgaris* L.), *Nutr. Rep. Int.*, 8, 873, 1988.
63. Hoseney, R. C., Varriano-Marston, E., and Dendy, D. A. V., Sorghum and millets, in *Advances in Cereal Sciences and Technology,* Vol. IV, Pomerancz, Y., Ed., American Association of Cereal Chemists, St. Paul, Minnesota, 1981, chap. 3.
64. Lorenz, K., Tannins and phytate content in proso millet *(Panicum milaceum), Cereal Chem.*, 60, 424, 1983.
65. Spanos, G. A. and Wrolstad, R. E., Phenolics of apple, pear, and white grape juices and their changes with processing and storage — a review, *J. Agric. Food Chem.*, 40, 1478, 1992.
66. Berry, R. E. and Tatum, J. H., Bitterness and immature flavor in grapefruit: analyses and improvement of quality, *J. Food Sci.*, 51, 1368, 1986.
67. Shaw, P. E. and Wilson, C. W., Debittering citrus juices with β-cyclodextrin polymer, *J. Food Sci.*, 48, 646, 1983.
68. Johnson, J. D., Viale, H. E., and Wait, D. M., U.S. Patent 4,126,709, Method for extracting carotenoid pigments from citrus oils, 1978.

Part F
Lectins (Hemagglutinins)

Pavel Kalač

Lectins appear to be one of the most deleterious antinutritional factors.[1] According to Kocourek and Hořejší as quoted by Etzler,[2] "lectins are proteins (or glycoproteins) of nonimmunoglobulin nature capable of specific recognition and reversible binding to carbohydrate moieties of complex carbohydrates without altering the covalent structure of any of the recognized glycosyl ligands." Lectins are usually detected in aqueous and saline extracts by their ability to agglutinate erythrocytes of various origin because of their specific recognition of and binding to well-defined carbohydrate structures on the surface of red cells (hemagglutination). Individual lectins frequently occur as a group of closely related proteins, designated as isolectins. Their synthesis is under direct genetic control.

CHEMISTRY

As mentioned above, lectins are proteins or glycoproteins. The carbohydrate moieties are not required for biological activity. Lectins are classified into four groups according to their binding to a carbohydrate structure:[3]

1. Mannose/glucose-binding lectins, such as concanavalin A (Con A).
2. *N*-Acetylglucosamine-binding lectins, mainly from Gramineae and Solanaceae families.
3. *N*-Acetylgalactosamine/galactose-binding lectins. This group contains the most active lectins. Two different but structurally related lectins are found in aqueous extracts of *Ricinus communis*: the highly cytotoxic ricin RCA_{II} and the powerful hemagglutinin RCA_{I}. Kidney bean lectins (PHA) comprise a family of five isolectins, the tetrameric glycoproteins with molecular weight of 118,000 Da, formed by two different subunits, erythroagglutinating and lymphoagglutinating, which have similar molecular weight of about 29,500 Da.
4. Fucose-binding lectins, such as that from furze seeds (*Ulex europaeus*).

Factors denaturating proteinaceous molecules of lectins decrease, but often not entirely eliminate their biological activities.

TOXIC EFFECTS

Antinutritional effects of dietary lectins and their immune and hormonal effects have been widely reviewed[1,2,4-8] in the past few years. Often lectins are not the only antinutritive factor in a diet. For instance, in raw soybean the effects of lectins, trypsin inhibitors, and some other antinutritional factors are additive and possibly synergistic.[9]

The antinutritive effects of the kidney bean lectin (PHA) are better known than any other edible plant lectins. This is due to its high concentration in the seed meal (10 to 15% of the total protein) and its well-known detrimental effects on both animals and humans who eat raw or inadequately cooked kidney beans. Similar nutritionally toxic lectins are present in the seeds of lima beans, tepary beans, jack beans (Con A), and runner beans. Purified lectins of these seeds are apparently toxic to animals at dietary concentrations of 0.5 to 0.6% (w/w). They prevent growth and/or at higher dietary concentrations cause rapid weight loss and in some cases death.[5]

Consumption of raw kidney beans causes gastroenteritis, nausea, and diarrhea in humans, and rapid weight loss and death in rats and quail.

Other commonly used legume seeds have detrimental effects on animal growth. Soybean lectin in raw meal or soy whey survives passage through the small intestine to a lesser extent than PHA or Con A. It is not toxic, but it is still a potent antinutrient as a growth retardant. Tomato, pea, and lentil lectins are apparently not toxic.

Some common features of the reaction mechanism of the nutritionally toxic food lectins have been summarized.[1,6] The level of toxicity observed upon consuming lectins appeared to be dependent on the dietary concentration of the lectin, the extent to which it survived gut passage, and the rate at which it was taken up into systemic circulation. It is therefore difficult to assess the potential toxicity of a particular lectin by *in vitro* methods. Thus all seed lectins should be considered potentially toxic.[5]

Celiac disease occurring in genetically predisposed individuals is a primary intolerance of the gastrointestinal tract to peptides originating from wheat glutens. The initial opinion that some components of the gluten and/or gliadin fraction of the wheat endosperm behave as polymannose-specific lectins was supplemented with data on the concentration of gluten proteins with wheat-germ agglutinin.[10] Both lectins perhaps operate simultaneously and immature enterocytes are damaged and their absorptive function is reduced.

Table 1 Sources of Main Plant Lectins

Source		Symbol of lectin (agglutinin)
Kidney bean (common bean)	*Phaseolus vulgaris*	PHA
Lima bean	*P. lunatus*	
Tepary bean	*P. acutifolius cv. latifolius*	
Runner bean	*P. coccineus*	
Soybean	*Glycine max*	SBA
Jack bean	*Canavalia ensiformis*	Con A (concanavalin A)
Winged bean	*Psophocarpus tetragonolobus*	
Broad bean	*Vicia faba*	VFL
Castor bean	*Ricinus communis*	RCA_{II} (ricin) RCA_{I} (hemagglutinin)
Pea seed	*Pisum sativum*	PSL
Wheat germ	*Triticum vulgare*	WGA
Tomato fruit	*Lycopersicon esculentum*	LEL

OCCURRENCE

Lectins are widely distributed in plants, animals, and microorganisms.[11] They are found in nearly all taxonomic groups of the plant kingdom, but they are particularly common to members of the Leguminosae and Gramineae families. Seeds are the richest source. The most common lectins are given in Table 1. They are also present in potato tubers, lentil seeds, rye, rice, and many other crops. Seed lectins in leguminous plants are mainly located in the cotyledons.

Two proposed functions in plants are currently attracting the most attention: (1) as mediators of symbiosis between plants and microorganisms, and (2) the role of natural pesticides for protection of plants against phytopathogens. Crop breeding aiming to decrease amounts of lectins may therefore negatively affect the agrobiological properties of plants.

Foods derived from seeds and vegetative parts of plants contain nutritionally significant amounts of highly reactive lectins. According to Nachbar and Oppenheim,[12] about 30% of the fresh and processed foods in the U.S. diet, including fruits, green salads, spices, dry cereals, and roasted nuts, contain lectins. The gut of humans and animals is continuously exposed to exogenous dietary lectins. Thus, as mentioned above, they constitute one of the major antinutritive factors in foods of plant origin, and their presence in foods may have very serious consequences for growth and health.[1]

CHANGES DURING FOOD PROCESSING AND STORAGE

Many studies dealing with different processing techniques for inactivation of both lectin and protease inhibitors in *Phaseolus vulgaris* seeds for feedstuffs are widely reviewed.[13]

Cooking of either soaked or unsoaked whole seeds for human consumption has been the most common processing method. Purified PHA is sensitive to thermal inactivation at temperatures of 70°C or greater (Figure l).[14] However, the stability of the native protein in the whole cotyledons is probably higher. Grant et al.[15] in their study abolished lectin activity of white, red, and black kidney beans by presoaking for 16 h and heating for 4 h at 90°C, 45 min at 90°C, or 4 to 10 min at 100°C. There were no detectable changes in the hemagglutinating activity (HA) of presoaked beans heated at 50, 65, and 70°C for 6 h. At 75, 80, and 85°C the HA was progressively reduced although not completely eliminated.

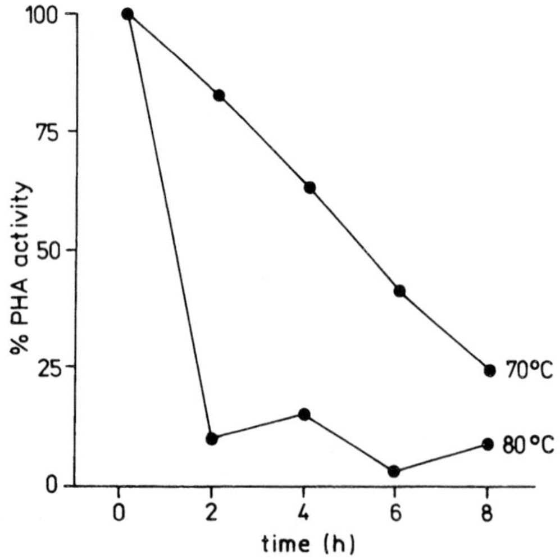

Figure 1 Effect of thermal treatment on hemagglutinating activity of purified PHA (250 μg protein) from red kidney beans cultivar Montcalm: $r = -0.999$ at 70°C, percent activity remaining = 102.18 – 9.87 (h at 70°C). (From Coffey, D. G., Uebersax, M. A., Hosfield, G. L., and Bennink, M. R., *J. Food Biochem.*, 16, 43, 1992. With permission.)

Coffey et al.[16] found that to reduce the HA 10-fold in an extract of whole dark red kidney beans, it was necessary to heat it for 12 min at 100°C, 62 min at 93°C, 136 min at 88°C, or 160 min at 82°C. Cooking for 14 h rendered the beans essentially free of PHA activity. HA was detected in beans held for 5 h or less at 91°C, but no HA was found after 6 h or more of heating.

Nevertheless, the genotype of *Phaseolus vulgaris* must be carefully considered. In a study by Dhurandhar and Chang,[17] the lectin activity in raw red kidney beans was twice as much as in navy beans (45,900 and 21,640 hemagglutinin units per gram bean flour on dry weight basis, respectively). Complete inactivation of lectin activity in red kidney beans was obtained by cooking at 94°C for 30 min, whereas 0.1% remained in similarly treated navy beans. In a more extensive study, Bonorden and Swanson[18] tested the thermal stability of five major groups of *Phaseolus vulgaris* cultivars, distinguished by their globulin-2/albumin polypeptides. Lectin concentrations of the representative cultivars were 15 to 30 $mg.g^{-1}$ of dry flour. The thermal processing time required for complete loss of lectin activity in unsoaked whole seeds at 89°C was between 60 and 130 min in the individual group representatives.

HA decreased only by some 5 and 3.7% in red and navy kidney beans,[17] respectively, presoaked for 16 h at 22 to 25°C, probably due to lectin extraction into the water. Presoaking was repeatedly proved to be an important factor for lectin loss during cooking. For instance, 90 min at 100°C was required to abolish the lectin activity of dry kidney beans as compared with 4 to 10 min in the beans presoaked for 16 h. This difference may be seen in Figure 2.[19] Dry heating is significantly less efficient than cooking. Specific lectin activity decreased by 99.8% in commonly cooked kidney beans, but only by 84% in the beans toasted for 15 min at 135°C.[20] About one-third of the lectin activity was retained in dehulled soybean extruded at temperatures of 150, 160, and 170°C, with a screw speed of 120 rpm and a moisture content of 16%. A quadratic equation for the effects of these three variables on HA was developed.[21]

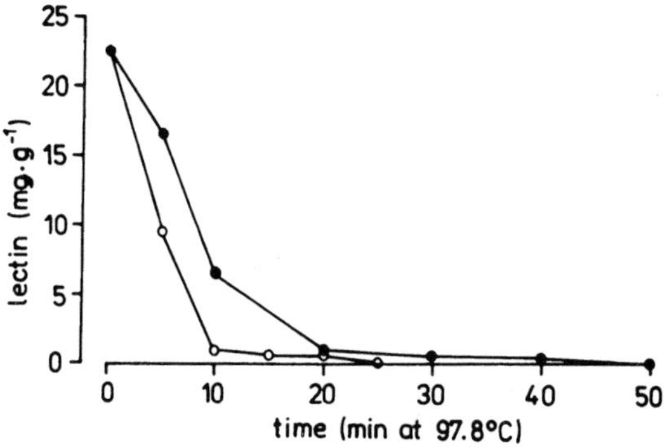

Figure 2 Dry weight basis concentrations of biologically active porcine thyroglobulin-binding lectins in flour prepared from whole black turtle soup beans (*Phaseolus vulgaris*) thermally processed at 97.8°C. ●, soaked, ○, unsoaked. (From Bonorden, W. R. and Swanson, B. G., *J. Sci. Food Agric.*, 59, 245, 1992. With permission.)

In conclusion, the most effective procedure to abolish the nutritional toxicity even of the most resistant lectins, such as PHA, is achieved by thorough soaking of the seeds, followed by cooking for 15 to 20 min at 100°C. The soaking and cooking water should be discarded. A prolonged cooking time must be used in places of high altitude. For instance, the boiling point of water in Mexico City is only 89°C.

As a result of kinetic studies, thermal inactivation of PHA at temperatures at or above 80°C is described as a biphasic, first-order reaction.[22,23]

The effects of three major processing factors on soybean lectin inactivation may be seen in Figure 3.[24]

The results of van der Poel et al.[25] indicate that autoclaving of dry common beans at 119°C for 5 or 10 min seems to be a good compromise in terms of both lectin and trypsin inhibitor inactivation and protein damage. HA decreased to 15 or 1.5% of the original value after 5 and 10 min, respectively. At 102°C a long processing time is necessary. HA decreased to 31% after 40 min and to nearly 0% after 80 min of autoclaving. Further research is needed to evaluate the effects of pressure-cooking at 136°C for less then 90 s.

Based on a comparison with raw beans, whole extruded kidney and black beans (150 to 180°C, 700 to 1000 psi) retained 82 to 88% of the original HA.[26]

No lectin was found in canned navy beans processed by two commonly used methods.[17]

Thermal treatment during substrate preparation of tempeh-type fermented products caused a decrease in the lectin concentration to such low levels that the effect of fermentation with *Rhizopus oligosporus* was negligible. This was true both for soybeans[27] and common beans.[28]

Purified PHA was observed to be stable to freezing and retained its full activity for at least 7 months when stored at –23°C (Figure 4). Treatment of purified PHA with 2 *M* sodium chloride or with HCl (pH 3.0) caused a slight decrease, while treatment with NaOH (pH 12) caused a 65% reduction of HA. PHA was sensitive to some enzymatic treatments. Proteolysis significantly reduced its agglutinating potential (Figure 5).

Changes in both lectins and other antinutritional factors during germination of legume seeds were reviewed.[29] Lectin activity is decreased by degradation caused by enzymes releasing peptides and amino acids necessary for sprouting. For instance, Nielsen and Liener[30] observed a gradual decrease in HA of common beans germinated at 25°C in the dark. By the 10th day HA was reduced to some 40 to 50% of the original activity.

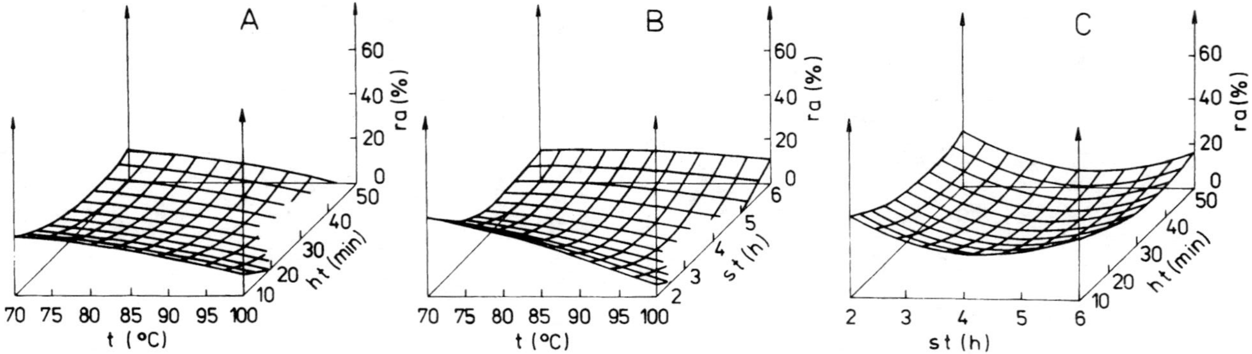

Figure 3 Remaining lectin activity (percent of the original value) in whole soybeans. (A) 4 h of soaking. (B) 30 min of heating. (C) heating at 85°C. *t*, temperature; ht, heating time; st, soaking time; ra, remaining activity. (From Petres, J., Senkalszky-Akos, E., and Czukor, B., *Nahrung,* 34, 905, 1990. With permission.)

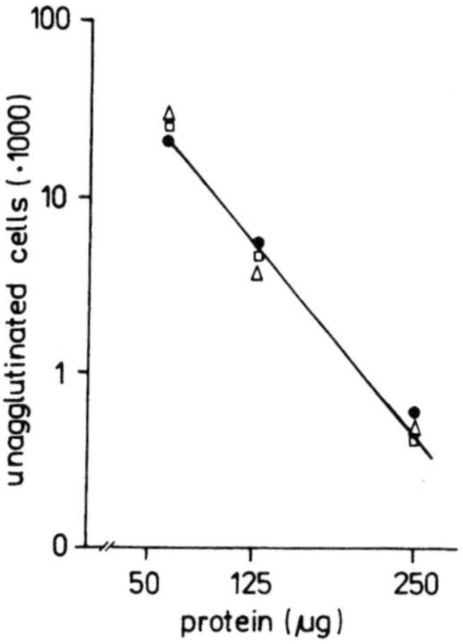

Figure 4 Effect of frozen storage (–23°C) on the hemagglutinating activity of purified PHA from red kidney beans cultivar Montcalm. ●, 0 months; △, 3 months; □, 7 months. (From Coffey, D. G., Uebersax, M. A., Hosfield, G. L., and Bennink, M. R., *J. Food Biochem.*, 16, 43, 1992. With permission.)

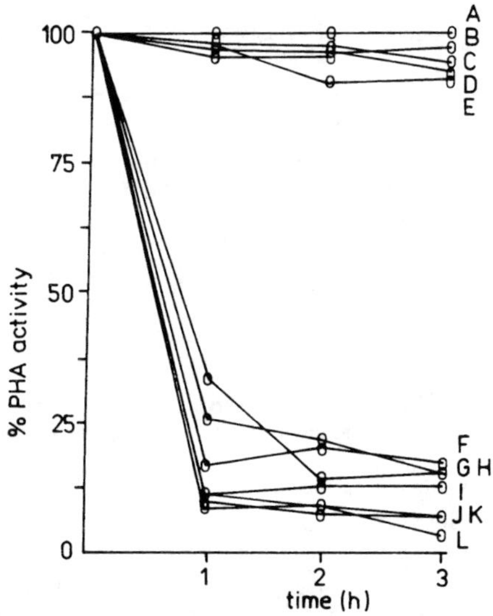

Figure 5 Effect of enzymatic digestion on the hemagglutinating activity of purified PHA (250 μg protein) from red kidney beans cultivar Montcalm at room temperature (enzyme concentration = 1% substrate concentration, 0.05 mg.ml^{-1}). (A) Control. (B) α-Amylase. (C) β-Amylase. (D) Neuraminidase. (E) α-Mannosidase. (F) Trypsin. (G) Chymotrypsin. (H) Pancreatin. (I) Pepsin. (J) Peptidase. (K) ALA-aminopeptidase. (L) Protease. (From Coffey, D. G., Uebersax, M. A., Hosfield, G. L., and Bennink, M. R., *J. Food Biochem.*, 16, 43, 1992. With permission.)

Sprouting time for at least 4 to 6 d seems to be necessary for efficient decrease in HA in different legume seeds.[29]

A survey of active soybean lectin in foods in Mexico[31] showed the significance of processing methods. Unprocessed defatted flour and raw beans contained 4,580 and 3,600 $mg.kg^{-1}$, respectively. Processing decreased these concentrations by 97 and 53%. While meat substitutes are free of active lectin, processed milk substitutes have very low levels of about 10 $mg.kg^{-1}$.

REFERENCES

1. Pusztai, A., Lectins, in *Toxicants of Plant Origin,* Vol. III, Cheeke, P. R., Ed., CRC Press, Boca Raton, Florida, 1989, 29.
2. Etzler, M. E., Plant lectins: molecular and biological aspects, *Annu. Rev. Plant Physiol.,* 36, 209, 1985.
3. Goldstein, I. J. and Poretz, R. D., Isolation, physicochemical characterization, and carbohydrate-binding specifity of lectins, in *The Lectins,* Liener, I. E., Sharon, N., and Goldstein, I. J., Eds., Academic Press, Orlando, Florida, 1986, 33.
4. Liener, I. E., Nutritional significance of lectins in the diet, in *The Lectins,* Liener, I. E., Sharon, N., and Goldstein, I. J., Eds., Academic Press, Orlando, Florida, 1986, 527.
5. Grant, G., Anti-nutritional effects of dietary lectins, *Aspects Appl. Biol.,* 19, 51, 1989.
6. Pusztai, A., Effects on gut structure, function and metabolism of dietary lectins. The nutritional toxicity of the kidney bean lectin, in *Advances in Lectin Research,* Vol. 2, Franz, H., Ed., VEB Verlag Volk und Gesundheit, Berlin, 1989, 74.
7. Pusztai, A., Plant and food lectins as metabolic signals for the gut, *Annu. Rep. Rowett Res. Inst.,* Aberdeen, 1990, 18.
8. Pusztai, A., Ewen, S. W. B., Carvalho, A. F. F. U., Grant, G., Stewart, J. C., and Bardocz, S., Immune and hormonal effects of dietary lectins, in *Effects of Food on the Immune and Hormonal Systems, Proc. Euro. Food Toxicology III,* Zurich, 1991, 20.
9. Grant, G., Anti-nutritional effects of soyabean: a review, *Progr. Food Nutr. Sci.,* 13, 317, 1989.
10. Sollid, L. M., Kolberg, J., Scott, H., Ek, J., Fausa, O., and Brandzaeg, P., Antibodies to wheat germ agglutinin in coeliac disease, *Clin. Exp. Immunol.,* 63, 95, 1986.
11. Lis, H. and Sharon, N., Lectins as molecules and as tools, *Annu. Rev. Biochem.,* 55, 35, 1986.
12. Nachbar, M. S. and Oppenheim, J. D., Lectins in the United States diet: a survey of lectins in commonly consumed foods and a review of literature, *Am. J. Clin. Nutr.,* 33, 2338, 1980.
13. Van der Poel, A. F. B., Effect of processing on antinutritional factors and protein nutritional value of dry beans (*Phaseolus vulgaris* L.). A review, *Anim. Feed Sci. Technol.,* 29, 179, 1990.
14. Coffey, D. G., Uebersax, M. A., Hosfield, G. L., and Bennink, M. R., Stability of red kidney bean lectin, *J. Food Biochem.,* 16, 43, 1992.
15. Grant, G., More, L. J., Mc Kenzie, N. H., and Pusztai, A., The effect of heating on the hemagglutinating activity and nutritional properties of bean (*Phaseolus vulgaris*) seeds, *J. Sci. Food Agric.,* 33, 1324, 1982.
16. Coffey, D. G., Uebersax, M. A., Hosfield, G. L., and Brunner, J. R., Evaluation of the hemagglutinating activity of low-temperature cooked kidney beans, *J. Food Sci.,* 50, 78, 1985.
17. Dhurandhar, N. V. and Chang, K. C., Effect of cooking on firmness, trypsin inhibitors, lectins and cystine/cysteine content of navy and red kidney beans (*Phaseolus vulgaris*), *J. Food Sci.,* 55, 470, 1990.
18. Bonorden, W. R. and Swanson, B. G., Analysis and thermal stability of porcine thyroglobulin-binding lectins in the major *Phaseolus vulgaris* L. G2/albumin groups, *J. Food Sci.,* 57, 1056, 1992.
19. Bonorden, W. R. and Swanson, B. G., Thermal stability of black turtle soup bean (*Phaseolus vulgaris*) lectins, *J. Sci. Food Agric.,* 59, 245, 1992.
20. Almeida, N. G., Calderón de la Barca, A. M., and Valencio, M. E., Effect of different heat treatment on the antinutritional activity of *Phaseolus vulgaris* (variety Ojo de Cabra) lectin, *J. Agric. Food Chem.,* 39, 1627, 1991.

21. Petres, J. and Czukor, B., Investigation of the effects of extrusion cooking on antinutritional factors in soybeans employing response surface analysis. II. Effect of extrusion cooking on urease and hemagglutinating activity, *Nahrung*, 33, 729, 1989.
22. Boufassa, C., Lafont, J., Rouanet, J. M., and Besancon, P., Thermal inactivation of lectins (PHA) isolated from *Phaseolus vulgaris*, *Food Chem.*, 20, 295, 1986.
23. Paredes-López, O., Schevenin, M. L., Guevara-Lara, F., and Barradas, I., Thermal inactivation of hemagglutinating activity of a normal and genetically improved common bean varieties: a kinetic approach, *Food Chem.*, 31, 129, 1989.
24. Petres, J., Senkalszky-Akos, E., and Czukor, B., Inactivation of trypsin inhibitor, lectin and urease in soybean by hydrothermal treatment, *Nahrung*, 34, 905, 1990.
25. Van der Poel, T. F. B., Blonk, J., van Zuilichem, D. J., and van Oort, M. G., Thermal inactivation of lectins and trypsin inhibitor activity during steam processing of dry beans (*Phaseolus vulgaris*) and effects on protein quality, *J. Sci. Food Agric.*, 53, 215, 1990.
26. Coffey, D. G., Uebersax, M. A., Hosfield, G. L., and Bennink, M. R., Thermal extrusion and alkali processing of dry beans (*Phaseolus vulgaris* L.), *Food Process. Preserv.*, 16, 421, 1993.
27. Suparmo and Markakis, P., Tempeh prepared from germinated soybeans, *J. Food Sci.*, 52, 1736, 1987.
28. Paredes-López, O. and Harry, G. I., Changes in selected chemicals and antinutritional components during tempeh preparations using fresh and hardened common beans, *J. Food Sci.*, 54, 968, 1989.
29. Savelkoul, F. H. M. G., van der Poel, A. F. B., and Tamminga, S., The presence and inactivation of trypsin inhibitors, tannins, lectins and amylase inhibitors in legume seeds during germination. A review, *Plant Foods Hum. Nutr.*, 42, 71, 1992.
30. Nielsen, S. S. and Liener, I. E., Effect of germination on trypsin inhibitor and hemagglutinating activities in *Phaseolus vulgaris*, *J. Food Sci.*, 53, 298, 1988.
31. Calderón de la Barca, A. M., Vásquez-Moreno, L., and Robles-Burgueno, M.R., Active soybean lectin in foods: isolation and quantification, *Food Chem.*, 39, 321, 1991.

Part G
Toxic Amino Acids and Lathyrogens

Pavel Kalač and Jiří Davídek

TOXIC AMINO ACIDS

CHEMISTRY

Toxic amino acids often bear structural analogy to the essential amino acids or to the transmitters of the central nervous system of humans and animals. They are invariably of the L-configuration. A systematic classification is difficult due to their diverse range and biological effects. They are therefore usually divided on the basis of their chemical structure or of their physiological properties.[1,2]

Some uncommon amino acids deleterious for humans are described elsewhere in this volume. Most of the other harmful amino acids are more important for animal than for human nutrition. They may be divided into three groups: analogs of sulfur-containing amino acids, antagonists and analogs of urea cycle substrates, and other toxic amino acids.

The structural analogs of methionine is *S*-methyl-L-cysteine sulfoxide. Djenkolic acid belongs to another sulfur-containing amino acid with toxic properties.[2] In many low-rainfall areas of the world selenoanalogs of sulfurous amino acids have been detected.

From the second group, antagonism with arginine was proved in canavanine, indospicine, and homoarginine.

Hypoglycin and its γ-glutamyl derivative are representatives of the third group (Figure1).

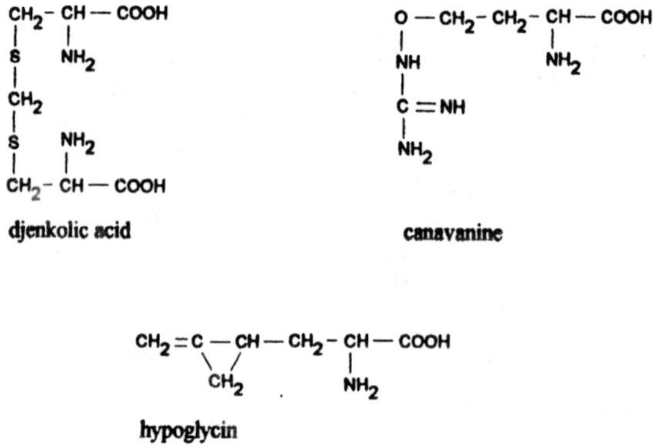

Figure 1 Some toxic free amino acids.

TOXIC EFFECTS

S-Methyl-L-cysteine sulfoxide and *S*-methyl-L-cysteine cause severe hemolytic anemia in ruminants, but they seem to be harmless to humans.[3]

Consumption of djenkol bean (*Pithecellobium lobatum*) causes acute kidney malfunction through precipitation of the amino acid in the body fluid. It has not been possible (except in China) to identify any specific definitive long-term health problems in humans,[4] but changes in nails and hair were noted after consumption of food with a high content of selenoanalogs of sulfurous amino acids.

Canavanine and other arginine analogs, such as indospicine and homoarginine, are of limited significance for human nutrition.

Hypoglycin causes an acute illness called vomiting sickness, occurring mainly in malnourished people, especially children. A comprehensive review was published by Kean.[5]

OCCURRENCE

There are over 700 natural amino and imino acids. Only a small group of them is normally described as having toxic and antinutritional properties to humans and/or animals. These amino acids are not normal components of proteins and usually occur in a free state. They are spread over a wide range of plants, particularly in leguminous species. Seeds generally contain the highest concentration. The presence of these amino acids in the genera *Lathyrus, Canavalia, Leucaena,* and *Indigofera* means that these plants have limited use as economically important plants for human and animal nutrition, particularly in developing countries. Plans for removal of them from crops by breeding techniques must also consider their roles for plant resistance to insects, fungi, and other predators.

S-Methyl-L-cysteine sulfoxide and *S*-methyl-L-cysteine are generally spread in *Brassica* crops. Djenkolic acid occurs at levels up to 2% in dry seeds of *Pithecellobium lobatum* (djenkol bean), much used in Indonesia. The leguminous plants *Canavalia ensiformis* (jack bean), *Indigofera spicata,* and others contain 1 to 12.5% of canavanine based on the dry weight.[2]

Unripe fruit of the ackee tree (*Blighia sapida*), often eaten by Jamaicans, contains hypoglycin.[5]

CHANGES DURING PROCESSING AND STORAGE

Canavanine is stable at temperatures up to 135°C. Extraction of whole jack beans in a large amount of water at 60°C reduced canavanine concentrations from around 50 to

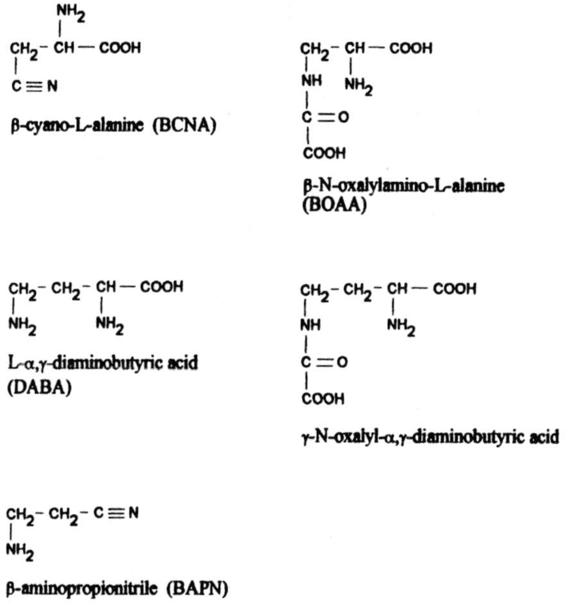

Figure 2 Lathyrogenic amino acids.

8.3 g.kg^{-1} dry matter, while extraction with smaller volumes of water at room temperature was less effective with concentrations averaging 26 g.kg^{-1} dry matter.[6]

Culinary practice with unripe fruit of the ackee tree (*Blighia sapida*) is to free the arils of any attached reddish pericarp and then boil them in water before consumption. The cooking water is discarded as unsafe. Importation of this fruit to some countries is allowed only as canned products. Chase et al.[7] found in the drained edible solid portion of the canned fruit an average of 94 (29 to 176) mg and in the salt liquid portion 110 (42 to 208) mg hypoglycin per 100 grams. Widely varying levels from can to can may be caused by variable ripeness of the fruits, since hypoglycin concentrations decrease considerably during ripening. Hypoglycin is soluble in water and is extracted into the liquid.

LATHYROGENS

CHEMISTRY

Neurotoxically active substances in seeds of the Viciaceae family consist of several free amino acids and one glutamyl dipeptide. From the genetically initial amino acid β-cyano-L-alanine, β-*N*-oxalylamino-L-alanine (BOAA, or often referred to as β-*N*-oxalyl-α,β-diaminopropionic acid, ODAP) and its α isomer are formed. Besides ODAP, L-α,γ-diaminobutyric acid (DABA) and its γ-*N*-oxalyl derivative also belong to the main neurotoxic amino acids (Figure 2).[8,9]

TOXIC EFFECTS

Lathyrogens have been implicated in a neurological disorder of humans and animals. Lathyrism or neurolathyrism occurs to a greater extent in the developing countries during periods of limited food sources. Neurolathyrism in humans generally appears after 3 to 6 months of consumption of a diet consisting of more than two-thirds of *Lathyrus sativus* seeds. Young men are the most susceptible group, and women are affected to a lesser degree. The disorder involves the central nervous system and is characterized by muscular rigidity, weakness, and paralysis of leg muscles, but rarely by death.

DABA, the lower homolog of ornithine, and its γ-*N*-oxalyl derivative also disturbs ornithine-urea cycle reactions, increasing the free ammonia concentration in the blood and brain.

A second disorder, osteolathyrism, may be induced experimentally in laboratory animals by feeding seeds of *L. odoratus* (sweet pea). This disorder of collagen and elastin metabolism is induced by β-aminopropionitrile (BAPN) (Figure 2) and its γ-glutamyl derivative. These compounds lack any toxic effect on the nervous system. There is no known relationship to human neurolathyrism.

OCCURRENCE

Seeds of *L. sativus* (chickling vetch or chickling pea), *L. cicera* (flat-podded vetch), and several other species of the genus *Lathyrus* are the main source of lathyrogens.

The ratio of β-*N*-oxalyl-L-α,β-diaminopropionic acid to its α isomers in *L. sativus* seeds is about 95 to 5, respectively.[10] These seeds contain 0.1 to 2.5% BOAA based on the dry weight, depending on a source. The amino acid was confirmed in over 20 species of *Lathyrus* genus.

Occurrence of *Vicia sativa* or other *Vicia* seeds in those of *Lathyrus*, containing α-glutamyl-β-cyano-L-alanine at some 0.5% of the dry matter, was considered for a period as the causative agent of the neurolathyrism. Nevertheless, the disorder in humans arises from *L. sativus* seeds free of *Vicia* contamination, or contaminated only slightly. L-α,γ-Diaminobutyric acid (DABA) and its γ-*N*-oxalyl derivative occur in a lot of *Lathyrus* seeds, namely, in *L. silvestris* (flat pea) and *L. latifolius* (perennial pea), at up to about 1.5% of the dry matter, but not in *L. sativus*.

CHANGES DURING PROCESSING AND STORAGE

There is no correlation between color, size, or physical properties and BOAA content in *L. sativus* seeds. Levels of BOAA may be significantly reduced by plant breeding, but a safe level has not been defined. Recommended methods to remove this amino acid from the seeds are cooking the pulp in an excess of water followed by draining, soaking the seeds in cold water overnight, and steeping the dehusked seeds in hot water.[9] At most 80% of BOAA can be reduced by any of these methods. This reduction may not be sufficient to reduce long-term toxic effects.

Ayyagari et al.[11] tested the effect on BOAA concentration of nine processing methods commonly used in Indian households for the preparation of foods from either dehusked *L. sativus* seeds or the powder of these seeds. A decrease of 95% of the initial value was observed both in soaking and pressure-cooking, followed by fermentation and steaming, while only a 42% decrease was observed after boiling. Drying in the sun combined with roasting had no effect, and drying in the sun followed by deep-fat frying caused only a very limited decrease, as did the deep-fat frying of wet dough. Roasting of whole seeds at 150°C for 20 min destroyed 85% of BOAA.[12] Jha[13] observed a decrease in BOAA concentration of some 69, 79, and 89% in the whole seeds of *L. sativus* after 1, 2, and 3 h of boiling without previous soaking, while in the *dhal* (split cotyledons) the decrease was 71, 79, and 88%, respectively. Nevertheless, complete loss of thiamine, riboflavin, and niacin and a very high decrease in protein and sugar content were found within the first hour of the treatment. The dhal, obtained by dehulling, is the most common form in which *L. sativus* seeds are used by consumers. The concentration of BOAA was found to be greatest in the germ of the seeds.[14] The germ is separated and removed during milling.

Deshpande and Campbell studied the effect of different solvents on protein recovery and neurotoxin and trypsin inhibitor contents of the grass pea (*L. sativus).*[15] Depending on the extractant used, BOAA associated with the various protein isolates ranged from 0.65 to 2.22 $g.kg,^{-1}$, which represented reduction of about 50 to 85% from the neurotoxin level in the whole *L. sativus* seeds, genotype LS 89039. Greater levels were extracted and recovered in protein isolates prepared under alkaline conditions. The greatest reduction was observed in the protein isolate prepared using the isoelectric precipitation technique.

REFERENCES

1. Rosenthal, G. A., *Plant Nonprotein Amino and Imino Acids,* Academic Press, New York, 1982.
2. D'Mello, J. P. F., Toxic amino acids, *Aspects Appl. Biol.,* 19, 29, 1989.
3. Benevenga, N. J., Case, G. L., and Steele, R. D., Occurrence and metabolism of *S*-methyl-L-cysteine and *S*-methyl-L-cysteine sulfoxide in plants and their toxicity and metabolism in animals, in *Toxicants of Plant Origin,* Vol. III, Cheeke, P. R., Ed., CRC Press, Boca Raton, Florida, 1989, 203.
4. Whanger, P. D., Selenocompounds in plants and their effects on animals, in *Toxicants of Plant Origin,* Vol. III, Cheeke, P. R., Ed., CRC Press, Boca Raton, Florida, 1989, 141.
5. Kean, E. A., Hypoglycin, in *Toxicants of Plant Origin,* Vol. III, Cheeke, P. R., Ed., CRC Press, Boca Raton, Florida, 1989, 229.
6. D'Mello, J. P. F. and Walker, A. G., Detoxification of jack beans (*Canavalia ensiformis*): studies with young chicks, *Anim. Feed Sci. Technol.,* 33, 117, 1991.
7. Chase, G. W., Jr., Landen, W. O., Jr., Gelbaum, L. T., and Soliman, A. G. M., Ion-exchange chromatographic determination of hypoglycin A in canned ackee fruit, *J. Assoc. Off. Anal. Chem.,* 72, 374, 1989.
8. Roy, D. N., Toxic amino acids and proteins from *Lathyrus* plants and other leguminous species: a literature review, *Nutr. Abstr. Rev.,* 51, 691, 1981.
9. Roy, D. N. and Spencer, P. S., Lathyrogens, in *Toxicants of Plant Origin,* Vol. III, Cheeke, P. R., Ed., CRC Press, Boca Raton, Florida, 1989, 169.
10. Roy, D. N. and Narasinga Rao, B. S., Distribution of α- and β-isomers of *N*-oxalyl-α,β-diaminopropionic acid in some varieties of *Lathyrus sativus, Curr. Sci. (India),* 37, 395, 1968.
11. Ayyagari, R., Narasinga, R., and Roy, D. N., Lectins, trypsin inhibitors, BOAA and tannins in legumes and cereals and the effects of processing, *Food Chem.,* 14, 229, 1989.
12. Padmanaban, G., Lathyrogens, in *Toxic Constituents of Plant Foodstuffs,* 2nd ed., Liener, I. E., Ed., Academic Press, New York, 1980, 239.
13. Jha, K., Effect of the boiling and decanting method of Khesari (*Lathyrus sativus*) detoxification, on changes in selected nutrients, *Arch. Latinoam. Nutr.,* 36, 101, 1987.
14. Prakash, S., Misra, B. K., Adsule, R. N., and Barat, G. K., Distribution of β-*N*-oxalyl-L-α,β-diaminopropionic acid in different tissues of aging *Lathyrus sativus* plant, *Biochem. Physiol. Pflanzen,* 171, 369, 1977.
15. Deshpande, S. S. and Campbell, C. G., Effect of different solvents on protein recovery and neurotoxin and trypsin inhibitor contents of grass pea (*Lathyrus sativus*), *J. Sci. Food Agric.,* 60, 245, 1992.

Part H

Biogenic Amines

Tomáš Davídek and Jiří Davídek

Food contains numerous amines, many of which are called biogenic amines, because of their biological activity and possible toxicity when present at high levels.[1] Chemically, biogenic amines have been defined as low-molecular-weight aliphatic, alicyclic, or heterocyclic organic bases.[2] They arise mainly from decarboxylation of the corresponding amino acids or transamination of aldehydes by amino acid transaminases (EC 2.6.1.1).[3] The reaction scheme is given in Figures 1 and 2. Amines derived from basic and aromatic amino acids belong to the most important groups and are listed in Table 1.

In addition to mono- and diamines derived from amino acids, the oligoamines spermidine and spermine are detected in many food materials. They are produced from putrescine by reaction with decarboxylated *S*-adenosylmethionine.[1]

The occurrence of biogenic amines in foods, the changes during storage, and the physiological effects and toxicity have been extensively studied and many reviews exist.[1,3-9]

CHEMISTRY

Biogenic amines are very reactive. They may be converted into aldehydes by oxidative deamination, and they may be further transformed into biologically active products such as serotonin or adrenaline. With lipids biogenic amines form amides on heating or prolonged storage; they may enter nonenzymatic browning reactions; they are oxidized into imines by hydrogen peroxide or lipid hydroperoxides. Secondary amines, as mentioned above, may produce nonvolatile nitrosamines by reaction with nitrites or nitrogen oxides (Figure 3).[10]

With proteins, biogenic amines such as phenylethylamine, putrescine, histamine, spermidine, and tyramine react, giving β-*N*-substituted diaminopropionic acid derivatives. The most probable mechanism for the formation of these amino acid derivatives is via β-elimination from the cysteine residue, followed by addition of the amine to the double bond of dehydroalanine as occurs when lysinoalanine is produced. For example, phenylethylamine is formed in this way from D,L-3-(*N*-phenylethylamino)alanine.[11,12]

TOXIC EFFECTS

Biogenic amines are needed for many critical functions such as regulation of nucleic acid function, protein synthesis, stabilization of membranes, control of gastric secretion, control of blood pressure, etc.[1] Though they are essential for many functions, high concentrations of these compounds cause an antinutritional or toxic effect. Biogenic amines may exert psychoactive as well as vasoactive effects or both. Psychoactive amines act on the neural transmitters in the central nervous system, while vasoactive amines act either directly or indirectly on the vascular system and can be divided into vasoconstrictors (e.g., tyramine) and vasodilators (e.g., histamine).[1,5,9] Symptoms that occur after excessive oral intake of biogenic amines are nausea, respiratory distress, hot flush, sweating, heart palpitation, headache, oral burning, and hyper- or hypotension.[4]

In the intestinal tract of mammals a fairly efficient detoxification system exists that metabolizes normal intakes of biogenic amines. The enzymes monoamine oxidase (MAO, EC 1.4.3.4) and diamine oxidase (DAO, EC 1.4.3.6) play an important role in the detoxification process. However, this system fails to eliminate high levels of biogenic amines.[9]

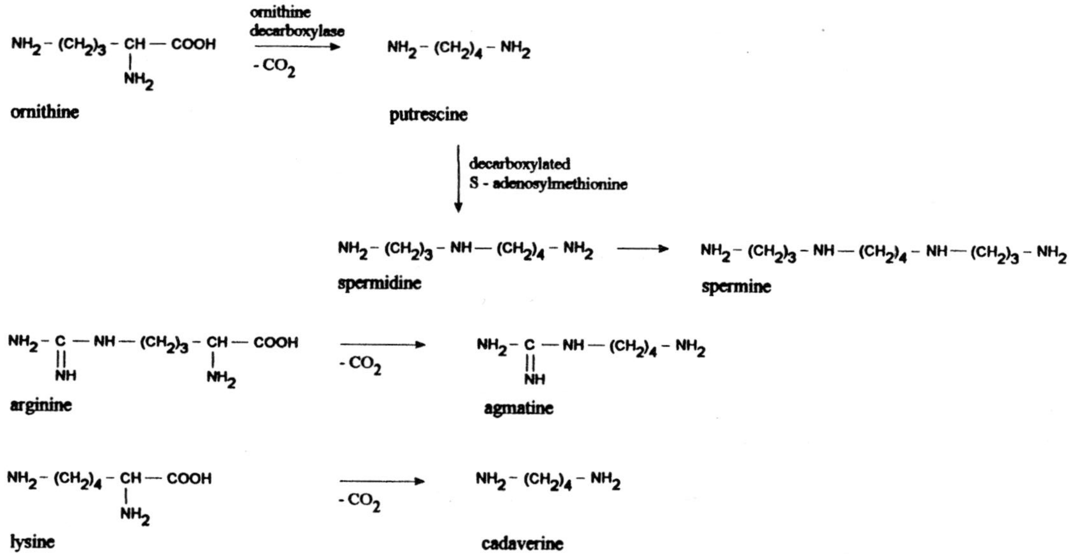

Figure 1 Formation of biogenic amines from aliphatic amino acids.

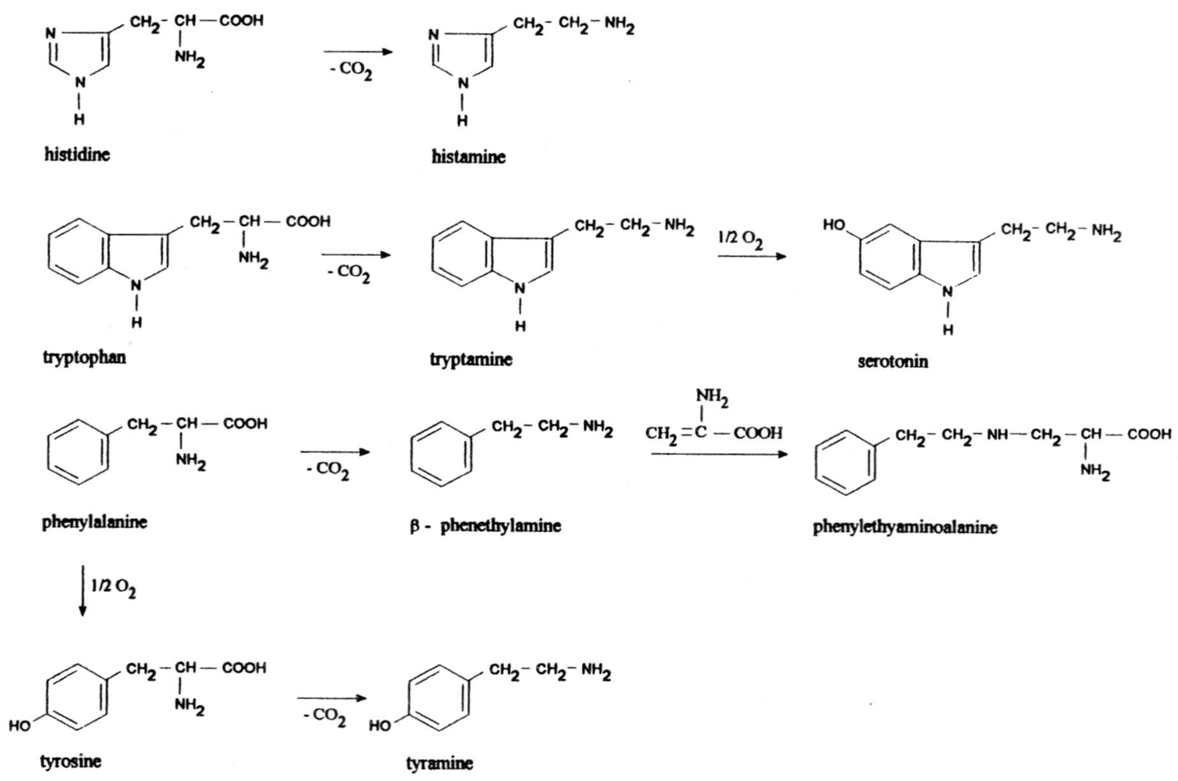

Figure 2 Formation of biogenic amines from aromatic and heterocyclic amino acids.

Table 1 Some Biogenic Amines Derived from Basic and Aromatic Amino Acids

Amino acid precursor	Corresponding amine
Ornithine	Putrescine
Lysine	Cadaverine
Arginine	Agmatine
Histidine	Histamine
Phenylalanine	Phenylethylamine
Tyrosine	Tyramine
Tryptophane	Tryptamine

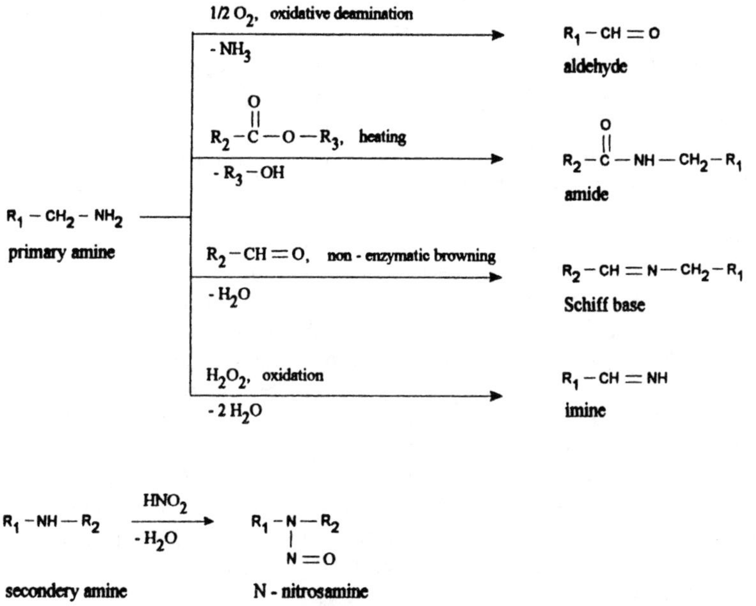

Figure 3 Reactions of biogenic amines.

A toxic dose of biogenic amines strongly depends on the efficiency of detoxification, which may vary considerably between individuals and which is influenced by many factors, such as presence of certain drugs (MAO inhibitors) or presence of potentiators, etc. Thus in considering the toxic levels of biogenic amines in foods one has to take into account not only one particular amine, but also the other factors as the amount of food consumed, the presence of other amines, the amine content of other dietary components, etc. Therefore, it is very difficult to determine the exact toxicity threshold of biogenic amines. Generally, histamine levels above 500 to 1000 $mg.kg^{-1}$ are considered potentially dangerous to humans.[9] A legal upper limit of 100 $mg.kg^{-1}$ in food and 2 $mg.dm^{-3}$ in alcoholic beverages has been suggested.[1] Even less is known about the toxic dose of other amines. Threshold values of 100 to 800 $mg.kg^{-1}$ for tyramine and 30 $mg.kg^{-1}$ for phenylethylamine have been reported.[1] It should also be stated that secondary amines can react with nitrites to form carcinogenic nitrosamines (page 229).

OCCURRENCE

Biogenic amines are natural constituents of many foods. Although foods normally contain small amounts of these amines, formation of higher amounts has been reported in some fruits and vegetables, in aged fermented products, or in products that have undergone spoilage.[1,3,5,9] The content of biogenic amines in some foods is listed in Table 2.

The biogenic amine levels in fresh fish are generally very low. For example only traces of histamine and tyramine were found in fresh anchovies, 0 to 10 $mg.kg^{-1}$ histamine and 0 to 2 $mg.kg^{-1}$ tyramine were detected in good-quality tuna, etc.[9,13] However, fish muscle is relatively rich in histidine. Tissue of so-called scombroid fish (the families Scomberesocidae and Scombridae, e.g., tuna, mackerel, skipjack) especially contains high levels of free histidine that can be converted to histamine by association and contamination with microflora. Thus, spoiled fish can contain high levels of histamine. Up to 8,000 and 3,000 $mg.kg^{-1}$ histamine were found in spoiled tuna and mackerel, respectively.[9] Nonscombroid fish such as herring and anchovies can also accumulate high amounts of histidine.[1,9,14] Tyramine, cadaverine, and putrescine are other biogenic amines that can arise in rather high quantities in fish. Tarjan et al. analyzed 57 samples of tuna for tyramine and found traces up to 1,060 $mg.kg^{-1}$ with an average of 574.6 $mg.kg^{-1}$.[2] Pechanek et al. found up to 447 $mg.kg^{-1}$ cadaverine and up to 200 $mg.kg^{-1}$ putrescine in canned tuna.[15] Fermented fish products such as fish paste tend to contain higher amounts of biogenic amines.[16]

Tyramine, histamine, tryptamine, putrescine, and cadaverine can be formed in high concentrations in various cheeses, especially in so-called blue-veined cheeses (Roquefort, Gorgonzola, Bleu) or well-matured cheeses such as cheddar (Table 2). As much as 4100 $mg.kg^{-1}$ histamine, 2,551 $mg.kg^{-1}$ tyramine, 1,100 $mg.kg^{-1}$ tryptamine were found in blue-veined cheeses, and some samples of Gorgonzola contained 1,245 $mg.kg^{-1}$ putrescine and 4,280 $mg.kg^{-1}$ cadaverine.[1,17] However, the content of biogenic amines in cheeses is generally low or even absent if they are prepared under good hygienic conditions.[18,19]

Fermented sausages may contain high levels of biogenic amines. In a survey of 390 samples of sausages, levels up to 550 $mg.kg^{-1}$ histamine have been reported in dry fermented sausages such as Italian dry salami or pepperoni.[20] Vandekerckhove found maximal amounts of 286 mg histamine, 396 mg putrescine, and 1,506 mg tyramine per kilogram of dry matter in dry fermented sausages.[21]

Biogenic amines occur in lactic fermented vegetables (e.g., sauerkraut) and in soybean fermented products such as miso or soy sauce.[4,9,22-27]

Some fruits and vegetables contain rather high amounts of biogenic amines. For example, up to 400 $mg.kg^{-1}$ histamine and 680 $mg.kg^{-1}$ tyramine were found in spinach and up to 1,200 $mg.kg^{-1}$ tyramine were found in tomato.[1,2] Walnut embryo is rich in serotonine (550 $mg.kg^{-1}$); banana pulp contains 78 $mg.kg^{-1}$ serotonine and 95 $mg.kg^{-1}$ tyramine.[1,2]

Occasionally, alcoholic beverages such as beer and wine can contain biogenic amines at levels that may exert a toxic effect.[1-3,5,9,28-33]

CHANGES DURING PROCESSING AND STORAGE

In nonfermented food, biogenic amines appear as a result of undesirable microbial activity, so that they can be used as indicators of freshness of seafood or meat. The contents of histamine, putrescine, and cadaverine usually increase during the decomposition of seafood, whereas spermidine and spermine levels decrease. In very badly decomposed seafood spermidine and spermine often disappear. These characteristics have been expressed by Karmas as a biogenic amine index (BAI):[34]

$$BAI = \frac{\text{histamine} + \text{putrescine} + \text{cadaverine}}{1 + \text{spermine} + \text{spermidine}}$$

where amine concentrations are given in $mg.kg^{-1}$.

According to Karmas, seafood products can be classified into acceptable, borderline, and unacceptable quality with BAI values $BAI < 1$, $1 < BAI < 10$, $BAI > 10$, respectively.

Many studies have been reported on the effect of storage temperature on biogenic amine formation (namely, histamine) in various types of fish. The majority of studies seem to indicate that histamine formation is negligible in fish stored at 0°C or below. However, the results concerning the optimal temperature for histamine formation in fish are quite variable (from 5 to 38°C).[6] The reason may be due to differences in type and level of microflora in fish used in various studies.

Storage on ice decreases the rate of formation of biogenic amines, but it is not sufficient to prevent the formation completely. Ababouch et al. followed the formation of biogenic amines in raw and salted sardines stored in ice and at ambient temperature (25 to 28°C).[35] Histamine, cadaverine, and putrescine accumulated rapidly, reaching levels of 2,350, 1,050, and 300 $mg.kg^{-1}$, respectively, in raw sardines after 24 h of storage at ambient temperature. Histamine and cadaverine reached similar levels in raw sardines stored in ice after 8 d, whereas putrescine formation was insignificant. Spermidine and spermine levels increased only slightly during storage at ambient temperature, reaching levels of 60 and 50 $mg.kg^{-1}$, respectively, after 24 h. Storage in ice inhibited formation of these amines. Addition of sodium chloride at 8% (w/w) did not affect the rate of formation of biogenic amines in sardines stored at ambient temperature. For the ice-stored sardines, histamine and cadaverine production was delayed by the presence of the salt for 60 to 70 h, but the rate of formation was very rapid after this. Consequently, after 8 d of storage histamine and cadaverine reached levels similar to those obtained in iced nonsalted sardines.[35]

Biogenic amines can be useful indicators of poor quality raw material in preserved and semi-preserved fish products as has been demonstrated, e.g., in smoked mackerels or vacuum-packed herrings. Mackerel that was immediately frozen after catch, then stored for 2 months, thawed, brined, and hot-air smoked contained only 1 $mg.kg^{-1}$ of histamine, whereas mackerel prepared in the same way but stored 48 h at 15°C before freezing contained 97 $mg.kg^{-1}$ of histamine.[11] Similarly vacuum-packed mattes herring fillets stored at 4 and 7°C accumulated within 10 d 11 to 47 and 46 to 89 $mg.kg^{-1}$ histamine, respectively, but the fillets contaminated with histidine-decarboxylating photobacteria accumulated 990 to 1,000 $mg.kg^{-1}$ histamine at 4°C within 10 d and 713 to 821 $mg.kg^{-1}$ of histamine at 7°C within 9 d.[11]

Aerobic storage of red meats leads to a distinct increase of putrescine and cadaverine. The sum of these diamines is used as a quality indicator of pork. Following aerobic storage of pork and beef, Shlemr et al. were able to classify pork into three classes according to the diamine level.[36] Fresh pork (first class) had a mean value of the sum of the parameters SUM (cadaverine + putrescine) of about 7 $mg.kg^{-1}$, whereas spoiled pork (third class) had a mean value of SUM (cadaverine + putrescine) of about 60 $mg.kg^{-1}$. The histamine concentration rose slightly and more slowly.[36] No changes were detected in polyamine concentrations in pork stored for 16 d at 4°C.[37]

Table 2 Biogenic Amine Content in Foods ($mg.kg^{-1}$)

Food	Hism	Tyrm	Phem	Putr	Cdv	Spm	Spd	Trpm	Agm	Sert	Ref.
Tuna	tr-8,000	tr-1,060	tr-45	tr-200	tr-447	tr-18.6	1-4.4				2,9,15,28,34
Mackerel	tr-3,000	tr-75	tr-126	tr-40	tr-226	tr-48	2-4				9,14,15,54
Herring	tr-1,300	0-3,000	tr	1-37	tr-34	tr-92	50-56				4,15,55,57
Anchovy	tr-935	tr-66	88	13	53	4					1,13,15,56
Sardine	4-2,350	1-68		4-300	18-1,050	35-65	4-60				35,56,57
Fermented fish paste	78-680	tr-38	tr-600		tr-35			tr-163			16
Cheddar	0-1,300	0-1,500	0-303	1-996	4-408			0-300			1,3,4,59,60
Ementhaler	tr-2,000	1-1,000	0-490	1-130	0-460			0-210			4,15,19,46
Gouda	0-850	0-670	0-46	1-200	1-140			10-200			1,4,9,58,64
Edam	0-88	tr-320		tr	tr						3,4,58
Camembert	0-480	20-2,000		605	1,180			10-70			1,3,4,58
Roquefort or Bleu	0-4,100	tr-1,350	10-25	44-830	42-905			10-1,100			1,17,28
Gorgonzola	nd-2,300	50-2,551		1,245	4,280			500			17,58
Gruyere	nd-200	41-516		100	57						3-5,28
Mozzarella	0-50	0-410		8-20	10-21						4,64
Sauerkraut	1-200	2-310	0-9	6-550	1-311						2,9,22
Soy sauce[a]	nd-274	nd-882	nd	nd-93				nd-100			5,24,25
Miso	nd-492	nd-1,011	nd-158	nd-134	nd-50	nd-39	nd-148	tr			27,49
Straw mushroom	nd-2	3-65	3-66	1-5	nd-23			nd-7			52
Beer[a]	0-200	1-177	tr	1-12	0-60				12-114		5,9,28,30
Wort[a]	1-4	9-28		4-10					23-117		50
Red wine[a]	0-30	0-90	tr	tr-6	0-47						2,5,28,10,33
White wine[a]	nd-20	nd-212		1-11	3-108						2,5,32
Sherry[a]	0-31	1-17	1	3-25	1						9,33
Pork	0-45	1-35		tr-702	0-171	1-177	tr-619	1-48			1,3,62
Pork, putrefied	45	22		1,494	250	8,060	3,399	48			3
Beef	0-217	tr-61		tr-26	0-27	4-382	tr-50		2-112		38,61
Chicken	1	23	tr	6	9	58					15
Ham	1-271	nd-618	tr-215	tr-598	tr-97	tr-331	13-72	8-67			1,15,62
Bacon	15	1-3		tr-8	tr-1	1-212	2-42	4			3,62

Sausage	tr-550	0-1,240	0-61	1-396	tr-298	16-241	23-137	29		1,5,9,21,47
Salami	tr-550	tr-663	tr-696	8-329	tr-787	tr-35		nd-3		15,20,60
Chocolate	0-10	0-2	0-27	0	0-8	nd-11	1-2	tr-1		1,9,59
Cacao	1	4-12	0-22	1		1	12	2		1,59,63
Green coffee				37,000-54,000		7,000-10,000	15,000-20,000			3,51
Roasted coffee				1,000-2,000						3,51
Banana (pulp)		7-95							12-78	1,4
Pineapple	2-65	0-4								1,4
Orange		1-10						0.1		1,4
Grape		0-1,400								1,2
Spinach	400	0-680								1,2
Walnut (embryo)									550	1
Tomato	tr-1	0-1,200						4	12	4,5

Note: tr, traces; nd, not detected; Hism, histamine; Tyrm, tyramine; Phem, phenylethylamine; Putr, putrescine; Cdv, cadaverine; Spm, spermine; Spd, spermidine; Trpm, tryptamine; Agm, agmatine; Sert, serotonin.

[a] Content in mg dm^{-3}.

Table 3 Effect of Storage and Cooking on the Content of Biogenic Amines in Ground Beef (in mg.kg^{-1})

	Time	Put		Hism		Cdv		Spm		Spd		Tyrm	
Temperature	(days)	Raw	Cooked	Raw	Cooked	Raw	Cooked	Raw	Cooked	Raw	Cooked	Raw	Cooked
4°C	0	10.7	10.4	23.0	20.6	nd	nd	382.2	440.4	38.6	55.6	7.8	25.1
	4	13.2	11.5	27.7	19.0	nd	nd	783.6	292.5	55.8	77.9	12.1	17.9
	8	46.2	42.1	28.6	9.7	nd	nd	519.5	407.3	54.3	65.2	15.9	11.9
	12	74.1	85.4	31.8	40.5	nd	nd	331.3	382.1	113.3	189.0	12.4	25.1
7°C	0	12.6	11.7	23.0	23.0	nd	nd	317.6	393.9	32.5	53.6	4.6	25.8
	4	17.3	19.1	28.1	41.1	nd	0.9	563.1	436.8	90.6	91.5	17.8	19.9
	8	94.1	106.7	25.0	52.2	1.8	4.0	524.4	359.7	156.6	215.7	89.4	35.8
	12	223.6	202.1	44.6	17.0	39.1	35.8	390.2	349.1	200.8	265.5	201.1	111.3
10°C	0	12.2	11.5	28.0	25.1	nd	nd	362.3	445.9	80.4	49.9	3.9	12.2
	4	68.7	59.7	35.9	42.8	1.6	1.9	517.2	317.0	131.2	128.3	12.4	27.1
	8	207.0	204.8	31.6	36.4	34.6	35.9	344.7	321.1	277.6	267.1	51.8	150.6
	12	368.1	277.1	28.7	12.1	107.6	100.0	445.8	360.6	176.7	274.1	333.1	224.1

Note: nd, not detected; Put, putrescine; Hism, histamine; Cdv, cadaverine; Spm, spermine; Spd, spermidine; Tyrm, tyramine.

Adapted from Sayem-El-Daher, N., Simard, R. E., and Fillion, J., *Lebensm. Wiss. Technol.*, 17, 319, 1984. With permission.

The effects of storage and cooking on the biogenic amine content in ground beef are listed in Table 3. Putrescine, cadaverine, and tyramine levels increased, with time and temperature of storage. Spermine declined after initial increase, and histamine fluctuated with time and temperature. Cooking had little effect on the amine concentration of ground beef. Spermine was the only amine partly destroyed during cooking.[38] On the other hand, it has been reported that cooking decreased the total amine content in pork (from 1,720 to 773 $mg.kg^{-1}$).[39] Spermine and putrescine were the amines that most significantly decreased. Similarly, spermidine, cadaverine, putrescine, and tryptamine levels decreased during the manufacture of bacon, but the histamine content increased threefold and tyramine content twofold.[40]

During the preparation of fermented foods the product is incubated for days, weeks, or even months to reach the desired degree of fermentation and maturation. Especially during the early stages of fermentation different kinds of microorganisms can grow. Hence biogenic amines can be expected to increase during preparation of fermented foods.

The situation during preparation of Dutch cheese has been extensively studied by Joosten et al.[18,41-44] Gouda and Maasdam cheese made from pasteurized milk using commercially available starter cultures did not contain either nonstarter bacteria or biogenic amines. Even after 1 year of ripening the amine content was still negligible (lower than 0.25 $mmol.kg^{-1}$).[18] In another experiment, the same laboratory investigated the role of nonstarter bacteria in biogenic amine formation. The presence of Gram-negative microorganisms in milk did not lead to amine formation in cheese if the pasteurization was performed properly. The investigated *Pediococci* were not able to cause amine formation in cheese. Contamination with *Bacillus proteliticum* gave slight putrescine formation (1.3 $mmol.kg^{-1}$) after 1 year. Enteroccocci caused tyramine formation, and if present in high densities, phenylethylamine was also found. Cheese contaminated with *Streptococcus faecalis* (2×10^9 $cfu.g^{-1}$) contained 9.5 $mmol.kg^{-1}$ tyramine and 12.8 $mmol.kg^{-1}$ phenylethylamine after 6 months of ripening. Representatives of *Enterobacteriaceae* caused mainly cadaverine and partly putrescine buildup. For example, cadaverine reached a maximal concentration of 5.9 $mmol.kg^{-1}$ if an inoculum of 1×10^5 cfu *Enterobacteriaceae* mixture per milliliter of cheese milk was used. Some lactobacilli formed biogenic amines as well (Table 4).[41] Tyramine, histamine, and putrescine were detected in some cheeses, while cadaverine was present only in cheese containing the salt-tolerant lactobacilli. Contamination of milk with a mixture of the salt-tolerant lactobacilli led to the formation of 29 $mmol.kg^{-1}$ cadaverine and 8.3 $mmol.kg^{-1}$ putrescine in a 1-year old-cheese. Salt-sensitive lactobacilli did not produce more than 10 mmol total amines per kilogram of cheese.[41]

Other parameters that govern formation of biogenic amines in cheese, such as pH, temperature, and salt concentration, have been studied as well.[42] Histamine concentration was strongly influenced by temperature. Cheese stored at 21°C accumulated 6.8 $mmol.kg^{-1}$ histamine during 1 year of ripening, while cheese stored at 9°C accumulated only 2.2 $mmol.kg^{-1}$. Similarly, a higher pH resulted in higher histamine formation. In the cheese with a pH value of 5.39 almost twice as much histamine was found after 1 year of storage at 14°C than in the cheese with a pH value of 5.19 (6.5 and 3.5 $mmol.kg^{-1}$, respectively; see Table 5).[42] Higher salt concentrations, on the other hand, resulted in lower histamine levels. After 6 months of storage, 3.5 $mmol.kg^{-1}$ of histamine was found in the cheese with low salt/water ratio (0.026) and 2.1 $mmol.kg^{-1}$ with high salt/water ratio (0.048).[42]

A similar effect of salt concentration was reported by Sumer et al. studying factors controlling histamine production in Swiss cheese inoculated with *Lactobacillus buchneri*.[45]

Table 4 Formation of Biogenic Amines in Cheese by *Lactobacilli*

Strain(s)[a]	Density in cheese milk (cfu.ml^{-1})	Age of cheese (days)	Amine content (mmol.kg^{-1}) Tyrm	Hism	Put	Cdv	Trypm	Phem
Lactobacillus brevis 2B5B	4,000	90	1.35	—[b]	—	—	—	—
		180	4.10	—	—	—	—	—
		365	5.55	—	—	—	—	—
L. brevis Hem 3	5,000	90	1.80	—	—	—	—	—
		180	3.95	—	—	—	—	—
		365	6.00	—	—	—	—	—
L. buchneri St2A	1,000	90	—	0.75	—	—	—	—
		180	—	1.45	—	—	—	—
		365	—	4.33	—	—	—	—
L. buchneri St2A	1,500	90	—	0.85	—	—	—	—
		180	—	1.70	—	—	—	—
		365	—	5.10	—	—	—	—
Lactobacillus sp. 4720-2	1,400	90	—	1.40	—	—	—	—
		180	—	1.30	—	—	—	—
		365	—	3.60	—	—	—	—
Mixture	9,000	90	1.45	—	—	—	—	—
		180	2.60	—	—	—	—	—
		365	4.35	—	—	—	—	—
Mixture	5,500	90	1.45	0.70	1.70	—	—	—
		180	2.35	1.80	2.50	—	—	—
		365	4.60	4.95	4.50	—	—	—
Mixture	8,000	90	—	0.75	0.70	—	—	—
		180	—	2.15	1.15	—	—	—
		365	0.30	6.00	1.30	—	—	—
Mixture of salt-tolerant strains	nd[c]	90	—	—	1.70	4.10	—	—
		180	—	—	4.10	13.40	—	—
		365	n.d.	0.45	8.30	>29	—	—

Note: Tyrm, tyramine; Hism, histamine; Put, putrescine; Cdv, cadaverine; Trypm, tryptamine; Phem, phenylethylamine.

[a] The lactobacilli were added to the cheese milk after pasteurization.

[b] Less than 0.2 mmol.kg^{-1} for Tyrm, Hism, Put and Cdv; less than 0.4 mmol.kg^{-1} for Trpm and Phem.

[c] nd; not determined.

Adapted from Joosten, H. M. L. J. and Northold, M. D., *Neth. Milk Dairy J.*, 41, 259, 1987. With permission.

The ability of *Lactobacillus buchneri* to form histamine decreased with increasing concentration of salt. Following the histamine production in cheese contaminated with different levels of *Lactobacillus buchneri,* the same authors found the histamine production to be proportional to inoculum level. The control cheeses with no *Lactobacillus buchneri* added did not develop detectable amounts of histamine over a 3-month storage period. In contrast, cheese made with 10^2 *Lactobacillus buchneri* per milliliter developed 150 mg histamine per kilogram cheese during 3 months of ripening, whereas cheese contaminated with 10^5 *Lactobacillus buchneri* per milliliter developed 250 mg histamine per kilogram cheese after 1 month of storage and 800 mg.kg^{-1} after 3 months of storage.[45]

All the above-mentioned data as well as other reported data clearly demonstrate that when sufficiently hygienic conditions are used, it is possible to prepare cheeses with a

Table 5 Influence of pH and Storage Temperature on the Formation of Histamine in Gouda Cheese Infected with *L. Buchneri* St2a

Cheese number	Milk lot[a]	Ripening temperature (°C)	pH[b]	Salt-water ratio[b]	Ripening time (months)	Histamine ($mmol.kg^{-1}$)
1	1	9	5.19	0.046	3	0.5
					6	1.1
					12	2.2
2	1	14	5.19	0.046	3	0.7
					6	1.4
					12	3.4
3	2	14	5.39	0.043	3	1.3
					6	2.4
					12	6.5
4	1	18	5.19	0.046	3	1.0
					6	2.2
					12	5.6
5	2	18	5.39	0.043	3	nd[c]
					6	4.7
					12	8.6
6	1	21	5.19	0.046	3	1.6
					6	3.7
					12	6.8
7	2	21	5.39	0.043	3	2.5
					6	6,8
					12	9.4

[a] About 2000 $cfu.dm^{-3}$ was added to the milk.
[b] The pH and salt and water content were determined after two weeks of ripening.
[c] n.d., not determined.

Adapted from Joosten, H. M. L. J., *Neth. Milk Dairy J.*, 41, 329, 1988. With permission.

negligible biogenic amine content, especially if all the technological parameters are carefully controlled.[19,46]

Another fermented product that may accumulate high levels of biogenic amines is fermented sausage. Initially a variable association of microflora is present and usually a starter culture is added. Thus the final amine content of the sausage depends not only on type and activity of starter culture, but also on the microbial composition of the original meat. Even two batches prepared by the same manufacturer with the same starter culture may vary considerably in levels of biogenic amines.[9] Changes in biogenic amine content during sausage preparation when two different starter cultures were used are shown in Table 6.[9] Fermentation took place for 2 d at 26°C, followed by smoking and drying at 15°C for 20 d. Only low levels of biogenic amines (mainly tyramine) were found in sausages prepared with a starter culture that did not possess amino acid decarboxylase activity (starter culture II). On the other hand, putrescine and tyramine were produced during the first day of fermentation in the sausages inoculated with the starter possessing tyrosine and ornithine decarboxylase activity (starter culture I). Cadaverine, phenylethylamine, and to a lesser extent histamine were produced during the second day of fermentation. Except for putrescine, the levels of biogenic amines further increased during the drying of sausages. Putrescine levels slightly decreased.[9]

Table 6 Changes in the Biogenic Amine Content During Sausage Fermentation (in mg.kg^{-1})

Starter	Time (days)	Put	Cdv	Hism	Tyrm	Phem
Starter I	0	1	1	3	2	2
	1	21	7	4	69	2
	2	18	35	5	95	9
	9	15	64	8	142	11
	21	13	84	6	120	11
Starter II	0	1	1	3	2	2
	1	1	1	3	2	2
	2	1	1	3	5	2
	9	2	1	4	20	2
	21	3	1	3	21	2

Note: Put, putrescine; Cdv, cadaverine; Hism, histamine; Tyrm, tyramine; Phem, phenylethylamine.

Adapted from Ten Brink, B., Damink, C., Joosten, H. M. L. J., and Huis in't Veld, J. H. J., *Int. J. Food Microbiol.*, 11, 73, 1990. With permission.

In another experiment, Rice et al. examined the production of biogenic amines by different starter cultures.[47] Lower tyramine levels (approximately 200 mg.kg^{-1}) were formed when *Pediococcus cerevisiae* and *Lactobacillus planarum* were used as starter cultures to prepare sausages than when *Streptococus* sp. were used (approximately 300 mg.kg^{-1}).

The formation of biogenic amines in other fermented foods such as sauerkraut, miso, soy sauce, etc. has also been studied. For example, Mayer et al. showed that the histamine level of sauerkraut increased throughout fermentation, reaching a peak of 160 mg.kg^{-1} after 10 weeks.[48]

Salt level was a significant factor in the formation of biogenic amines in miso.[49] The misos with a low salt formulation (5% NaCl) had an average level of 314 mg.kg^{-1} tyramine, whereas misos with a higher salt formulation (10% NaCl) had an average level of 176 mg.kg^{-1}. Similarly, much higher histamine levels were found in low-salt formulation (>100 mg.kg^{-1}) than in high-salt formulation (<50 mg.kg^{-1}) misos. The tryptamine content was slightly higher in low-salt than in high-salt formulation misos, and a trace of phenylethylamine was found only in low-salt misos. Incubation temperatures within the range of 25 to 35°C had only a negligible effect on biogenic amine formation. The studies on the raw material for miso preparation showed that putrescine, cadaverine, spermidine, and spermine in miso originated from the raw materials. On the other hand, tyramine, histamine, and phenylethylamine were not detected in the raw materials and were formed during miso fermentation.[26,27]

Amine production in beer has been shown to be related both to the nature of the adjuncts used and to microbial contamination of wort.[50] Putrescine level was twice as high, tyramine levels three times higher, and agmatine level half as high in worts inoculated with *Lactobacillus brevis* than in worts noninoculated or inoculated with *Saccharomyces uvarum*. *S. uvarum* did not produce biogenic amines. Partial substitution of malt by adjuncts, in particular by rice, resulted in a lower amine content in fermented worts.[50]

The formation of histamine and tyramine in Spanish beer was followed by Izquierdo-Pulido et al.[29] The formation of these two amines was different. Formation of histamine was negligible throughout the entire brewing process (from 0.6 to 0.8 $mg.dm^{-3}$), whereas the formation of tyramine was observed (from 2.5 to 40 $mg.dm^{-3}$). The highest level of tyramine was observed during the first 5 d of fermentation. A gradual increase in tyramine was observed during secondary fermentation (from 35.7 to 40.5 $mg.dm^{-3}$). The final filtration had practically no effect on the level of either amine.

In coffee, a decrease in putrescine, spermine, and spermidine levels occurs during roasting.[51] The putrescine level decreased to about 2 to 6% of its original value, and spermidine with spermine disappeared completely during roasting.

Cooking (5 min in boiling water) leads to a significant decrease of tryptamine, phenylethylamine, putrescine, cadaverine, histamine, and tyramine in the straw mushroom *Volariella volvacea.* The total amount of these six amines in fresh mushroom was reduced from 147.7 to 28.1 $mg.kg^{-1}$, a reduction of about 80%. This reduction can be attributed to the loss into water during cooking. On the other hand, storage of fresh mushrooms at 4 and 25°C markedly increased levels of biogenic amines. The total amine content increased from 133 to 878 $mg.kg^{-1}$ during 5 d of storage at 4°C and to 2,384 $mg.kg^{-1}$ during 5 d of storage at 25°C.[52]

At present some technological processes exist for reducing the biogenic amine content in certain foods. These processes are both enzymatic and nonenzymatic. The enzymatic processes are based on the oxidative deamination using diamino oxidase (DAO). The nonenzymatic ones use the nonenzymatic browning reactions between biogenic amines and sugars.[53] In some cases the biogenic amine content can be reduced during other processes such as cooking (via loss into water) as shown above. However, often the level of biogenic amines once formed is not reduced and might even increase during processing. Therefore, prevention of the formation of biogenic amines is the best way to produce foods with a low biogenic amine content. Proper storage temperature and good hygienic care seem to be the most important factors for this prevention.

REFERENCES

1. Smith, T. A., Amines in foods, *Food Chem.*, 6, 169, 1981.
2. Tarjan, V. and Janossy, G., The role of biogenic amines in foods, *Nahrung*, 22, 285, 1978.
3. Maga, J. A., Amines in foods, *Crit. Rev. Food Sci. Nutr.*, 10, 373, 1978.
4. Rice, S. L., Eitenmiller, R. R., and Koehler, P. E., Biologically active amines in food: a review, *J. Milk Food Technol.*, 39, 353, 1976.
5. Stratton, J. E., Hutkins, R. W., and Taylor, S. L., Biogenic amines in cheese and other fermented foods: a review, *J. Food Prot.*, 54, 460, 1991.
6. Taylor, S. L., Histamine food poisoning: toxicology and clinical aspects, *Crit. Rev. Toxicol.*, 17, 91, 1986.
7. Smith, T. A., Phenethylamine and related compounds in plants, *Phytochemistry,* 16, 9, 1977.
8. Smith, T. A., Tryptamine and related compounds in plants, *Phytochemistry*, 16, 171, 1977.
9. Ten Brink, B., Damink, C., Joosten, H. M. L. J., and Huis in't Veld, J. H. J., Occurrence and formation of biologically active amines in foods, *Int. J. Food Microbiol.*, 11, 73, 1990.
10. Davídek, J., Pokorný, J., and Velišek, J., *Chemical Changes during Food Processing, Developments in Food Science 21,* Elsevier, Amsterdam, 1990.
11. Jones, G. P., Rivett, D. E., and Tucker, D. J., The reaction of biogenic amines with proteins, *J. Sci. Food Agric.*, 32, 805, 1981.
12. Tucker, J. D., Jones, G. P., and Rivett, D. E., Formation of beta-phenylethylaminoalanine in protein foods heated in the presence of added amine, *J. Sci. Food Agric.*, 34, 1427, 1983.

13. Veciana-Nogués, M. T., Vidal-Carou, M. C., and Mariné-Font, A., Histamine and tyramine during storage and spoilage of anchovies, *Engraulis encrasicholus*: relationships with other fish spoilage indicators, *J. Food Sci.*, 55, 1192, 1990.
14. van Spreekens, K. J. A., Histamine production by psychrophilic flora, in *Seafood Quality Determination*, Kramer, D. E. and Liston, J., Eds., Elsevier, New York, 1987, 309.
15. Pechanek, U., Phannhauser, W., and Woidich, H., Determination of the content of biogenic amines in four groups of the Austrian marketplace, *Z. Lebensm. Unters. Forsch.*, 176, 335, 1983.
16. Fardiaz, D. and Markakis, P., Amines in fermented fish paste, *J. Food Sci.*, 44, 1562, 1979.
17. de Boer, E. and Kuik, D., A survey of the microbiological quality of blue-veined cheeses, *Neth. Milk Dairy J.*, 41, 227, 1987.
18. Joosten, H. M. L. J. and Stadhouders, J., Conditions allowing the formation of biogenic amines in cheese. 1. Decarboxylative properties of starter bacteria, *Neth. Milk Dairy J.*, 412, 247, 1987.
19. Antila, P., Antila, V., Matilla, J., and Hakkarainen, H., Biogenic amines in cheese. II. Factors influencing the formation of biogenic amines, with particular reference to the quality of milk used in cheese making, *Milchwissenschaft,* 39, 400, 1984.
20. Taylor, S. L., Leatherwood, M., and Lieber, E. R., A survey of histamine levels in sausages, *J. Food Prot.*, 41, 634, 1978.
21. Vandekerckhove, P., Amines in dry fermented sausage, *J. Food Sci.*, 42, 283, 1977.
22. Mayer, K. and Pause, G., Biogene amine in sauerkraut, *Lebensm. Wiss. Technol.*, 5, 108, 1972.
23. Taylor, S. L., Leatherwood, M., and Lieber, E. R., Histamine in sauerkraut, *J. Food Sci.*, 43, 1030, 1978.
24. Chin, K. D. H. and Koehler, P. E., Identification and estimation of histamine, tryptamine, phenethylamine and tyramine in soy sauce by thin-layer chromatography of dansyl derivatives, *J. Food Sci.*, 48, 1826, 1983.
25. Yamamoto, S., Wakabayashi, S., and Makita, M., Gas-liquid chromatographic determination of tyramine in fermented food products, *J. Agric. Food Chem.*, 28, 790, 1980.
26. Ibe, A., Nishima, T., and Kasai, N., Formation of tyramine and histamine during soybean paste (miso) fermentation, *Jpn. J. Toxicol. Environ. Health*, 38, 181, 1992.
27. Ibe, A., Tamura, Y., Kamimura, H., and Tabata, S., Determination and contents of non-volatile amines in soybean paste and soy sauce, *Jpn. J. Toxicol. Environ. Health*, 37, 379, 1991.
28. Ingles, D. L., Back, J. F., Gallimore, D., Tindale, R., and Shaw, K. J., Estimation of biogenic amines in foods, *J. Sci. Food Agric.*, 36, 402, 1985.
29. Izquierdo-Pulido, M. L., Vidal-Carou, M. C., and Mariné-Font, A., Histamine and tyramine in beers. Changes during brewing of a Spanish beer, *Food Chem.*, 42, 231, 1991.
30. Zee, A. J., Simard, R. E., and Desmarais, M., Biogenic amines in Canadian, American and European beers, *Can. Inst. Food Sci. Technol. J.*, 14, 119, 1981.
31. Vidau, Z., Gonzales, E., and Garcia Roché, M. O., Some considerations about the tyramine content of some Cuban beers and wines, *Nahrung*, 33, 793, 1989.
32. Baucom, T. L., Tabacchi, M. H., Cottrell, T. H. E., and Richmond, B. S., Biogenic amine content of New York state wines, *J. Food Sci.*, 51, 1376, 1986.
33. Ough, C. S., Measurement of histamine in California wines, *J. Agric. Food Chem.*, 19, 241, 1971.
34. Karmas, E., Biogenic amines as indicators of seafood freshness, *Lebensm. Wiss. Technol.*, 14, 273, 1981.
35. Ababouch, L., Afilal, M. E., Benabdeljelil, H., and Busta, F. F., Quantitative changes in bacteria, amino acids and biogenic amines in sardine (*Sardina pilcharus*) stored at ambient temperature (25–28°C) and in ice, *Int. J. Food Sci. Technol.*, 26, 297, 1991.
36. Slemr, J. and Beyermann, K., Concentration profiles of diamines in fresh and aerobically stored pork and beef, *J. Agric. Food Chem.*, 33, 336, 1985.
37. Nakamura, M., Naoka, N., Sawaya, T., Takahashi, T., and Kawabata, T., Polyamine content of pork products. *Kanagara-ken Eisei Kenkyusho Kenkyu Hokoku*, 7, 35, 1977.,(*Chem. Abs.*, 91, 54766, 1979).
38. Sayem-El-Daher, N., Simard, R. E., and Fillion, J., Changes in amine content of ground beef during storage and processing, *Lebensm. Wiss. Technol.*, 17, 319, 1984.
39. Lakritz, L., Spinelli, A. M., and Wasserman, A. E., Determination of amines in fresh and processed pork, *J. Agric. Food Chem.*, 23, 344, 1975.
40. Spinelli, A. M., Lakritz, L., and Wasserman, A. E., Effects of processing on the amine content of pork bellies, *J. Agric. Food Chem.*, 22, 1026, 1974.

41. Joosten, H. M. L. J. and Northolt, M. D., Conditions allowing the formation of biogenic amines in cheese. 2. Decarboxylative properties of some non-starter bacteria, *Neth. Milk Dairy J.*, 41, 259, 1987.
42. Joosten, H. M. L. J., Conditions allowing the formation of biogenic amines in cheese. 3. Factors influencing the amounts formed, *Neth. Milk Dairy J.*, 41, 329, 1988.
43. Joosten, H. M. L. J., The biogenic amine contents of Dutch cheese and their toxicological significance, *Neth. Milk Dairy J.*, 42, 25, 1988.
44. Joosten, H. M. L. J. and Boekel, M. A. J. S., Conditions allowing the formation of biogenic amines in cheese. 4. A study of the kinetics of histamine formation in an infected Gouda cheese, *Neth. Milk Dairy J.*, 42, 3, 1988.
45. Summer, S. S., Roche, F., and Taylor, S. L., Factors controlling histamine production in Swiss cheese inoculated with *Lactobacillus buchneri*, *J. Dairy Sci.*, 73, 3050, 1990.
46. Antila, P., On the formation of biogenic amines in cheesemaking, *Kiel. Milchwirtsch. Forschungsber.*, 35, 373, 1977.
47. Rice, S. L. and Koehler, P. E., Tyrosine and histidine decarboxylase activities of *Pediococcus cerevisiae* and *Lactobacillus* species and the production of tyramine in fermented sausages, *J. Food Milk Technol.*, 39, 166, 1976.
48. Mayer, K., Pause, G., and Vetsch, U., Fermentation characteristics and histamine formation in sauerkraut production, *Mitt. Geb. Lebensmittelunters. Hyg.*, 65, 234, 1974.
49. Chin, K. D. H. and Koehler, P. E., Effect of salt concentration and incubation temperature on the formation of histamine, phenethylamine, tryptamine and tyramine during miso fermentation, *J. Food Prot.*, 49, 423, 1986.
50. Zee, J. A., Simard, R. E., Vaillancourt, R., and Boudreau, A., Effect of *Lactobacillus brevis, Saccharomyces uvarum* and grist composition on amine formations in beers, *Can. Inst. Food Sci. Technol. J.*, 14, 321, 1981.
51. Amorim, H. V., Basso, L. C., Crocomo, O. J., and Teixeira, A. A., Polyamines in green and roasted coffee, *J. Agric. Food Chem.*, 25, 957, 1977.
52. Yen, G. C., Effect of heat treatment and storage temperature on the biogenic amine contents of straw mushroom (*Vollvariella volvacea*), *J. Sci. Food Agric.*, 58, 59, 1992.
53. Pavelka, J., Methods of histamine incidents prevention and elimination on food products, *Prům. Potravin.*, 43, 272, 1992.
54. Klausen, N. K. and Lund, E., Formation of biogenic amines in herrings and mackerel, *Z. Lebensm. Unters. Forsch.*, 182, 459, 1986.
55. Askar, A., El-Saidy, S., Ali, A., Sheheta, M. I., and Bassiouny, S. S., Biogenic amines in fish products, *Dtsch. Lebensm. Runds.*, 82, 188, 1986.
56. Veciana-Nogues, M. T., Vidal-Carou, M. C., and Marine-Font, A., Histamine and tyramine in preserved and semipreserved fish products, *J. Food Sci.*, 54, 1653, 1989.
57. Lebiedzinska, A., Lamparczyk, H., Genowiak, Z., and Eller, K. I., Differences in biogenic amine patterns in fish obtained from commercial sources, *Z. Lebensm. Unters. Forsch.*, 192, 240, 1991.
58. Viogt, M. N., Eitenmiller, R. R., Koehler, P. E., and Hamdy, M. K., Tyramine, histamine and tryptamine content of cheese, *J. Milk Food Technol.*, 37, 377, 1974.
59. Baker, G. B., Wong, J. T. F., Coutts, R. T., and Pasutto, F. M., Simultaneous extraction and quantitation of several bioactive amines in cheese and chocolate, *J. Chromatogr.*, 392, 317, 1987.
60. Koehler, P. E. and Eitenmiller, R. R., High pressure liquid chromatographic analysis of tyramine, phenethylamine and tryptamine in sausage, cheese and chocolate, *J. Food Sci.*, 43, 1245, 1978.
61. Sayem-El-Daher, N., Simard, R. E., Fillion, J., and Roberge, A. G., Extraction and determination of biogenic amines in ground beef and their relation to microbial quality, *Lebensm. Wiss. Technol.*, 17, 20, 1984.
62. Zee, J. A., Simard, R. E., and L'Heureux, L., Evaluation of analytical methods for determination of biogenic amines in fresh and processed meat, *J. Food Prot.*, 46, 1044, 1983.
63. Kenyhercz, T. M. and Kissinger, P. T., Tyramine from *Theobroma cacao*, *Phytochemistry*, 16, 1602, 1977.
64. Staruszkiewicz, W. F., Jr. and Bond, J. F., Gas chromatographic determination of cadaverine, putrescine, and histamine in foods, *J. Assoc. Off. Anal. Chem.*, 64, 584, 1984.

Part I

Marine Toxins

Jana Dostálová and Jan Pokorný

Acute poisoning after consumption of fish and shellfish has been well known for many centuries. The oldest documents are from Egypt (2700 BC), Greece (Aristotle, 384 to 322 BC), Japan (400 AD), and China (618 to 907 AD).[1-3]

A variety of fish and other marine animals contain toxic components that may produce poisoning in man and animals. These organisms are scattered throughout various animal phyla, from single-celled protozoa *(Dinoflagellates)* through *Colenterata* (hydroids, jellyfish, coral, sea anemones), *Echinodermata* (sea urchins), *Mollusca* (univalves, shellfish, octopus), *Annelida* (worms) to *Chordata* (fishes, reptiles).[4] The number of poisonous animals is not exactly known. Data in the literature[2,5] for poisonous fish varies between 500 and 1000 species, respectively. They belong to *Agnatha, Chondroichthyes,* and *Osteichthyes.*

Marine toxins of fanerotoxic animals are found in various surface structures of some jellyfish and *Octopus* species and in the venom organs of various fish (approximately 200 species, most of them having a variety of spines on the body). Toxins of cryptotoxic *Tetraodontidae*, from the genera *Tetraodon* and *Fugu* (90 species) and in more than 300 species of animals, are located in flesh, liver, gonads, roe, intestine, skin, etc. (over 500 species).[6,7] Fish and shellfish belong to this group. The most important toxic fish species are from the family of *Tetraodontidae,* from the genera *Tetraodon* and *Fugu* (90 species), and more than 300 species have been found to produce ciguateratoxin (ichyosarcotoxin).[4]

Paralytic shellfish poison occurs primarily in temperate seas, the western Pacific coasts of the U.S. (including Alaska) and Canada, the North Sea, and the Chilean and Japanese coasts. However, outbreaks of shellfish poisoning have been reported in recent years in warmer waters as well, for example, the coasts of the Philippines, Malaysia, Indonesia, Guatemala, and Venezuela.[8,9] Ciguatera poisoning is most frequently associated with tropical fish species that inhabit reefs and shallow water (65 m or less) in Caribbean and Pacific island communities.[7] *Tetraodontidae* live in tropical and subtropical seas, especially in Japanese seas.[10]

The toxicity of most shellfish and fish appears to result from feeding habits and, therefore, it exhibits a seasonal effect.

In the South Pacific region the total number of reported illnesses, due to marine toxins increased from just under 2,000 in 1984 to almost 5,000 cases in 1987. In a household survey in the Virgin Islands, the annual incidence of ciguatera poisoning was found to be 7.3/1,000, and in another study, an incidence as high as 30/1,000 was suggested.[11] There are about 1,600 cases of paralytic shellfish poisoning reported, with 300 deaths worldwide each year.[12]

Outbreaks and cases of illness due to marine toxins in the U.S.A., for 1973 to 1987 are shown in Table 1. Sources of illness due to seafood toxins are evident from Table 2.

The chemical composition of different marine toxins differs considerably.[13] They are complex organic molecules, found in various parts of the organism.

A variety of types of poisoning occur after ingestion of marine animals. Fairly common examples include diarrhetic shellfish poisoning, resulting from okadaic acid, ciguatera fish poisoning, brevetoxin-produced neurotoxic shellfish poisoning, palytoxin poisoning, paralytic shellfish poisoning associated with saxitoxin and gonyautoxin, and puffer fish and scombroid poisoning.[14] It is interesting to note that, unlike the others, scombroid and, probably, puffer fish toxins are of bacterial origin.

Table 1 Outbreaks and Cases of Illness Due to Marine Toxins[a]

Marine toxins	Number of outbreaks	Percent[b]	Number of cases	Percent[b]
Ciguateratoxin	234	8	1,052	1
PSP	21	1	160	<1
Histamine fish poisoning	202	7	1,216	1

[a] U.S., 1973 to 1987.

[b] Expressed in percent of total foodborne diseases.

Adapted from Bean, N. H. and Griffin, P. M., *J. Food Prot.*, 48, 659, 1985.

Table 2 Sources and Causes of Illnesses Through Seafood Toxins

Environmental sources	Dinoflagellates, diatoms, bacteria
Food sources	Fish, shellfish
Important factors influencing the outbreak of illness	Heat resistance of toxins Lack of specific taste and appearance imparted by marine toxins The presence of toxins is unpredictable The degree of toxicity is determined by environmental conditions

Adapted from Nriagu, J. O. and Simmons, M. S., Eds., *Food Contamination from Environmental Sources*, John Wiley & Sons, New York, 1990, chap. 22.

TETRODOTOXIN

CHEMISTRY

In 1964 Woodward[15] determined the structure of tetrodotoxin as *O*-methyl-*O′*,*O″*-isopropylidene tetrodotoxin hydrochloride. Nakamura and Yasumoto[16] isolated various natural tetrodotoxin derivatives from *Fugu* fish. They were identified by NMR and mass spectrometry as follows: tetrodic acid, 4-epitetrodotoxin, and anhydrotetrodotoxin. Apart from these natural derivatives, there exist various tetrodotoxin analogs. Structures of different tetrodotoxin derivatives are summarized in Figure 1.

TOXIC EFFECTS

Tetrodotoxin is a neurotoxin, death following generalized paralysis. Approximately 60% of cases result in death.

OCCURRENCE

Tetrodotoxin is found in certain puffer fish (*Tetraodontidae*). There are over 90 species of these fish, highly prized by gourmands in Japan. Puffer fish belong to the genera *Tetraodon* and *Fugu*. The toxins are found only in the roe, liver, intestines, and skin, but not in meat. Only specially trained individuals are allowed to prepare this fish for consumption, but in some instances, errors are made, and human poisoning results. Illnesses are highest during the spawning season because the flavor is then better, and this is just the season when fish are most likely to feed on poisonous organisms. Therefore, puffer fish are toxic only in certain places and seasons.

Cultured specimens of puffer fish *Fugu rubripes* have no toxicity, regardless of the collection site, age, or tissue selection, and have high resistance to tetrodotoxin.[17] These

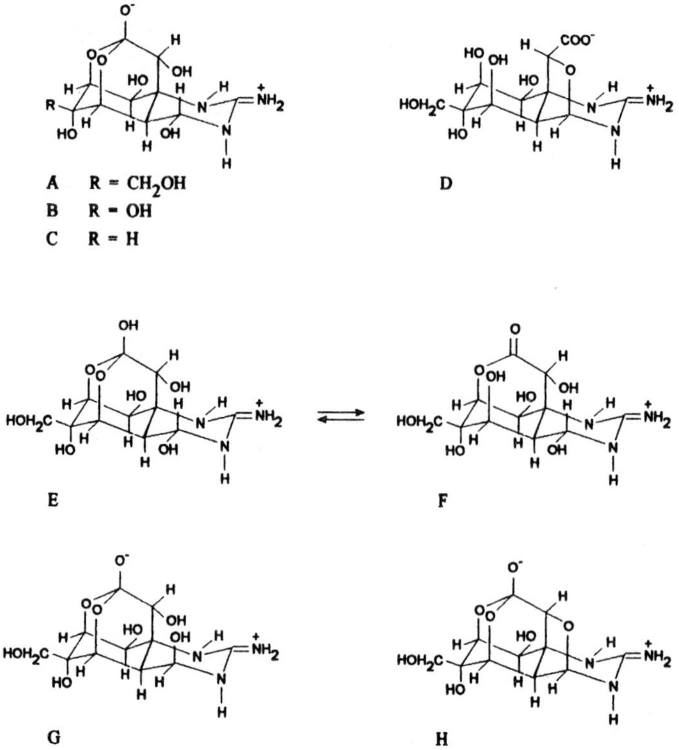

Figure 1 Structures of tetrodotoxin and related natural compounds. A, tetrodotoxin; B, nortetrodotoxin; C, nortetrodotoxin-alcohol; D, tetrodonic acid; E,F, hemilactal tautomers of tetrodotoxin salts; G, 4-epitetrodotoxin; H, anhydrotetrodotoxin.

results support the view that puffer fish are exogenously toxified through the food chain. It is believed that *Pseudomonas* species produce tetrodotoxin, which is transmitted to the fish through the skin surface.[18]

CHANGES DURING PROCESSING AND STORAGE

The toxicity of puffer roe pickled in rice bran may be reduced by extraction with water,[19] which is more efficient than extraction with 0.1% acetic acid or with methanol acidified to pH 4.0 with acetic acid. The toxicity of puffer roe may be reduced by treatment with alkali, the most effective being sodium bicarbonate. In a laboratory experiment, the toxicity markedly decreased during 9 months, but a less dramatic toxicity reduction was obtained in plant-scale experiments.[20] Some tetrodotoxin could be eliminated simply by pressing the material and washing. Further tetrodotoxin was extracted during subsequent heating to 100°C. The remaining tetrodotoxin showed a series of gradual structural changes to the less toxic anhydro-tetrodotoxin, which was further converted to the nontoxic tetrodonic acid.[21] The toxicity of puffer fish liver was reduced to less than 5 MU (mouse units) per gram by a cooking procedure comprising repeated rinsing and boiling in water (sodium bicarbonate was added to the boiling water before each treatment was completed).[22]

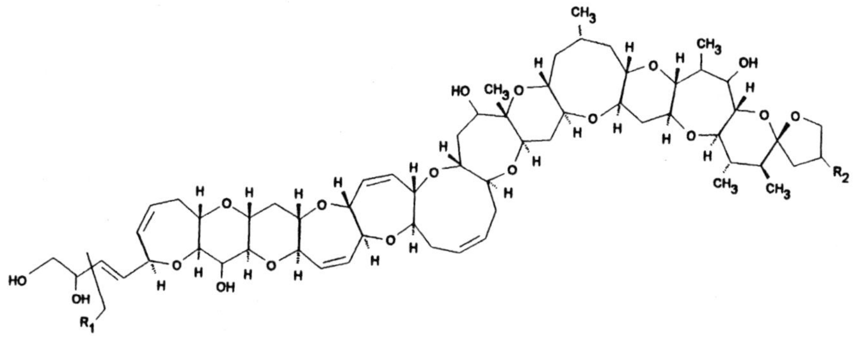

A R_2 = OH

B R_1 = $CH_2{=}CH$

R_2 = H

Figure 2 Structure of ciguatoxin. A, isolated from *Gymnothorax javanicus*; B, isolated from *Gambierdiscus toxicus.*

The toxification of the muscle of *Fugu niphobles* occurs due to migration of the toxin from skin and viscera. No significant differences were observed between slowly and quickly frozen specimens. The toxin did not migrate into muscles in only partially thawed specimens, but the muscle of most specimens was found to be toxic immediately after the first thawing (up to 58 MU/l g). The toxin migration proceeded gradually with time. Several specimens become strongly toxic after 24 to 48 h from the end of thawing.[23]

CIGUATERA TOXIN

CHEMISTRY

The chemical structure of the toxin is not yet known, but it probably belongs to the polyethers, containing several hydroxyl groups, and possibly sulfate and nitrogen groups. They are related to okadoic acid (Figure 2).

TOXIC EFFECTS

The symptons are gastrointestinal, occurring a few hours after consumption of a toxic fish, followed by neurological problems; muscle pains, pruritus, weakness, reduced blood pressure, and altered pulse may also occur. Although the mortality rate is low (about l to 7%),[4,24] the number of cases worldwide may be over 50,000 each year.

OCCURRENCE

Poisoning from ciguatera toxin is the most common form of seafood poisoning. More than 300 fish species have been found to produce ciguatera toxin. Apparently, any fish may acquire the toxicity, which appears to be a result of feeding habits. The toxin originates from the dinoflagellates *Gambierdiscus toxicus* and *Prorocentrum* sp. and occurs primarily in fish feeding on marine algae and the detritus of coral reefs.[25,26] It is transmitted to larger predator fish, which feed on the reef fish. It is difficult to know whether a fish is safe to eat because a species and the fishing spot can change erratically from safe to toxic. There is some evidence that the toxin is more likely acquired if the reef ecology has been disturbed. More outbreaks occur during the late spring and summer.

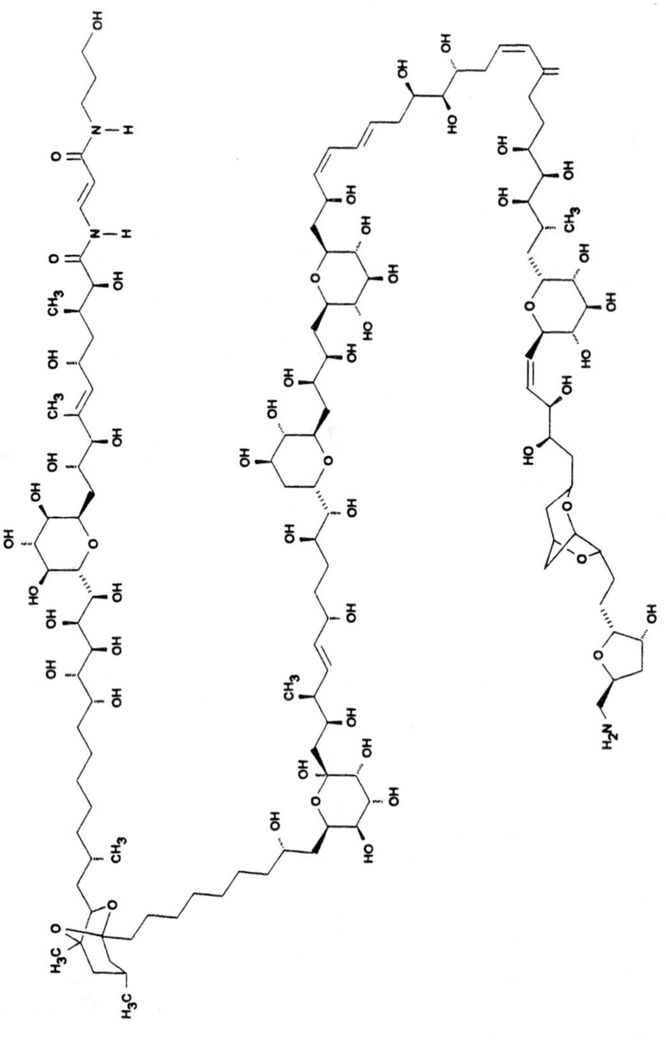

Figure 3 Structure of palytoxin.

CHANGES DURING PROCESSING AND STORAGE

The ciguatera toxin is of particular concern, because it is heat stable and is not destroyed by cooking, drying, or freezing. Therefore, it is difficult to remove it from fish meat. Soaking meat in water up to several days and discarding the toxin-containing water has been advocated as a means for preparing fish safe for human consumption.[4]

It is not possible to detect the toxin on the basis of flavor or odor characteristics, excepting perhaps a slight metallic taste in toxic fish.[7]

Because there is no way to eliminate ciguatera toxin from fish once they are caught, commercial fishing in ciguatera areas should cease. For monitoring the incidence of toxic fish, quick, easy, and cheap methods should be used. Immunological methods, sumarized in a review by Hokama and Smith,[14] belong to these methods.

PALYTOXIN

CHEMISTRY

Palytoxin is a group of lipophilic compounds, the exact structure of which was discovered only recently (Figure 3). The molecular formulas for this toxin are $C_{129}H_{221}N_3O_{54}$ and $C_{129}H_{223}N_3O_{54}$ for the toxins of a Tahitian *Palythoa* species and *P. toxica*[27], respectively, suggesting that only minor differences exist between species.

TOXIC EFFECTS

Palytoxin is an extremely poisonous compound, with clinical signs resembling those of tetrodotoxin and paralytic shellfish poisoning. According to Fukui et al.,[28] palytoxin also has carcinogenic properties.

OCCURRENCE

Palytoxin was first isolated in 1969 by Hashimoto et al.[29] from intestines of *Alutera scripta* which contained the reef fragments of *Palythoa tuberculosa.* It was recently isolated from viscera, meat, and intestines of *Melichthys vidua,* and from crabs.[30]

Palytoxin is present in the liver of parrot fish *(Ypsiscarus ovifrons)*, which are consumed as a delicacy in Japan. There have been 52 cases reported of poisoning caused by toxic liver.[31]

Fukui et al.[28] found only residues of red algae and no coelenterates in intestines of toxic crabs, and therefore red algae are suspected as a further source of palytoxin.

CHANGES DURING PROCESSING AND STORAGE

Palytoxin seems to be a relatively stable group of substances, and no literature data are available on changes occurring during cooking, heating, or storage.

SAXITOXIN

CHEMISTRY

Saxitoxin is a polycyclic compound with several nitrogen atoms in the molecule (Figure 4). The presence of amido and imine groups suggests some sensitivity on heating due to reactions with other components of fish meat.

TOXIC EFFECTS

Saxitoxin belongs to the neurotoxins. Sodium conductance in nerve and muscle membranes is blocked by these, causing paralysis of muscles. Even with adequate health care the case fatality rate is about 8.5%.

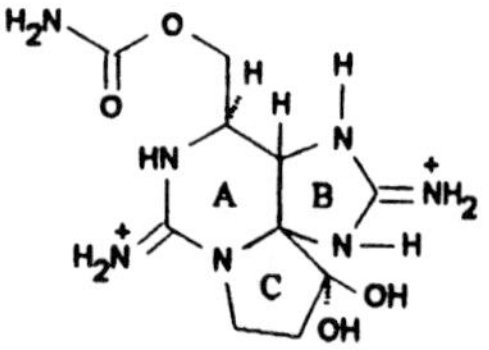

Figure 4 Structure of saxitoxin.

OCCURRENCE

Saxitoxin is a component of paralytic shellfish poison (PSP), which occurs primarily in temperate seas. The predominant food sources that have caused most outbreaks in these areas are shellfish, particularly clams, oysters, mussels, cockles, scallops, and whelks. The poison is accumulated in shellfish from the dinoflagellates *Protogonyoaulax* and *Pyrodinium,* which occur naturally in these areas and are capable of producing a variety of related neurotoxins, called saxitoxins. For marine life to be toxic, dinoflagellate blooms are normally necessary. These tend to be seasonal, at least in temperate waters, and depend on water temperature, salinity, amount of sunshine, and upwelling of cold, nutrient-rich water, winds, tides, and elimination of toxic metal ions.[8]

CHANGES DURING PROCESSING AND STORAGE

A large percentage of the incidents of PSP illness have been related to the ingestion of cooked shellfish and therefore, according to some authors, the toxin is heat stable and cannot be destroyed by cooking or pickling. They believe there is no way of eliminating the toxin from the seafood once it has been harvested. In many regions, shellfish are carefully monitored, and areas may be closed or opened depending on the results.

Nevertheless, some evidence exists about possible partial detoxification of marine food infested by the toxin. Prakash et al.[32] reported that the total toxicity in the scallop was reduced by about 90% during canning. Noguchi et al.[33,34] also demonstrated that a significant reduction of toxicity in the Japanesse scallop *Patinopecten yessoensis* occurred during retorting, and slow but steady reduction of the remaining toxicity in canned scallop proceeded during storage. Dassow[35] reported that 10 min steaming followed by a 75 min processing at 250°F (121°C) resulted in a reduction of toxin by up to 93%.

The effects of pH and heating on the PSP were examined by Asakawa and Takagi.[36] About 40 to 50% of toxicity of the diluted extract from *Protogonyaulox tamarensis* was decomposed in the pH range 6 to 8 at ambient temperature, while 87% of PSP toxicity was decomposed at pH 8 and 110°C for 30 min. In a dilute solution containing egg albumin, the degradation of PSP by heating at lower pH was depressed, due to the protective effect of protein. Gill et al.[37] studied the thermal resistance of paralytic shellfish poison present in toxic soft-shell clams *Mya arenaria* and determined that the thermal-time destruction curve was linear ($r^2 = 0.97$), indicating that the PSP destruction followed zero order kinetics.

The components of PSP have various stabilities against heat and chemical or biochemical reduction. Saxitoxin is more stable than other components, e.g., gonyautoxin.[38,39]

Some fish species, e.g., finfish, are unable to accumulate toxins in their flesh, so that there seems to be no problem about its suitability for human consumption, except possibly, when whole fish is consumed without processing.[40]

Adductor muscles of scallop *Patinopecten yessoensis* were nontoxic if the digestive gland toxicities did not exceed the range of 1,000 to 2,900 MU.g^{-1}, but in the case of

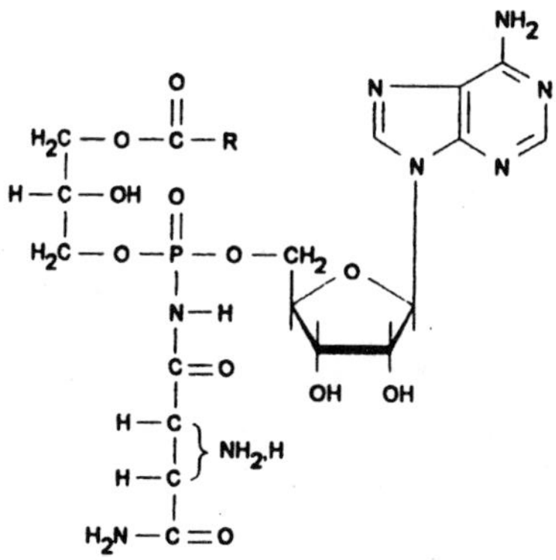

Figure 5 Structure of dinogunellin. R, residue of a fatty acid.

higher values, there was some toxicity. The toxicity was raised by freeze-thaw cycles, indicating migration of toxins (PSP) between tissues.[41]

ICHTHYOOTOXIN

CHEMISTRY

Ichthyootoxin belongs to lipoproteins. Asano and Itoh[42] isolated three lipoproteins from roe of *Stichaeus grigorjewi* — α-, β- and γ-lipostichaerin. In addition to neutral lipids, they contain a specific phospholipid, dinogunellin, containing adenosin and 2-aminosuccinamide (Figure 5).

TOXIC EFFECTS

The toxin acts principally on the central nervous system.The maximum toxicity is reached in the spawn time from March to June. Poisonings due to ichthyootoxic fish have been recorded in Europe, Asia, and America, but they are rare. In most cases, patients get well within several days.

OCCURRENCE

Ichthiootoxin was isolated from roe of various fish species. Only the roe of these fish is toxic and other parts of their body are edible.[1,43,44] The habitat of ichthyootoxic fish is in fresh waters in Europe, Asia, and America, and in seas all over the world. The toxin acts principally on the central nervous system. In most cases, patients get well within several days.

CHANGES DURING PROCESSING AND STORAGE

Lipoproteins are easily denatured by heat, but the toxic substance seems to be dinogunellin, which is rather heat stable. However, it may be hydrolyzed by enzymes. Nevertheless, no data on the existence of specific enzymes have been reported.

ICHTHYOHEMOTOXIN

CHEMISTRY

The chemical composition and structure of ichthyohemotoxin are not exactly known. The toxic substance is insoluble in 90% aqueous alcohol, it is not dialyzable, it is thermolabile, and it is destroyed both by organic and inorganic acids and alkalis. Some authors presume ichthyotoxin to be a protein, possibly albumin.[45,46]

TOXIC EFFECTS

The degree of toxicity of eel blood is individual and dependent on the season.The highest toxicity has been reported in summer, during the spawn time.

Poisonings with ichthyohemotoxins are very rare because eel blood is perorally toxic only in large quantities. Cases of poisoning were reported only when eel blood was ingested in a mixture with wine as an antialcoholic treatment. The toxins influence the nervous system. Contact of eel blood with mucous membranes and eyes caused inflammation.[1]

OCCURRENCE

Ichthyohemotoxins are present in the blood of some fish species, most of all, eels (families *Anguillidae* and *Congridae*). The habitat of the family *Anguillidae* is in rivers and seas of Europe, Japan, China, Korea, and at the Atlantic coast of Mexico. *Congridae* live in the tropic Atlantic Ocean and in the Mediterranean Sea.

CHANGES DURING PROCESSING AND STORAGE

The detoxification can be effected by heating to temperatures over 70°C or by exposure to ultraviolet irradiation. The toxicity is also destroyed by digestive fluids and by proteolytic enzymes.[45,46]

ICHTHYOCRINOTOXINS

CHEMISTRY

The structure depends on the origin. Thompson et al.[47] isolated a poisonous secretion from *Pardachirus pavoninus,* consisting of three peptides with 33 amino acids and having a molecular weight of 2800 Da. These peptides were named pardaxin-1, pardaxin-2, and pardaxin-3. Six *N*-acetylglucosaminid steroids,[48] pavonins 1 to 6 were also isolated (Figure 6). Five mosesins were isolated from the lipophilic fraction of the secretion from *Pardachirus marmoratus.*[49]

The skin secretion of *Arius bilineatus* contains proteins (85%), lipids (triacylglycerols, phospholipids, and glycolipids (13%) and a negligible amount of carbohydrates.[50] One fraction possessed strong hemolytic activity.[51]

Boylan and Scheuer[52] isolated the toxic substance from skin secretion of *Ostracion lentiginosus* — pahutoxin. It was found to be the choline ester of 3-acetoxyhexadecanoic acid. The skin secretion of *Ostracion immaculatus* contains two toxins, pahutoxin and homopahutoxin, which are choline diesters of 3-propionylhexadecanoic acid.[53]

Ichthyocrinotoxins of other fish belong to polypeptides, such as ryptisin, grammistin, etc.

TOXIC EFFECT

The skin excretions have a strong hemolytic activity. Poisoning in humans is not known. These fish are ichthyotoxic to various species of fish, molluscs, and other marine animals. Antibiotic activities of the secretions have been described in various bacteria yeasts.

OCCURRENCE

Ichthyocrinotoxins are produced by some groups of fish in their skin secretion as a defence system against carnivorous fish and microorganisms.[54] Ichthyocrinotoxic fish pardaxin P-1 : Gly-Phe-Phe-Ala-Leu-Ile-Pro-Lys-Ile-Ile-Ser-Ser-Pro-Leu-Phe-Lys-Thr-Leu-Leu-Ser-Ala-Val-Gly-Ser-Ala-Leu-Ser-Ser-Ser-Gly-Glu-Gln-Glu

pardaxin P-2 : Gly-Phe-Phe-Ala-Leu-Ile-Pro-Lys-Ile-Ile-Ser-Ser-Pro-Ile-Phe-Lys-Thr-Leu-Leu-Ser-Ala-Val-Gly-Ser-Ala-Leu-Ser-Ser-Ser-Gly-Gly-Gln-Glu

pardaxin P-3 : Gly-Phe-Phe-Ala-Phe-Ile-Pro-Lys-Ile-Ile-Ser-Ser-Pro-Leu-Phe-Lys-Thr-Leu-Leu-Ser-Ala-Val-Gly-Ser-Ala-Leu-Ser-Ser-Ser-Gly-Glu-Gln-Glu

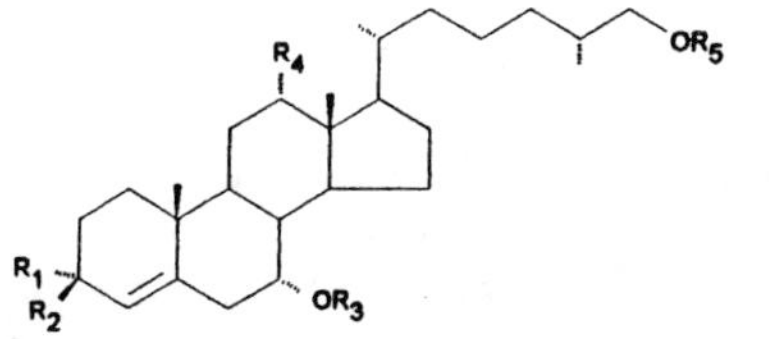

mosesin - 1 : R_1 = OH, R_2 = H, R_3 = a, R_4 = OH, R_5 = $OCCH_3$

mosesin - 5 : R_1 = OH, R_2 = H, R_3 = b, R_4 = OH, R_5 = $OCCH_3$

pavoninin 1 : R_1 = R_2 = O, R_3 = d, R_4 = H, R_5 = OCCH3

pavoninin 2 : R_1 = R_2 = O, R_3 = d, R_4 = H, R_5 = H

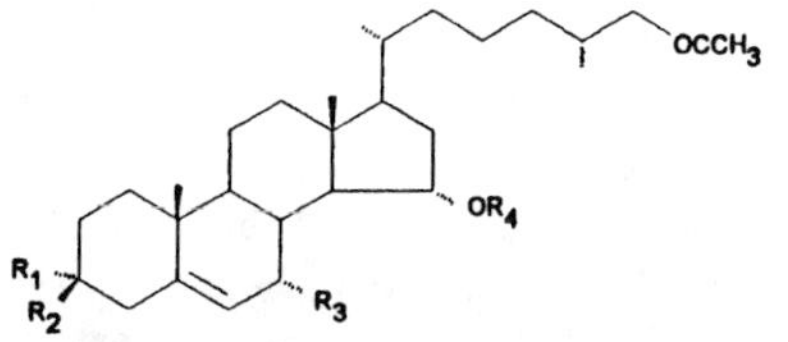

mosesin - 2 : R_1 = H, R_2 = OH, R_3 = O-b, R_4 = H

pavoninin 3 : R_1 = OH, R_2 = H, R_3 = H, R_4 = d

pavoninin 5 : R_1 = H, R_2 = OH, R_3 = H, R_4 = d

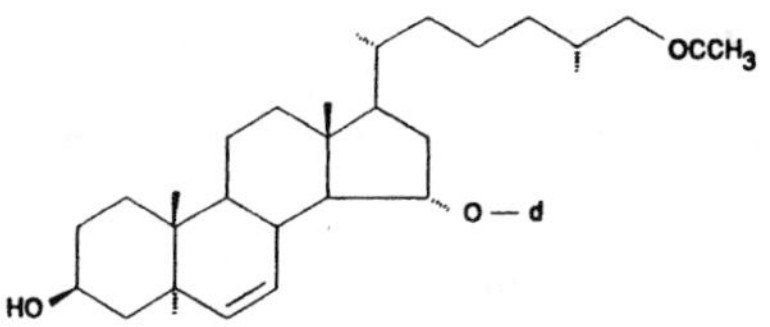

pavoninin 6

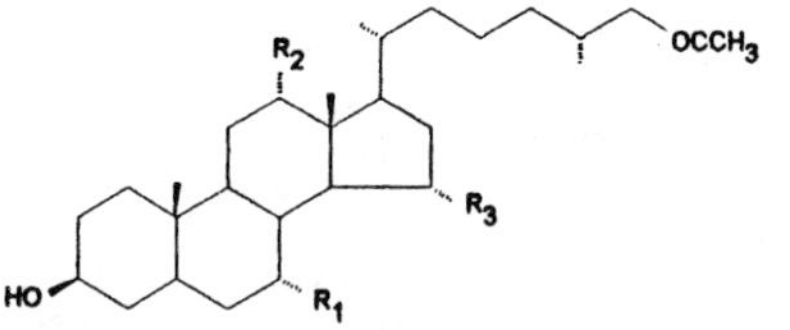

mosesin - 3 : R_1 = O-a, R_2 = OH, R_3 = H

mosesin - 4 : R_1 = O-b, R_2 = OH, R_3 = H

pavoninin 4 : R_1 = H, R_2 = H, R_3 = O-d

a = 6-acetyl-β-D-galactose

b = β-D-galactose

d = N-acetyl-β-D-glucosamin

Figure 6 Structures of toxins from the skin secretion of *Pardachirus.*

belong to various families (*Soleidae, Ariidae, Ostraciontidae, Grammistidae, Tetraodontidae, Gobiidae, Gobiesocidae, Batrachoididae,* and *Muraenidae).* These families are widespread in seas and oceans throught the world, particularly in tropic areas and Japan.

CHANGES DURING PROCESSING, AND STORAGE

The taste of most ichthyocrinotoxins is very unpleasant, bitter or sharp, so that the skin is not edible. Being mostly polypeptides, ichthyocrinotoxins are thermolabile and can be easily destroyed by cooking.[55] The toxicity is eliminated by proteolytic enzymes as well.

TOXINS OF FISH POISON APPARATUS

Fish poison apparatus consists of a variety of spines on the body and only some several species have poisonous teeth. A common characteristic of the toxins is their relative instability at room temperature or even on freeze-drying of freshly prepared extracts. For this reason, the structure of many toxins is unknown, but the main components are probably proteins, sometimes with enzymic activity.

Heat lability also complicates the study of toxic properties, but it is a helpful tool that may be exploited in the treatment of poisoned individuals or in the detoxication of food.

HALLUCINOGENS

Some species of the order *Perciformes* contain toxins which evoke hallucination.[1,56] The fish containing hallucinogens occur in tropical areas, and the toxicity is seasonal and regional. For instance, there are only two islands of the Hawaiian archipelago where fish are toxic from June to August.

Brain is more toxic than meat. Clinical signs (hallucination and depression, mostly with gastrointestinal symptoms) begin very quickly after ingestion, and last only for a short time.

The chemical structure of these compounds is not known.

BIOGENIC AMINES, HISTAMINE

The poisoning caused by histamine is known as scombroid fish poisoning (page 108).

VITAMIN A HYPERVITAMINOSIS

Livers of some fish species, e.g., *Scomberomorus niphonius, Petrus repestris, Arctoscopus japonicus, Stereolopsis ischinagai,* and *Hippoglossus hippoglossus* are occasionally toxic, due to a high content of vitamin A. Cases of hypervitaminosis were reported after ingestion of liver of these fishes. The vitamin content is seasonal, and the vitamin is present in higher quantities in older fish.[1,57]

REFERENCES

1. Halstead, B. W., *Poisonous and Venomous Marine Animals of the World,* 2nd ed., Darwin Press, New Jersey, 1988.
2. Southcott, R. V., Australian venomous and poisonous fishes, *Clin. Toxicol.*, 10, 291, 1977.
3. Tsuda, K., Über Tetrodotoxin, Giftstoff der Bowlfische, *Naturwissenschaften,* 53, 171, 1966.
4. Doull, J., Klaassen, C. D., and Amdur, M. O., *Casarett and Doull's Toxicology, The Basic Science of Poisons,* 2nd ed., Macmillan, New York, 1980, 557.
5. Russell, F. E., Marine toxins and venomous and poisonous marine animals, *Adv. Mar. Biol.*, 3, 255, 1965.
6. Russell, F. E., Venom poisoning, *Ration. Drug Ther.*, 5, 1, 1971.
7. Jones-Miller, J., *Food Safety,* Eagon Press, St. Paul, 1992.
8. White, A. W., Toxic red tides and shellfish toxicity in South-East Asia, Proc. Meeting Southeast Asian Fisheries Devel. Centre, Singapore, September 11th to 14th, 1984, White, A. W., Anraku, M., and Hooi, K., Eds., Southeast Asian Fisheries Development Centre, Bangkok and International Development and Research Centre, Ottawa, Canada, p. 1.
9. Yentsch, C. M., Paralytic shellfish poisoning: an emerging perspective, in *Seafood Toxins,* Ragelis, E. P., Ed., ACS Symp. Ser. 262, American Chemical Society, Washington, D.C., 1984, 9.

10. Krebs, S., Tox*ine und Wehrsekrete bei Fischen,* Tierärztliche Hochschule, Hannover, 1990, 20.
11. *Protecting Consumers through improved Food Quality and Safety* (Theme Pap. No. 2), Prepcom/ ICN/92/INF/7, FAO and WHO, Rome, 1992, p. 7.
12. Halstead, B. W. and Schantz, E. J., *Paralytic Shellfish Poisoning,* Offset Publ. No. 79, WHO, Geneva, 1984.
13. Russell, F. E., Pharmacology of toxins in marine organisms, in *Pharmacology and Toxicology of Naturally Occurring Toxins,* Vol. 2, Rašková, H., Ed., Pergamon Press, New York, 1971, 3.
14. Hokama, Y. and Smith, S., Immunological assessment of marine toxins, *Food Agric. Immunol.,* 2, 99, 1990.
15. Woodward, R. B., The structure of tetrodotoxin, *Pure Appl. Chem.,* 9, 49, 1964.
16. Nakamura, M. and Yasumoto, T., Tetrodotoxin derivatives in puffer fish, *Toxicon,* 23, 271, 1985.
17. Saito, T., Marayama, J., Kanoh, S., Jeon, J. K., Noguchi, T., Harada, T., Murata, O., and Hashimoto, K., Toxicity of cultured puffer fish *Fugu rubripes* and its resistance to tetrodotoxin, *Bull. Jpn. Soc. Sci. Fish.,* 50, 1573, 1984.
18. Yotsu, M., Yamazaki, T., Meguro, Y., Endo, A., Murata, M., Naoki, H., and Yasumoto, T., Production of tetrodotoxin and its derivatives by *Pseudomonas sp.* isolated from the skin of a pufferfish, *Toxicon,* 25, 225, 1987.
19. Ozawa, C., Studies on detoxification of poisonous puffer roe pickled in rice bran, I. Toxicity of puffer roe pickled in rice bran, *J. Food Hyg. Soc. Jpn.,* 24, 258, 1983.
20. Ozawa, C., Studies on detoxification of poisonous puffer roe pickled in rice bran, II. Effect of the presence of alkalis during salting on the toxicity of puffer roe, *J. Food Hyg. Soc. Jpn.,* 24, 263, 1983.
21. Fuchi, Y., Noguchi, T., Saito, T., Morisaki, S., Nakama, S., Shimazaki, K., Hayashi, K., Ohtomo, N., and Hashimoto, K., Mechanisms involved in detoxification of puffer-fish liver during traditional cooking, *J. Food Hyg. Soc. Jpn.,* 29, 320, 1988.
22. Tsubone, N., Fuchi, Y., Morisaki, S., Mizokoshi, T., Shuto, M., Fuji, M., Yamada, K., and Hayashi, K., Removal of toxicity from puffer fish liver by cooking, *J. Food Hyg. Soc. Jpn.,* 27, 561, 1986.
23. Shiomi, K., Tanaka, E., Kumagai, I., Kikuchi, T., and Kawabata, T., Toxification of muscle after thawing of frozen puffer fish, *Bull. Jpn. Soc. Sci. Fish.,* 50, 341, 1984.
24. Ragelis, E. P., Ciguatera seafood poisoning-overview, in: *Seafood Toxins,* ACS Symp. Ser. 262, Ragelis, E. P., Ed., American Chemical Society, Washington, D.C., 1984, 25.
25. Bagnis, R., Chanteau, S., Chungue, E., Hurtel, J. M., Yasumoto, T., and Inoue, A., Origins of ciguatera fish poisoning: a new dinoflagellate, *Gambierdiscus toxicus* Adachi and Fukuyo definitely involved as a causal agent, *Toxicon,* 18, 199, 1980.
26. Tindall, D. R., Dickey, R. W., Carlson, R. D., and Morey-Gaines, G., Ciguatoxigenic dinoflagellates from the Caribbean sea, in *Seafood Toxins,* ACS Symp. Ser. 262, Ragelis, E. P., Ed., American Chemical Society, Washington, D.C., 1984, 225.
27. Moore, R. E. and Bartolini, G., Structure of palytoxin, *J. Am. Chem. Soc.,* 103, 2491, 1982.
28. Fukui, M., Murata, M., Inoue, A., Gawel, M., and Yasumoto, T., Occurrence of palytoxin in the trigger fish *Melichthys vidua, Toxicon,* 25, 1121, 1987.
29. Hashimoto, Y., Fusetani, N., and Kimura, S., Aluterin: a toxin of filefish, Alutera scripta, probably originating from a zoanthrian, *Palythoa tuberculosa, Bull. Jpn. Soc. Sci. Fish.,* 35, 1086, 1969.
30. Fukui, M., Yasumara, D., Murata, M., Alcala, A. C., and Yasumoto, T., The occurrence of palytoxin in crabs and fish, *Toxicon,* 26, 20, 1988.
31. Fusetani, N., Sato, S., and Hashimoto, K., Occurrence of water soluble toxin in a parrotfish *Ypsiscarus oviforns* which is probably responsible for parrotfish liver poisoning, *Toxicon,* 23, 105, 1985.
32. Prakash, A., Medcof, J. C., and Tennant, A. D., Paralytic shellfish poisoning in Eastern Canada, *Fish. Res. Bd. Can. Bull.,* 177, 1, 1971.
33. Noguchi, T., Ueda, Y., Onoue, Y., Kono, M., Koyama, K., Hashimoto, K., Seno, Y., and Mishima, S., Reduction in toxicity of PSP infested scallops during canning process, *Bull. Jpn. Soc. Sci. Fish.,* 46, 1273, 1980.
34. Noguchi, T., Ueda, Y., Onoue, Y., Kono, M., Koyama, K., Hashimoto, K., Takeuchi, T., Seno, Y., and Mishima, S., Reduction in toxicity of highly PSP-infested scallops during canning process and storage, *Bull. Jpn. Soc. Sci. Fish.,* 46, 1339, 1980.

35. Dassow, J., in *Proc. Joint Semin. North Pacific Clams,* Alaska Dept. Health Welfare, Public Health Service, U.S. Dept. Health, Education and Welfare, 1966, 34.
36. Asakawa, M. and Takagi, M., Effects of pH and heating on PSP, relating to boiling or canning process of toxic scallops, *Bull. Fac. Fish. Hokkaido Univ.*, 34, 260, 1983.
37. Gill, T. A., Thompson, J. W., and Gould, S., Thermal resistance of paralytic shellfish poison in soft-shell clams, *Food Protection,* 48, 659, 1985.
38. Asakawa, M., Takagi, M., Iida, A., and Oishi, K., Studies on the chemical-reductive conversion of paralytic shellfish poison (PSP) components in bivalves, *J. Hyg. Chem.*, 32, 212, 1986.
39. Asakawa, M., Takagi, M., Iida, A. and Oishi, K., Studies on the conversion of paralytic shellfish poison (PSP) components by biochemical reducing agents, *Jpn. J. Toxicol. Environ. Health*, 33, 50, 1987.
40. White, A. W., Paralytic shellfish toxins and finfish, in *Seafood Toxins,* ACS Symp. Ser. 262, Ragelis, E. P., Ed., American Chemical Society Washington, D.C., 1984, 171.
41. Noguchi, T., Nagashima, Y., Maruyama, J., Kamimura, S., and Hashimoto, K., Toxicity of the adductor muscle of markedly PSP-infested scallop *Patinopecten yessoensis, Bull. Jpn. Soc. Sci. Fish.,* 50, 517, 1984.
42. Asano, M. and Itoh, M., Lipoproteins (lipostichaerins) in the roe of a blenny, *Stichaeus grigorjewi* Herzenstein, *Tohoku J. Agric. Res.*, 16, 299, 1966.
43. Kamiya, H., Hatano, M., and Hashimoto, Y., Screening of ichthyootoxin, *Bull. Jpn. Soc. Sci. Fish.*, 43, 1461, 1977.
44. Fuhrman, F. A., Fuhrman, G. J., Dull, D. L. and Mosher, H. S., Toxins from eggs of fishes and amphibia, *J. Agric. Food. Chem.,* 17, 417, 1969.
45. Mosso, U., Un venin dans le sang des murenides, *Arch. Ital. Biol.*, 10, 141, 1988.
46. Mosso, U., Recherches sur la nature du venin qui se trouve dans le sang de l´anguille, *Arch. Ital. Biol.*, 12, 229, 1989.
47. Thompson, S. A., Tachibana, K., Nakanishi, K., and Kubota, I., Melittin-like peptides from the shark-repelling defense secretion of the sole *Padachirus pavoninus, Science,* 233, 341, 1986.
48. Tachibana, K., Sakaitani, M., and Nakanishi, K., Pavoninins, shark-repelling and ichthyotoxic steroid *N*-acetylglucosaminides from the defense secretion of the Pacific sole *Padachirus pavoninus* (Soleidae), *Tetrahedron,* 41, 1027, 1985.
49. Tachibana, K. and Gruber, S. H., Shark repellent lipophilic constituents in the defense secretion of the Moses sole *(Padachirus marmoratus), Toxicon*, 26, 839, 1988.
50. Al-Hassan, J. M., Thomson, M., Criddle, K. R., Summers, B., and Criddle, R. S., Catfish epidermal secretions in response to threat or injury: a novel defense response, *Mar. Biol.*, 88, 117, 1985.
51. Al-Lahham, A., Al-Hassan, J. M., Thomson, M., and Criddle, R. S., A haemolytic protein secreted from epidermal cells of the Arabian Gulf catfish, *Arius thalassinus* Ruppell, *Comp. Biochem. Physiol.*, 87 B, 321, 1987.
52. Boylan, D. B. and Scheuer, P. J., Pahutoxin: a fish poison, *Science,* 155, 52, 1967.
53. Fusetani, N. and Hashimoto, K., Occurrence of pahutoxin and homopahutoxin in the mucus secretion of the Japanese boxfish, *Toxicon,* 25, 459, 1987.
54. Cameron, A. M. and Endean, R., Epidermal secretions and the evolution of venom glands in fishes, *Toxicon*, 11, 401, 1973.
55. Clark, E. and Chao, S., A toxic secretion from the Red Sea flatfish *Padachirus marmoratus* Lacepede, *Sea Fish Res. St. Haifa Bull.,* 60, 53, 1973.
56. Helfrich, P. and Banner, A. H., Hallucinatory mullet poisoning: a preliminary report, *J. Trop. Med. Hyg.*, 63, 86, 1960.
57. Nater, J. P. and Douglas, H. M. G., Halibut liver poisoning in 11 fishermen, *Acta Derm. Vener.,* 50, 109, 1970.

Part J

Mushroom Toxins

Jana Hajšlová

Thanks to their special, delicious flavor, mushrooms have been used for preparation of various meals for ages. The popularity of mushrooms in the diet is, besides their attractive organoleptic properties, based on their low energy content, due to a typically low amount of lipids, and that they are a good source of dietary fiber and minerals.

Unfortunately, many wild and even some cultivated mushrooms contain toxic compounds.[1,2] Extremely (deadly) poisonous protoplasmic toxins are represented by so-called amanita toxins, to which belong phalloidin, phalloin, α-amanitin, and β-amanitin (the most toxic amatoxin). These chemically similar cyclopeptides possessing relatively high temperature stability occur in *Amanita phalloides, A. verna, A. virosa,* and related species.

Certain false morels (e.g., *Gyromitra esculenta,* syn. *Helvella esculenta*) contain another type of protoplasmic toxin. Gyromitrin, the main toxic principle, is metabolized by methylating agents, which exert many toxic effects including carcinogenicity. Agaritine, another N-N bond-containing substance with potentially cancer inducing properties, was found in mushrooms of the *Agaricus* genus.

Substances occurring in *Amanita muscarina* and *A. pantherina* exert neurological (psychotropic) effects. Muscarine, the main representative of these compounds, was found also in species of *Inocybe, Boletus, Clitocybe, Hebeloma, Lepiota, Russula,* etc. Substituted derivatives of tryptamine, psilocyn, and psilocybin were reported to be present in some species of *Conocybe, Panaeolus, Psilocybe, Psathyrella,* and *Russula.*

Physiological symptoms similar to those known as the alcohol-disulfiram syndrome can be encountered when ingestion of *Coprinus atramentarius* (and possibly other mushrooms) is followed by the intake of alcoholic beverages.

Many other mushrooms were recognized to contain substances with an irritating action upon the gastrointestinal tract. The above-mentioned muscarine together with muscaridine and choline are, e.g., supposed to cause vomiting after ingestion of *Rhodophyllus rhodopolius.* Resin-like substances are assumed to be the toxic (irritating) principle of species of *Agaricus, Boletus, Cantharellus, Clavaria, Clitocybe, Lactarius, Lepiota, Paxillus, Rhodophyllus, Russula,* etc.

A detailed discussion of all the mushroom toxins is beyond the focus of this section. Attention will be paid to potentially cancer-inducing toxins contained in edible mushrooms — agaritine and gyromitrin, to which humans can be exposed via their diet.

The demand for edible mushrooms is tremendous nowadays and is still growing. Market needs are saturated predominantly by commercially cultivated species — their total annual production is estimated to be well over 1.2 million tons,[3-5] of which *Agaricus bisporus* forms more than half the world's annual production.

Approximately 1 million people in Europe and 100 thousand people in the U.S. are supposed to consume *Gyromitra esculenta* annually.[6] False morels have considerable commercial value, especially in some Nordic countries; e.g., in Finland the amount of false morels picked for marketing is estimated to be close to 10,000 kg/year.[7]

AGARITINE

CHEMISTRY

Levenberg [8,9] in 1960 isolated from common champignon mushrooms (in levels up to 0.04%) a naturally occurring hydrazine compound, β-*N*-/γ-L(+)glutamyl/-4-(hydroxymethyl) phenylhydrazine, which is now known as agaritine (Figure 1).

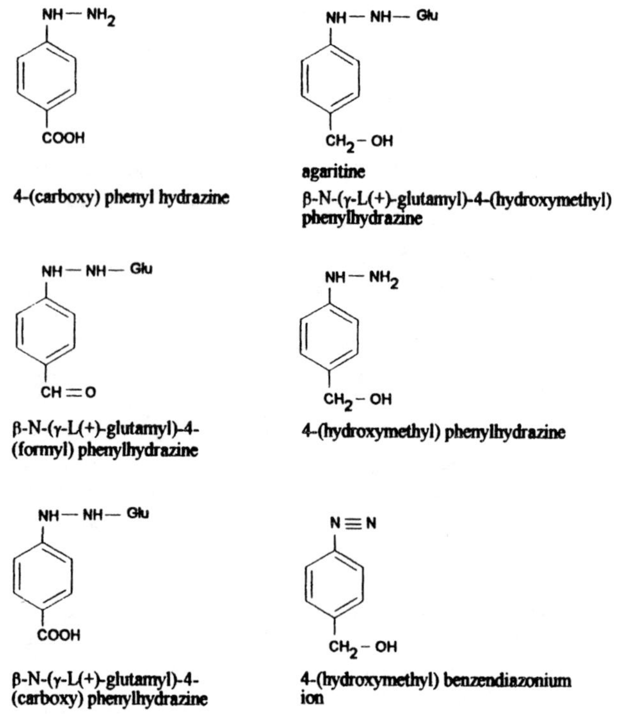

Figure 1 Hydrazines present in the genus *Agaricus.*

Besides agaritine, which is essentially a phenylhydrazine derivative, several other chemically related nitrogen-containing compounds have been isolated from mushrooms of the genus *Agaricus* (Figure 1). 4-(Carboxy) phenylhydrazine and β-*N*-(γ-L(+)-glutamyl)-4-(carboxy) phenylhydrazine were postulated as possible biosynthetic precursors of agaritine,[10,11] whereas others are degradation products.[12-15] Hydrolysis of agaritine (resulting in formation of 4-(hydroxymethyl) phenylhydrazine) is catalyzed by γ-glutamyl transferase (EC 2.3.2.1).[16] In general, most of these hydrazines are senzitive to oxidation and 4-(hydroxymethyl) phenylhydrazine easily decomposes by elimination of water.

TOXICITY

The results of short-term tests indicate mutagenity of extracts prepared from *Agaricus* as well as of some hydrazine derivatives occurring in these mushrooms.[17,18] Several long-term studies were carried out by Toth and Erickson.[19] Raw mushrooms and 4-(carboxy)phenylhydrazine, β-*N*-(γ-L(+)-glutamyl)-4-(carboxy) phenylhydrazine, 4-(hydroxymethyl) phenylhydrazine and 4-(hydroxymethyl)benzenediazonium ion (Figure 2) were proved to be carcinogenic after peroral administration to mice. However, the experimental conditions applied in this study were quite unusual, so that secondary effects on the tumor incidence cannot be excluded. It should also be mentioned that agaritine, the parent hydrazine compound, was not demonstrated to induce malignant tumors.

To evaluate the human health risk related to the consumption of champignons, studies carried out in accordance with modern test guidelines together with information on the concentration of hydrazine derivatives in mushrooms used for experiments as well as epidemiological data are needed.[20]

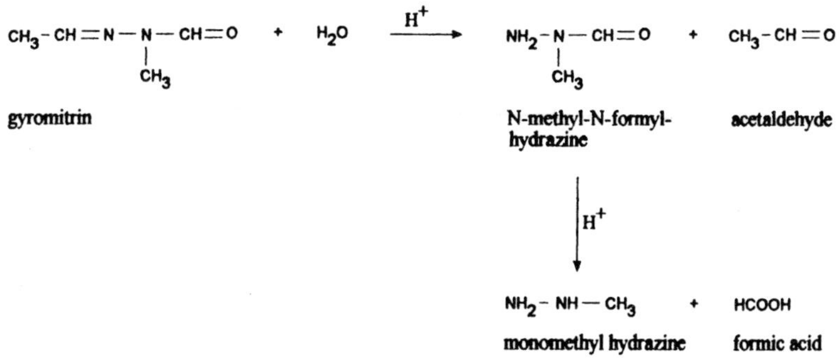

Figure 2 Degradation of gyromitrin.

OCCURRENCE

The presence of agaritine seems to be limited to the *Agaricus* genus. Reported levels of agaritine in fresh mushrooms vary considerably; nevertheless, completely agaritine-free easily cultivatable mushrooms are not known.

Liu et al.[13] found levels of agaritine to range from 330 to 1,730 $mg.kg^{-1}$ in 14 lots of button mushrooms from 10 different commercial growers in Pennsylvania. According to other studies, the agaritine content was from 440 to 720 $mg.kg^{-1}$ in two different mushroom batches,[14] from 160 to 650 $mg.kg^{-1}$ in four varieties of white champignons and from 240 to 650 $mg.kg^{-1}$ in brown ones,[21] from 80 to 250 $mg.kg^{-1}$ in two different strains.[22] In the last study, agaritine levels were found to be slightly higher in cup as opposed to the button mushrooms, which was attributed to the different content of solids. In general, higher levels of agaritine can be expected in young still-closed mushrooms. Enzymatic breakdown of agaritine yielding 4-(hydroxymethyl)hydrazine is considered to be responsible for its lower content of parent compound in older mushrooms.[13]

Limited data are available on levels of related hydrazines that are presented in Figure 1. The average concentrations 10.7 $mg.kg^{-1}$ of 4-(carboxy) phenylhydrazine, 40 $mg.kg^{-1}$ of β-*N*-(γ-L(+)-glutamyl)-4-(carboxy) phenylhydrazine and 0.6 $mg.kg^{-1}$ of 4-(hydroxymethyl)benzenediazonium ion were reported to be present in *A. bisporus.* The presence of β-*N*-(γ-L(+)-glutamyl)-4-(formyl)phenylhydrazine was proved only in *A. campestris.*[23]

An extensive study by Speroni et al.[24] showed that all the production steps — composting as well as spawning and cropping — influence the levels of agaritine. It should be mentioned that a very interesting and agriculturally unique phenomenon occurs during cultivation of champignons. Rhythmic 3- to 5-day harvests, constituting a single flush or break, are followed by periods when few or no mushrooms are available for harvest. It was recognized that agaritine levels varied considerably in mushrooms harvested from the peak days of different flushes. Champignons collected later in the cropping cycle were more likely to have higher agaritine levels than those harvested earlier. A general increase of toxin content in the later flushes is attributed to the changed metabolic interaction between a compost and mushrooms. Agaritine levels were found to be lower in mushrooms grown on natural composts (containing mostly horse manure) than in the case of blended or synthetic composts.

CHANGES DURING PROCESSING AND STORAGE

The content of agaritine in champignons stored at 2°C and 12°C was reduced significantly — about 32% of the original concentration remained after 5 d at both temperatures. The main decrease of toxin levels occurred after 4 d. These results are consistent with the study carried out by Ross et al.[14] Reduction of agaritine by 2 to 47% was observed in mushrooms stored at 4°C for 1 week. After 2 weeks of storage, the decrease ranged from 36 to 76%. Remarkable changes of agaritine were observed in frozen (–25°C, 30 d) and then thawed mushrooms, in which the losses were about 74%. The decrease of agaritine is assumed to be due to its breakdown by γ-glutamyl transferase (EC 2.3.2.1), yielding 4-(hydroxymethyl)phenylhydrazine and L-glutamic acid. The enzyme is allowed to come into contact with the substrate, after its separation from disrupted cellular structures in the course of freezing and following thawing. Lowered agaritine content caused by these processes was also observed by other authors;[21] while 400 to 700 $mg.kg^{-1}$ of toxin was contained in fresh mushrooms, only 75 to 300 $mg.kg^{-1}$ was found in frozen samples. Nevertheless, the freezing process itself (when thawing is not considered) does not appear likely to affect significantly the agaritine content.

Relatively high levels of agaritine were reported in dry powdered and sliced mushrooms which are used as a seasoning for soups (1,000 to 2,500 $mg.kg^{-1}$). Fischer et al.[25] observed the average agaritine content in dried commercial mushrooms to be 4,600 $mg.kg^{-1}$.

The influence of various types of heat processing was investigated in several laboratories. Blanching in boiling water for 5 to 7 min led to leaching of approximately one half of the agaritine into the blanch-water; nevertheless, the total content (i.e., in water and mushrooms together) was not altered in this experiment.[25] Liu et al.[13] reported that blanching for 5 min reduced the original content of agaritine by 57 and 75% in brown and white strains, respectively. These differences were attributed to unequal weight losses during blanching as well as to a different amount of agaritine in fresh tissue (429 $mg.kg^{-1}$ and 920 $mg.kg^{-1}$ in the brown and white strains, respectively).

Very low levels of agaritine were found in canned products. The remaining agaritine (expressed in percent of original content) ranged from 5.9 to 6.5 and from 7.3 to 7.8 in mushrooms, canned and in brine, respectively. In this case, only slight differences occurred in the extent of thermal destruction of agaritine occurred in brown and/or white champignons. This may be due to an apparent equilibrium developed between a solid tissue and a brine liquor. As was shown from a U.K. survey of the occurrence of agaritine in retail processed and cooked mushroom products, only low levels of toxin were found in tins containing large sliced champignons, in which the content of agaritine was 6 $mg.kg^{-1}$ and 20 $mg.kg^{-1}$ in brine and mushrooms, respectively.[21] In another study, the agaritine content in canned mushrooms was found to be in the range 1 to 55 $mg.kg^{-1}$ drained weight, with 3 to 103 $mg.kg^{-1}$ in the liquor.[26] In canned mushroom soup, Ross et al.[14] were even not able to detect the presence of agaritine. The thermal destruction of toxin by sautéing (in olive oil for 7 min) resulted in the 32% loss of agaritine.

It can be generally concluded that processed and cooked mushrooms are not likely to be a significant route of dietary exposure to agaritine.

GYROMITRIN

CHEMISTRY

In 1967, List and Luft[27] recognized acetaldehyde *N*-methyl-formylhydrazone (AMFH), so called gyromitrin, to be the main toxic principle of false morel, *Gyromitra esculenta.* This compound is easily oxidized by air at room temperature. It decomposes to *N*-methyl-*N*-formylhydrazine (MFH), which is more stable than gyromitrin.[28,29] Nevertheless, under the acid conditions (both *in vivo* and *in vitro*) it yields monomethylhydrazine (MMH)(Figure 2).

It was estimated that 25 to 30% of gyromitrin can be transformed via MFH to MMH *in vivo*. Liver microsomal monooxygenases also transform gyromitrin to the highly reactive *N*-nitroso-*N*-methylformamide (NMFA).[30] Production of another methylating agent, diazomethane, is also assumed.

TOXICITY

False morels containing toxic gyromitrins (even after processing) are considered to be edible mushrooms in some countries, especially in northern and eastern Europe. In this respect, *Gyromitra esculenta* appeared to be the most dangerous fungus, being the cause of several cases of death.[31,32]

Clinical data are characterized primarily by vomiting and diarrhea followed by jaundice, convulsion, and coma. Frequent consumption of false morels can cause hepatitis and neurological diseases. MFH and MMH originating from the parent compound are hazardous chemicals with hepatotoxic and even carcinogenic potency.[20]

OCCURRENCE

Gyromitrin is the most abundant toxic hydrazone in false morel. Up to 1,600 $mg.kg^{-1}$ of this compound were found in freshly picked mushrooms. According to other studies,[34] the levels of toxin range up to 3,000 $mg.kg^{-1}$; the content of MFH could reach 500 $mg.kg^{-1}$. The concentrations of MMH reported by several authors[35] ranged from 40 to 350 $mg.kg^{-1}$. A great part of gyromitrine and MFH in false morel is probably chemically bound (as glycosides) to higher molecular weight molecules.[36,37]

In addition to gyromitrin, eight other homologous *N*-methyl-*N*-formylhydrazones were identified in *Gyromitra esculenta*.[38] They contain the following higher aldehydes: propanal, *n*-butanal, 3-methylbutanal, *n*-pentanal, *n*-hexanal, *n*-octanal, *trans*-2-octenal, and *cis*-2-octenal. The weight ratio of gyromitrin to the total content of these hydrazones was found to be approx. 88:12.

CHANGES DURING PROCESSING AND STORAGE

Recent results suggest that drying of false morel is an inadequate way of detoxification.[37] Although reduction of free gyromitrin was recorded, this process does not eliminate all the precursors that can be hydrolyzed to MMH. The concentrations of MMH in mushrooms dried in the open air at room temperature for 3 months were 410 to 610 $mg.kg^{-1}$ (in dried tissue), which represented 30 to 71% of the original content. In some commercial dried false morels, levels of even 1,000 to 3,000 $mg.kg^{-1}$ of this hydrazine were reported.[31,33] Quick drying by applying infrared radiation for 30 min resulted in only a slight reduction of MMH levels.[37]

A significant decrease of hydrazines can be achieved by boiling. In experiments in which false morels were boiled for two periods of 5 min with a change of water, reduction of MMH content to 20 to 30 $mg.kg^{-1}$ occurred (corresponding to 12 $mg.kg^{-1}$ in fresh specimens).[37] On average, only 10 to 15% of MMH remained after boiling. When repeated boiling for five periods of 5 min was applied, the decrease of MMH was approximately 93% of the original content.[38] Speroni et al.[39] investigated the kinetics of agaritine in model systems (mushroom puree in buffer). Agaritine decomposition could be modeled by first order kinetics. Mushrooms processed for 68 min at 115°C contained 23% less agaritine than those held 11 min at 127°C.

The concentrations of MMH in drained canned mushrooms varied from 6 to 65 $mg.kg^{-1}$, which corresponds to 3 to 30 $mg.kg^{-1}$ in fresh tissue.[37] The average level of MMH in canned false morels was 23 $mg.kg^{-1}$,which is equivalent to 12 $mg.kg^{-1}$ in the fresh specimen.[38]

REFERENCES

1. Claus, E. P., Tyler, V. E., and Brady L. R., *Pharmacognosy*, 6th ed., Lea and Febiger, Philadelphia, 1977.
2. Tyler, V. E., Jr., in *Progress in Chemical Toxicology*, Vol 1., Stolman, A., Ed., Academic Press, New York, 1963.
3. Breene, W. M., Nutritional and medicinal value of specialty mushrooms, *J. Food Protect.*, 53, 883, 1990.
4. Hadar, Y. and Dosoretz, C. G., Mushroom mycelium as a potential source of food flavour, *Trends Food Sci. Technol.*, Elsevier Science Publishers, U.K., 1991, p. 214.
5. Chang, S. T., World production of cultivated mushrooms, *Mush. J. Tropics*, 7, 17, 1987.
6. Braun, R., The toxicology of 1-acetyl-2-methyl-2-formyl-hydrazine (ac-MFH), *Toxicol. Lett.*, 9, 271, 1981.
7. Nagel, D., Formation of methylhydrazine from acetadehyde *N*-methyl-*N*-formylhydrazine, a component of *Gyromithra esculenta, Cancer Res.*, 37, 9, 1977.
8. Levenberg, B., Structure and enzymatic cleavage of agaritine, a phenylhydrazide of L-glutamic acid isolated from Agaricaceae, *J. Biol. Chem.*, 83, 503, 1961.
9. Levenberg, B., Isolation and structure of agaritine, a γ-glutamyl-substituted aryl-hydrazine derivate from *Agaricaceae, J. Biol. Chem.*, 239, 2267, 1964.
10. Chauhan, Y., Nagel, D., Issenberg, P., and Toth, B., Identification of *p*-hydrazinobenzoic acid in the commercial mushroom *Agaricus bisporus, J. Agric. Food Chem.*, 32, 1067, 1984.
11 Chauhan, Y., Nagel, D., Gross, M., Cerny, R. and Toth, B., Isolation of N^2-[γ-L-(+)-glutamyl]-4-carboxyphenylhydrazine in the cultivated mushroom *Agaricus bisporus, J. Agric. Food Chem.*, 33, 817, 1985.
12. Chauhan, Y. P., Lawson, T., and Toth, B., Additional studies on hydrazines of *Agaricus bisporus:* analysis, metabolism and carcinogenesis, *Eur. J. Cancer Clin. Oncol.*, 21, (11), 1375, 1985.
13. Liu, J. W., Beelman, R. B., Lineback, D. R., and Speroni, J. J., Agaritine content of fresh and processed mushrooms, *J. Food Sci.*, 47, 1542, 1982.
14. Ross, A. E., Nagel, A. E., and Toth, D. L., Occurrence, stability and decomposition of β-N [γ-L(+)-glutamyl]-4-hydroxymethylphenylhydrazine (agaritine) from the mushroom *Agaricus bisporus, Food Chem. Toxicol.*, 20, 903, 1982.
15. Ross, A. E., Nagel, D. L., and Toth, B., Evidence for the occurrence and formation of diazonium ions in *Agaricus* mushrooms and its extracts, *J. Agric. Food Chem.*, 30, 521, 1982.
16. Gigliotti, H. J. and Levenberg, B., Studies on the γ-glutamyl-transferase of *Agaricus bisporus, Biol. Chem.*, 239, 2274, 1964.
17. Friederich, U., Fischer, B., Lüthy, J., Hann, D., Schlatter, C. and Würgler, F. E., The mutagenic activity of agaritine — a constituent of the cultivated mushroom *Agaricus bisporus* — and its derivates detected with the *Salmonella* mammalian microsome assay (Ames test), *Z. Lebensm. Unters. Forsch.*, 183, 85, 1986.
18. Pool, B. L., Schmezer, P., Sinrachatanant, Y., Reinhart, K., Martin, R., Klein, P., and Tricker, T., *Agaricus bisporus:* assessment of genotoxic potential. Mutagens and carcinogens in the diet, *A Satellite Symp. 5th Int. Conf. Environ. Mutagens*, Madison, Wisconsin, 1989.
19. Toth, B. and Erickson, J., Cancer induction in mice by feeding of the uncooked cultivated mushroom of commerce *Agaricus bisporus, Cancer Res.*, 46, 4007, 1986.
20. Schlatter, C., Toxicological significance of some hydrazines in food (cycasin, gyromitrin and agaritine), *Proc. Euro Food Tox II*, Zurich, 1986, 333.
21. Stijve, T., Fumeaux, T., and Philippossian, G., Agaritine, a *p*-hydroxymethylphenyl hydrazine derivative in cultivated mushrooms (*Agaricus bisporus*) and in some of its wild-growing relatives, *Dtsch. Lebensm. Rundsch.*, 82, 243, 1986.
22. Sharman, M., Patey, A. L., and Gilbert, J., A survey of the occurrence of agaritine in U.K. cultivated mushrooms and processed mushroom products, *Food Addit. Contam.* 7, 649, 1990.
23 Chulia, A. J., Bernillon, J., Favre-Bonvin, J., Kaouadji, M., and Arpin, N., Isolation of β-*N*-(γ-glutamyl)-4-formylphenylhydrazine (agaririnal) from *Agaricus campestris, Phytochemistry*, 27, 929, 1988.
24. Speroni, J. J., Beelmann, R. B., and Schisler, L. C., Factors influencing the agaritine content in cultivated mushrooms, *Agaricus bisporus, J. Food Protec.*, 46, 506, 1983.

25. Fischer, B., Lüthy, J., and Schlatter, C., Gehaltsbestimmung von Agaritin im Zuchtchampignon (*Agaricus bisporus*) mittels Hochleistungsflüssigchromatographie (HPCL), *Z. Lebensm. Unters. Forsch.*, 179, 218, 1984.
26. Sastry, S. K., Beelman, R. B., and Speroni, J. J., A three-dimensional finite element model for thermally induced changes in food: application to degradation of agaritine in canned mushrooms, *J. Food Sci.*, 50, 1293, 1985.
27. List, P. H., and Luft, P., Gyromitrin, das Gift der Frühjahrslorchel *Gyromitra (Helvella) esculenta* FR., *Tetrahedron Lett.*, 20, 1893, 1967.
28. Pyysalo, H., Niskanen, A., and Von Wright, A., Formation of toxic methylhydrazine during cooking of false morels, *Gyromitra esculenta, J. Food Safety*, 1, 295, 1978.
29. Coulet, M., Poisoning by *Gyromitra*: a possible mechanism, *Med. Hypotheses*, 8, 325, 1982.
30. Braun, R., Indications for nitrosamide formation from the mushroom poison gyromitrin by rat liver microsomes, *Xenobiotica*, 10, 557, 1980.
31. Hude, W., On the mutagenicity of metabolites derived from the mushroom poison gyromitrin, *Toxicology*, 26, 155, 1933.
32. Michelot, D. and Toth, B., Poisoning by *Gyromitra esculenta* — a review, *J. Appl. Toxicol.*, 11, 235, 1991.
33. Stijve, T., Ethylidene gyromitrine and *N*-methyl-*N*-formylhydrazine in commercially available dried false morels, *Trav. Chim. Aliment. Hyg.*, 69, 492, 1978.
34. Pyysalo, H. and Niskanen, A., On the occurrence of *N*-methyl-*N*-formyl-hydrazones in fresh and processed false morel, *Gyromitra esculenta, J. Agric. Food Chem.*, 25, 644, 1977.
35. Toth, B., Actual new cancer causing hydrazines, hydrazides and hydrazones, *J. Cancer Res. Clin. Oncol.*, 97, 97, 1980.
36. Simons, D. M., The mushroom toxins, *Del. Med. J.*, 43, 177, 1971.
37. Larsson, B. K. and Eriksson, A. T., The analysis and occurrence of hydrazine toxins in fresh and processed false morels, *Gyromitra esculenta, Z. Lebensm. Unters. Forsch.*, 189, 438, 1989.
38. Larsson, B. K., Methylhydrazin i stenmurkla, *Var Foda*, 41, 75, 1989.
39. Speroni, J. J., Sastry, S. K., and Beelman, R. B.,Thermal degradation kinetics of agaritine in model systems and agaritine retention in canned mushrooms, *J. Food Sci.*, 50, 1306, 1985.

Part K
Other Toxic Compounds

Richard Koplík, Jaroslav Prugar, and Jiří Davídek

Attention in Part K will be focused on toxic minerals, mineral binding compounds, nitrates, and nitrites. Their presence in food as a result of man's activities during processing, or as unwanted contaminants resulting from careless handling, spoilage, or some other uncontrolled or uncontrollable circumstances, will be not covered. This is especially important for toxic minerals, because in most cases, their presence in foodstuffs in concentrations above legislative limits comes from contamination. For this reason, only such elements as can be accumulated in plants or animals due to their genetic ability will be covered.

TOXIC ELEMENTS

Toxic metals such as lead, cadmium, and mercury are mostly considered to be food contaminants. However, their trace presence in foodstuffs can be explained in some cases as a result of bioaccumulation of metals in individual parts of a food chain. Therefore, it is often possible to detect toxic metals even in plant and animal tissues from unpolluted areas or surroundings. Examples given are focused on possibilities of reducing the toxic metal content in food during processing.

CADMIUM AND LEAD

Chemistry

Because of the differing position of cadmium and lead in the periodic table, their chemical properties are somewhat different.[1]

Unlike mercury and lead, cadmium compounds[1,2] exist only in oxidation state II and its organometallic compounds are unstable. In the presence of ligands such as Cl^-, Br^-, I^-, SCN^-, CN^-, NH_3, RNH_2, etc., cadmium forms complexes. In contrast to lead, cadmium (like mercury) shows a greater affinity to sulfur-containing ligands than to oxygen-containing ligands.

In the biochemistry of cadmium, the most important compounds are the polypeptides metallothioneins. Their biological function is not yet been fully understood, but it is assumed to play some role in detoxification processes.

Lead[1,3] shows the oxidation state II or IV in its compounds. Inorganic Pb(IV) compounds are powerful oxidizing agents and are less stable than Pb(II) compounds.

Many lead (II) compounds are either of low solubility or almost insoluble. The solubilization of slightly soluble lead compounds can be achieved by acidification or formation of complexes such as chloro- and hydroxo-complexes or complexes with organic ligands.

Organolead compounds contain at least one covalent lead-carbon bond. The most important organolead compounds, tetraethyl- and tetramethyl-lead, are used as antiknock substances in gasoline. This use of lead compounds results in a wide distribution of lead in the environment.

Toxic Effects

The toxic effects of lead and cadmium on humans are well known.[1,4,5] Both elements are accumulated in kidney and liver tissue. Cadmium and lead poisoning can result in a damage to kidneys, the cardiovascular system, the hemopoietic system, the reproductive system, the nervous system, and bones. Lead is an inhibitor of 5-aminolevulinic acid dehydrase (EC 4.2.1.24), the enzyme necessary for biosynthesis of heme and other porphyrins. Therefore, increased lead levels in blood cause anemia. Furthermore, cadmium shows carcinogenic, mutagenic, and teratogenic effects. Acceptable dietary intakes of Cd and Pb for adults are approximately from 60 to 70 and 400 μg/d, respectively.[6]

Occurrence

A number of studies have been focused on the Cd and Pb content in food and on their respective dietary intakes.[7-10] Some data concerning Cd and Pb levels in foodstuffs in the U.S. have been reviewed.[11-14] Increased levels of Cd and Pb in some food commodities are caused by bioconcentration of metals in some organisms, e.g., accumulation from the soil by mushrooms[15,16] or vegetables[17,18] such as lettuce, spinach, carrot, and endive, or by accumulation from sea-water by shellfish[19,20] (e.g., average Cd and Pb concentrations in spinach as a typical accumulator plant are 0.065 and 0.045 $mg.kg^{-1}$, respectively, but in onion only 0.011 and 0.005 $mg.kg^{-1}$, respectively). Terrestrial animals concentrate Cd and Pb from the absorbed feed mainly in their kidneys and livers, and metal content in these organs increases with the age of the animal[21](e.g., Cd concentrations in kidney tissue of 3.5-month-old calf and 5-year-old cow were 0.245 and 1.917 $mg.kg^{-1}$, respectively). Therefore, offal contributes significantly to the intake of Cd and Pb arising from the consumption of food of animal origin.

Changes during Processing and Storage

The content of Cd and Pb in foodstuffs can be to a certain extent influenced by the processing of agricultural products. Also, cooking may lead to some changes of metal

Table 1 Changes of Cd and Pb Content in Vegetables and Potatoes During Kitchen Preparation

Step of preparation	Cd (µg.kg^{-1})	Pb (µg.kg^{-1})	Cd (µg.kg^{-1})	Pb (µg.kg^{-1})
	Product			
	Green beans		**Carrots**	
Crude material — original content	6	45	27	60
Cleaned (mechanically)	5	40	28	44
Cleaned and washed	5	25	25	45
Peeled and washed	—	—	22	34
Scraped off and washed	—	—	21	29
Boiled[a]	5	28	—	—
Boiled[b]	—	—	19	36
	Cauliflower		**Brussels sprouts**	
Crude material — original content	9	61	19	94
Cleaned (mechanically)	9	31	22	42
Cleaned and washed	9	28	17	34
Boiled[a]	10	26	15	31
	Turnip cabbage		**Potatoes**	
Crude material — original content	14	41	35	299
Cleaned by washing	—	—	32	72
Cleaned and washed	12	27	—	—
Peeled and washed	13	23	32	24
Boiled[a]	—	—	29	27
Boiled[b]	16	23	22	24

[a] Boiled with the peel and then peeled.
[b] Boiled without the peel.

concentrations. These alterations may take place because of a heterogeneous distribution of metals in individual parts of food materials, when inedible parts are removed. Sometimes these operations cause a significant drop in metal levels. Another cause of metal loss can be seen in leaching during boiling of foodstuffs. A comprehensive study concerning variations of heavy metals in vegetables and potatoes during home cooking was made by Schelenz et al.[22] (Table 1).

While cleaning, washing, and peeling cause a substantial decrease in metal concentrations, boiling leads to less significant changes.

On the other hand, some technological processes may lead to an increase of metal levels in foodstuffs compared to starting materials (e.g., Cd level increases during production of soy-based food from 0.06 mg.kg^{-1} in whole soybeans to 0.19 mg.kg^{-1} in soy protein isolate as a result of Cd binding with proteins).[23]

MERCURY

Chemistry

Mercury compounds[1] may exist in oxidation states I and II. They have a great affinity to S^{2-} ions and compounds containing SH groups.

Organomercury compounds are relatively stable. Methylmercury compounds are naturally present in the aquatic enviroment and in bodies of animals as a result of biological methylation. A number of bacteria (e.g., *Clostridium, Enterobacter, Escherichia coli, Pseudomonas* etc.) and fungi (e.g., *Aspergillus, Neurospora,* etc.) can transform inorganic mercury compounds to the methylated ones.

Toxic Effects

Mercury probably represents the most dangerous heavy metal occurring in the environment[24] and in food.

Individual chemical forms of mercury substantially differ in the degree of their toxic effects. The order of decreasing toxicity is: alkylmercury, Hg metal vapor, Hg^{2+} salts, and phenylmercury and methoxymercury salts.[24] Generally, mercury and its compounds have nephrotoxic teratogenic and neurotoxic effects. Inorganic mercury compounds cause kidney damage, while organomercurials are typical neurotoxins. Acute poisoning by inorganic mercury salts may lead to a renal failure. The course of severe methylmercury poisoning is characterized by loss of sensation on the skin followed by loss of coordination in movement, loss of hearing, restricted visual field, blindness, coma, and death. It should be noted that intoxication by mercury from a normal diet is very unlikely. The acceptable daily intake (ADI)[27] of total Hg for adults is 50 μg and that of methylmercury is 30 μg.

Occurrence

The main nonanthropogenic sources of mercury emissions are rock weathering, geysers, forest fires, and volcanic activity.[1] Some organisms accumulate significant quantities of mercury in their bodies.[25] This is evident in aquatic animals such as fish and shellfish. For example, the Hg content of muscle tissue of freshwater fish is relatively high (for omnivore roach 0.09 to 0.44 and for carnivore species pike, eel, and silver salmon 0.2 to 2.87, 0.17 to 2.40 and 0.36 to 2.10 $mg.kg^{-1}$, respectively). On the other hand, Hg concentrations in muscles of terrestrial animals are significantly lower (for cattle 0.01 to 0.04 $mg.kg^{-1}$).[25] A great deal of mercury in aquatic organisms is represented by the highly toxic methylmercury.[26]

In total diet studies,[28-30] the actual dietary intakes of mercury were found to be well below the ADI value (e.g., in the U.S. 3.23 μg/d).A substantial portion of dietary Hg is accounted for by fish consumption (contribution 84 to 100%).[28,29]

Changes during Processing and Storage

The mercury content of foodstuffs can be slightly decreased by leaching, or due to its high volatility, by thermal processing. Valuable data concerning changes of mercury content in fish during various cooking processes were published by Hernandez Garcia et al.[31] Results are summarized in Table 2.

OTHER TOXIC ELEMENTS

Arsenic

Arsenic[1] is a nonmetallic element similar in its chemical properties to phosphorus. The degree of arsenic toxicity depends on the chemical form. The sequence of decreasing toxicity is arsine, arsenites, arsenates, and organoarsenicals (e.g., cacodylic acid, methylarsonic acid, arsenobetaine). The acceptable daily intake of arsenic is estimated to 120 μg. Higher arsenic concentrations in food are typical of fish and shellfish (e.g., herring, 0.8 to 1.43; cod, 0.6 to 7.29; shrimps, 3.2 to 25.7; and lobster, 1.5 to 122 $mg.kg^{-1}$).[32] Arsenic distribution in food shows that most of the arsenic in the diet is accounted for by low toxic organoarsenic compounds.[33]

Arsenic levels in vegetables and potatoes are substantially affected by various procedures of kitchen food preparation.[34] Peeling, cleaning, and boiling lead to a significant loss of arsenic in the final food (70% decrease for vegetables and almost complete elimination in the case of potatoes).

Table 2 Influence of Various Cooking Processes on the Mercury Content in Fish

Fish species	Type of processing	Hg content (μg.g⁻¹) Original sample	Processed sample
Anchovies	Frying	0.200 ± 0.022	0.117 ± 0.021
	Pickling in vinegar	0.200 ± 0.022	0.130 ± 0.031
Sardines	Roasting	0.310 ± 0.045	0.107 ± 0.046
Tuna	Frying	0.380 ± 0.110	0.290 ± 0.130
	Mixing with tomatoes and frying	0.380 ± 0.110	0.260 ± 0.080

From Hernandez Garcia, M. T., Martinez Para, M. C., and Masoud, T. A., *Anal. Bromatol.*, 40, 291, 1988. With permission.

Aluminum

Aluminum has been long considered to be a nonessential and nontoxic element. In humans aluminum toxicity is manifested in skeletal, hematological, and neurological systems. Because aluminum represents 8% of the earth's crust, this element can be regarded as a typically naturally occurring toxic metal in foods.

Foodstuffs of animal origin except kidney, liver, and brain contain only traces of aluminum. On the other hand, some herbs, spices, and tea leaves are very rich in aluminum (hundreds of $mg.kg^{-1}$). The most significant sources of aluminum in the diet are cereals containing from 2 to 50 $mg.kg^{-1}$ of aluminum. The dietary intake of aluminum for adults in the U.S. is 14 μg/day.[35]

Thallium

Thallium is a rare, toxic metal. It is toxic to the gastrointestinal tract and the central nervous system. Some mushrooms and *Brassicaceae* family plants[36] (e.g., cabbage, radish, and rape) regularly contain higher amounts of thallium than do other crops. Animals accumulate thallium contained in feed in their muscle tissue, the liver, and the kidney. Despite these facts, the normal thallium concentrations in foods are very low ($\mu g.kg^{-1}$ levels), and thallium dietary intake in the UK is estimated at 5 μg/day.

Selenium

Selenium[37] belongs to both essential and toxic trace elements if it is present in food at higher concentrations. Recommended dietary allowances of selenium for adult males and females are 70 and 55 μg/day, respectively.

The biological importance of selenium[38] is due to the fact that it is a substantial component of the enzyme glutathione peroxidase (EC 1.11.1.9), protecting tissues from oxidative damage. Selenium also moderates the toxic effects of heavy metals such as mercury and cadmium and enhances the biological effect of vitamin E.

Some plant species (e.g., *Astragalus, Haplopappus, Aster)* concentrate appreciable amounts of selenium from the soil, mostly in the form of the selenium analog of sulfur amino acids (page 103) The toxic effects of selenium are known in animals (namely, livestock) consuming these seleniferous plants. The occurrence of poisoning is limited only to areas with elevated selenium levels in the soil and vegetation. Typical examples of selenium toxicity in animals are alkali disease and blind staggers.

Selenium concentrations in food are greatly dependent on the food origin, namely, the agricultural production area (e.g., in the U.S. there are noticeable regional differences in Se content in food).[37]

The changes in the Se content of food as a result of cooking were studied by Higgs.[39] Selenium tends to be partially lost during thermal processing of food owing to the volatility of some Se compounds. Various kinds of processing (e.g., drying, boiling, etc.) were tested as factors influencing the Se content in several foods. Major sources of Se in the diet (meat, fishes, eggs, and cereal products) do not lose appreciable amounts of Se in the course of cooking. Only vegetables such as asparagus and mushrooms lose selenium significantly during cooking.

MINERAL BINDING COMPOUNDS

Mineral elements occur in food in a number of chemical forms, including their salts with organic acids and complexes with organic ligands. Proteins, peptides, amino acids, porphyrins, flavonoid compounds, hydroxycarboxylic acids, and sugar derivatives represent important components which are able to bind metal ions. Physiological and nutritional consequences of these binding effects are in most cases either beneficial or unknown.

On the other hand, there are two main organic substances which reduce the biological availability of nutritionally essential minerals and trace elements from the diet. They are phytic acid and oxalic acid.

PHYTIC ACID, PHYTIN, AND PHYTATES

Chemistry

Phytic acid[40] is a hexaphosphorylated compound derived from the cyclic alditol inositol (1,2,3,4,5,6-hexakis(dihydrogen phosphate) *myo*inositol). Phytin is the calcium-magnesium salt of phytic acid, phytates are anions of phytic acid or salts and complexes of phytic acid with a metal ion. In addition to phytic acid, less phosphorylated esters of inositol also exist.[41]

Antinutritional Action

In some crops, the fraction of phytate phosphorus represents up to 60% of the total phosphorus content, and this portion is poorly available. Biological availability[40] of metals, such as Zn, Fe, Ca, and Mg bound to phytate, can also be reduced to a certain extent, but it should be noted that results of several studies concerning metal absorption are contradictory. Strong toxic effects of phytic acid are not known.

Occurrence

Phytic acid is widely distributed in food of plant origin, especially in cereals, legumes, nuts, and oilseeds.[40] Certain other foodstuffs (potatoes, artichokes, carrots, broccoli, strawberries, blackberries, figs) contain small to moderate amounts of phytate, while anothers do not contain any phytate (lettuce, spinach, onions, mushrooms, celery, citrus fruits, apples, pineapple, bananas).[40] Table 3 summarizes the amounts of phytic acid in some crops. In the case of wheat and rice the concentration of phytic acid is considerably higher in the outer layers of the grain than in the whole grain.

Changes during Processing and Storage

Phytic acid and phytates form reaction products with proteins. Great attention was focused on phytate interaction with soybean proteins.[47] At low pH proteins are bound to phytate through cationic groups (lysyl, arginyl, and histidyl residues and terminal aminogroups). Binding of phytate to soy proteins is minimal at pH 5, being approximately equivalent to the respective isoelectric point. In slightly alkaline conditions, multivalent

Table 3 Content of Phytic Acid in Some Crops

Crop	Phytic acid content (% on dry weight basis)	Ref.
Barley	0.97–1.08	42
Oat	0.84–1.01	42
Wheat		
Whole grain	1.14	43
Grain Fraction	0.004–4.14	43
Bran portion	4.59–5.52	42
Rice		
Whole grain	0.8	
Germ	3.48	44
Endosperm	0.01	
Dry beans	0.54–1.58	45
Soybeans	1.00–1.47	42
Rapeseed	3–5	46

cations such as calcium and magnesium appear to chelate with the phytate, and this complex binds to the protein.

Phytic acid as an undesirable food component may be partially removed in the course of food processing. In the preparation and production of soya protein isolates and concentrates it is possible to utilize dialysis or ultrafiltration.[47] Another approach[48] is based on the significantly lower solubility of phytate at pH 11.5 in the presence of 10 $mmol.dm^{-3}$ of Ca^{2+}, whereas the protein yield is high. Extraction of soy flour with a 10% solution of NaCl at pH 8 also leads to low phytate concentration in the extract. Using a combination of selective protein extraction with dialysis or ultrafiltration, it is possible to reduce the high phytate content in initial defatted soy flour (1.5%) to a very low level in the final isolate (0.05 to 0.07%).[48]

In an analogous way as with proteins, phytates form compounds with acidic phospholipids.[49] Crude soybean oil contains 48.9 to 339.4 $mg.kg^{-1}$ phytates. Most phytates are removed in the course of degumming (the degummed oil contains only 3.9 to 50.9 $mg.kg^{-1}$ phytates) and they pass into the crude lecithin.[50] Binding of metals, expecially iron and copper, by phytic acid present in oil contributes to improvement of oxidative stability of the oil.

Thermal treatments also lead to a partial destruction of phytic acid in processed food. Considerable reduction of phytate content was reported after coffee roasting.[51] Boiling of defatted soy flour causes 22 to 23% losses of phytate.[52] Similarly, 15 min of microwave heating results in a 46% loss of phytate in defatted soybeans.[53] Cooking rice with an original phytate content 0.14 to 0.19% (in dry matter) in tap water results in a substantial lower amount in the cooked product, ranging from 0.042 to 0.054% (in dry matter).[15]

Chemical destruction of phytic acid during food processing and storage may occur as a result of enzyme-catalyzed hydrolysis of phytate to form myoinositol (or lower myoinositol phosphates) and phosphoric acid. The respective enzyme, phytase[40] (EC 3.1.3.26), occurs widely in plant material such as seeds and grains. Phytase activity in food material depends on the temperature, pH, and humidity. During bread making, the phytate content is reduced as the enzyme hydrolysis takes place. Breakdown of phytate is more effective under sourdough fermentation of dough. The phytate level can be lowered by one third to a half.[55] Chemical changes and interactions of phytic acid with food components are shown in Figure 1.

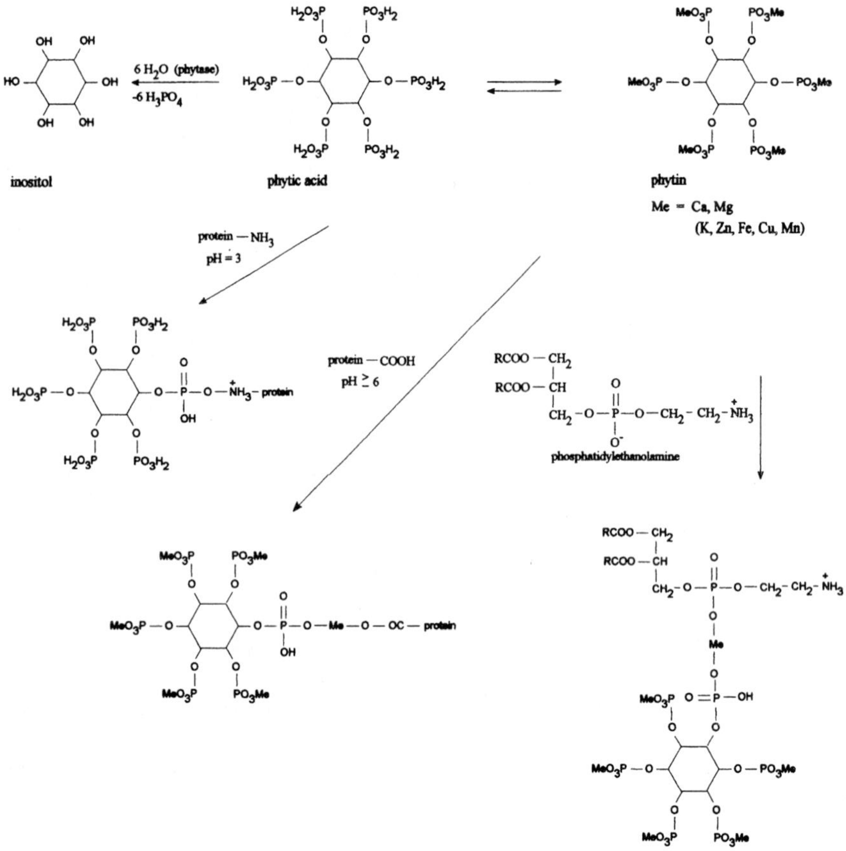

Figure 1 Reaction of phytin, phytic acid, and phytates.

OXALIC ACID AND OXALATES

Chemistry

Oxalic acid is the simplest dicarboxylic acid. It occurs both as a soluble form and as insoluble calcium oxalate. With respect to the low solubility of calcium oxalate (pKs = 8.58), a low ratio of calcium vs. oxalate in the diet may cause chronic calcium deficiency.[56] The solubility of zinc is also influenced by the presence of oxalic acid.[57]

Toxic effects

Acute oxalic acid poisoning[58] is manifested by a local corrosive action in the mouth and gastrointestinal tract, effects on the nervous system, decreased blood coagulability, and renal insufficiency. There are also some connections among high oxalate consumption and arthritis and formation of urinary stones. Long-term oxalate exposure leads to a chronic deficiency of calcium and other minerals. Consumption of high-oxalate food such as spinach or rhubarb by children may lead to acute poisoning. The toxicity of rhubarb may be also due to the presence of anthraquinone glycosides.

Occurrence

Oxalic acid is a normal component of some vegetables and fruits[58] (Table 4). The most significant dietary source of oxalic acid is probably tea beverage,[58] containing 50 to 260 $mg.dm^{-3}$.

Table 4 Oxalic Acid Content in Food

Food	Oxalic acid content (%)	Ref.
Tea	0.651–0.697	59
Cofee	0.058	59
Sorghum	0.144	59
Rice	$2.9.10^{-3}$	59
Orange juice	$4.4.10^{-3}$	59
Barley malt	$(5.6–22.8).10^{-3}$	60
Wheat malt	$(22.1–50.1).10^{-3}$	60
Cocoa	0.338–0.443	61
Chocolate	$(1.6–50.8).10^{-3}$	61
Rhubarb	0.29–0.64	62
	4.7–9.6[a]	63
Spinach	6.63[a]	64
	5.4–9.8[a]	65

[a] In dry matter.

Changes during Processing and Storage

The amount of oxalic acid in some vegetables can be reduced by blanching. A large excess of water is convenient for effective leaching of oxalate from spinach. Repeated blanching of spinach in hot water decreases the oxalic acid content to 75% of the original amount.[66] In broad beans and okra, during blanching (5 min at 100°C) the oxalate level was reduced by 57 and 44%, respectively. In dry legume seeds such as beans, lentils, and peas, the processes of decortication, steeping, stewing, boiling, and baking significantly reduce the oxalate level.[67] To lower the oxalic acid content in beer, calcium precipitation is applied. Another approach is based on enzymatic decomposition of oxalate by oxalate decarboxylase[68] (EC 4.1.1.2).

NITRATES AND NITRITES

During the last 30 years, the problem of nitrate, nitrite, and *N*-nitroso compounds in the food chain has become urgent because of their possible deleterious effects on human health.

CHEMISTRY

Nitrates and nitrites are natural components of the environment, being part of the nitrogen pool in nature. Nitrates and nitrites, and specifically nitric oxide, may react in living organism or in foods, forming toxic substances such as methemoglobin or nitrosamines (page 229). They are also used as a food additives in the meat industry for improving the color stability of meat products.

Nitrites absorbed into the blood through intestinal walls may cause methemoglobinemia. It is caused by oxidation of the bivalent Fe ion to trivalent Fe of hemoglobin in the course of transformation of red hemoglobin to dark brown methemoglobin (Figure 2).

Nitrates and nitrites are used in the meat industry together with salt in curing mixtures when preparing meat for further processing, such as smoking. They are added in order to increase stability, to preserve or improve color, and to protect against *Clostridium botulinum*, the bacterium producing the highly toxic botulinum toxin.

Another useful effect of curing salts is their antioxidant activity and inhibition of undesirable bacteria that could otherwise influence the storage of the products.

$$HNO_2 \longrightarrow NO^+ + OH$$
$$Fe^{2+} + NO^+ \longrightarrow Fe^{3+} + NO$$
$$4\,HNO_2 + HbO_2 + 2\,H_2O \longrightarrow 4\,HNO_3 + 4\,MetHbOH + O_2$$

Figure 2 Formation of methemoglobin. Hb = hemoglobin, MetHb = methemoglobin.

$$H^+ + Mb + NO_2^- \longrightarrow NO + MetMb^+(OH^-)$$
$$Mb + NO \longrightarrow MbNO$$
$$MetMb + AA \longrightarrow Mb + DAK$$

Figure 3 Reaction of nitrites with myoglobin. Mb = myoglobin, MetMb = metmyoglobin, MbNO = nitroxymyoglobin, AA = ascorbic acid, DAK = dehydroascorbic acid.

The pink color of corned meat and meat products is caused by the reaction of nitrite with the heme, inhibiting the oxidation of Fe atom during further processing.

The reaction of nitrites contributing to the pink color can be simply explained as follows: first, the nitrite is reduced to nitric oxide (NO) by the myoglobin in an acidic environment, and NO thus formed reacts with a further molecule of myoglobin, leading to the formation of nitroxymyoglobin. To prevent the formation of metmyoglobin due to partial oxidation of myoglobin, ascorbic acid may be added, which reduces metmyoglobin back to myoglobin (Figure 3).

During the thermal treatment or due to acidification, globin is separated from nitroxsyheme and a further NO molecule is bound to the vacant 5th coordination position of the heme, giving rise to nitroxyhemochrome (also dinitroxyhemochrome) (Figure 4). The latter is stable to oxidation in the dark, even at a high temperatures. Under the action of light, dissociation of stabilizing NO molecules occurs, and the heme formed is quickly oxidized to hemin or, as the case may be, a further dissociation occurs. Cut meat products become grey and pale.

A part of the nitrite from the curing salt forms colored compounds and the remainder reacts with other meat components. In manufactured products therefore, nitrite occurs in different forms.

Nitrate does not react directly with heme coloring substances; it must first be converted to nitrite or nitric oxide via the nitrate-reducing microflora (bacteria of the genus *Micrococcus, Streptococcus,* etc.).

Basic components of curing salts — nitrates and nitrites — are progressively decomposed during the curing of meat products.[69]

TOXIC EFFECTS

Nitrates in low concentrations and in a nonreducing environment are not dangerous for a healthy adult, because they are relatively quickly reduced in the kidney. The acceptable daily dose, safe even for long-term consumption, was fixed in 1974 by the World Health Organization at 5 mg $NaNO_3$ (3.5 mg NO_3^-) per 1 kg body weight.

The potential toxicity of nitrates in food consists in their possible reduction to a lower oxidation state (nitrites) which can cause some serious health problems not only in children, but also in adults.

Nitrates are reduced by nitrate reductase enzymes (EC 1.7.7.1), both exogenously and endogenously. The first case, for instance, occurs during transport, storage, and processing

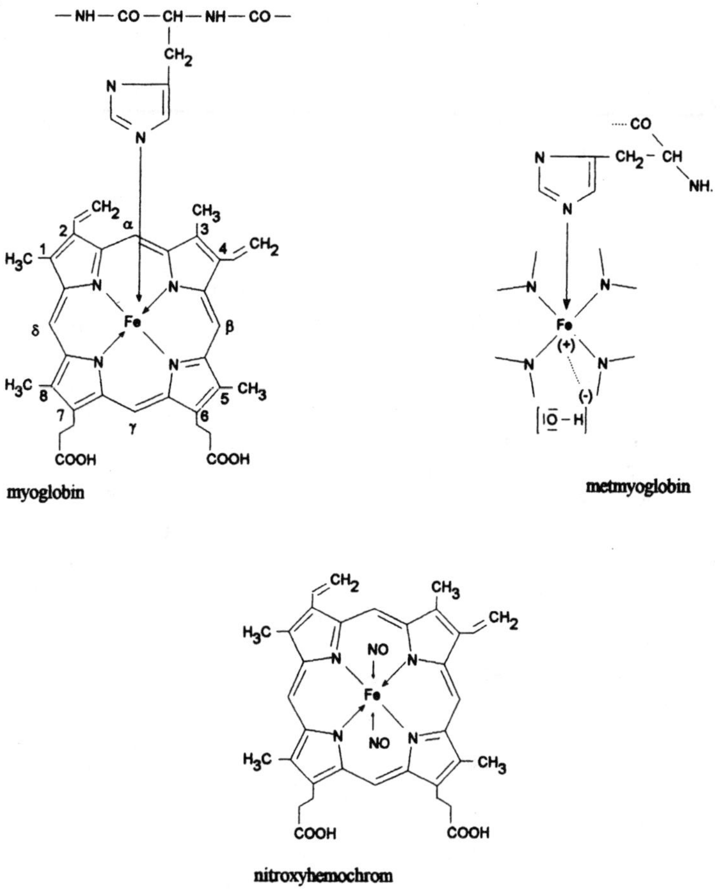

Figure 4 Heme-coloring substances.

of agricultural products and food. Unsuitable storage of prepared vegetable or vegetable-meat meals with a high nitrate content is particularly dangerous, especially when food is kept under warm conditions for a long time.

Nitrites can arise endogenously in the gastrointestinal tract or in the mouth. According to Spiegelhalder,[70] 6 to 7% of consumed nitrates are converted to nitrites within 24 h. Nitrates are absorbed and transferred into the blood stream and into tissues. After 4 to 12 h, most of the nitrate is eliminated by the kidneys (about 80% for young and 50% for old people). The rest remains in the body. Through blood circulation, nitrates return to salivary glands where they concentrate and return to the oral cavity. The consumed quantity of nitrates is proportional to their concentration in the saliva, which is quantitatively connected to the nitrite formation.

Reduction of endogenous nitrates to nitrites may take place in the oral cavity. There is a linear relation between the quantity of nitrate consumed in food and the quantity secreted into the saliva, as well as the degree of nitrite formation in saliva, which has been proved experimentally.[73] A certain threshold concentration seems to be needed for the nitrates to be secreted to the oral cavity and for their consequent reduction to nitrites (50 mg NO_3^-). If the quantity of nitrate consumed is less than that level, it should not initiate the formation of nitrite or *N*-nitro compounds. Large differences occur between individuals.

Under normal physiologic conditions, about 2% of the oxidized hemoglobin cannot transfer oxygen. Red globule reductases of an adult are able to transform the methemoglobin back to hemoglobin.

Nitrites represent an acute danger for young babies. In the first 2 to 4 months of life, their own enzymatic system is not yet sufficiently developed in the erythrocytes to reverse the reduction of methemoglobin to hemoglobin. Fetal F hemoglobin in newborn children (its part being about 85% at the moment of birth) is more predisposed to oxidation by nitrites than in the A hemoglobin of an adult. In addition, in the stomach of very young babies, there is a lower acid concentration, which means a higher pH than in later years, and for that reason some microorganisms, normally nonpathogenous, can proliferate there as well as in the upper parts of the intestinal tract. These microorganisms reduce nitrates to nitrites before the nitrates can be absorbed in the normal way. This happens with dyspepsias and similar digestion troubles, when the intestinal microflora are displaced to upper parts of the digestive tract where some of the nitrates are not yet absorbed. Nitrites get into blood and affect a number of organs causing mainly methemoglobinemia.

The external manifestation of this disease is a gray-blue or blue-violet coloring of the mucous membranes and skin of peripheral parts of body, mainly the lips (so-called cyanosis), accompanied by a fall of blood pressure, a higher pulse frequency, and shortness of breath. The first symptoms appear at a 6 to 7% concentration of methemoglobin in the blood. A concentration of 10 to 20% causes some problems, and at a level of 20 to 40% more serious ones occur, while at over 40% it can lead to death. At levels over 50%, the physiological ratio of both basic components of hemoglobin is totally disturbed.

Until recently, methemoglobinemia was considered to be dangerous only for children of a very young age, but it has now been proved that an asymptomatic form of methemoglobinemia may occur with older children and even with adults. Nitrates in higher concentrations may influence enzymes in the digestive organs, resorption of certain nutrients, metabolism of vitamin A, and the thyroid gland function. Symptoms of nitrate and/or nitrite poisoning may also cause changes in electrocardiogram values and in the central nervous system. In experiments with animals, changes in electrical activities of brain, memory, and behavior troubles, as well as a reduction of motor activities, have been observed due to increased nitrate levels in food. Epidemiological research done in the former Soviet Union on a group of children consuming water high in nitrates for a long time indicate a reduced acquisition of conditioned reflexes and reduced response to visual and auditive stimulations.[71] A possible connection between a higher nitrate content in certain susceptible individuals and the appearance of alimentary pseudoallergies is being admitted. According to some recent data, an increased intake of nitrates (that are transformed to nitrites) by the human body may weaken the immune system.[72]

Medical research has recently been aimed at the effect of nitrates and nitrites on the formation of N-nitroso compounds (page 229).

OCCURRENCE

Nitrates may get into food from several sources. They are, in low concentrations, a natural component of the environment, being part of the nitrogen pool in nature. They often occur in soil in increased concentrations and from there they get into water and plants. Nitrates and nitrites are used as additives for maintaining the natural color of final products and for inhibiting certain microbial processes in the processing some raw materials of animal origin in the food industry.

Table 5 Average Daily Nitrate and Nitrite Consumption per Capita from Different Food Groups

Sample	Nitrate (mg)	Nitrite (mg)
Vegetables and potatoes	40.0–80.0	0.1–0.3
Fruits	1.0–4.0	Traces
Cereals	1.5–2.5	0.2–0.4
Meat and meat products	5.5–12.5	0.4–1.0
Milk and milk products	0.2–0.5	Traces

The total daily intake of nitrates per person varies according to individual dietary habits. In Europe and North America, on average 75% of total intake is consumed with vegetables and potatoes, about 15% with meat and meat products, and the rest with other foodstuffs. Individual differences may nevertheless be considerable[73] (Table 5).

Occurrence in Foodstuffs of Plant Origin

The nitrate content of plants is influenced by the environmental conditions in which the plant is grown and ripened. The nitrate pool is very labile and dynamic, and for that reason the environmental effects may exert a very strong influence upon the variability of their content.

In general, nitrates accumulate in plants in higher quantities when the nitrogen cannot be utilized by the plant and when the plant cannot reduce nitrates in its metabolism to a more assimilable ammonia form. This may, for instance, be due to improper thermal, humidity, and especially light conditions inducing a deficiency in carbon compounds necessary for the transformation of accumulated nitrate nitrogen into amino acids with consecutive protein synthesis.[74]

Data about consumption of nitrates in foodstuffs show that vegetables and potatoes are the main source. There are great differences between different vegetable species as to their ability to accumulate nitrates. From that point of view, they may approximately be classified into three groups:

1. Species with a high content (over 1,000 mg $NO_3^-.kg^{-1}$ of fresh matter): lettuce, spinach, mangold, endive, beetroot, white and black radish, different forms of garden radish, Chinese cabbage, Pekinese cabbage, kohlrabi, celery, rhubarb, garden cress, sweet fennel, corn salad, and purslane.
2. Species with a middle content (250 to 1000 mg $NO_3^-.kg^{-1}$ of fresh matter): white and red cabbage, savoy cabbage, kale, cauliflower, leek, eggplant, parsley, celeriac, carrot, parsnip, forced cucumber, muskmelon, watermelon, zucchini, squash, pumpkin, broccoli, chives, garlic, swede, turnip, horseradish, snap bean, and potato.
3. Species with a low content (under 250 mg $NO_3^-.kg^{-1}$ of fresh matter): Brussels sprouts, onion, sweet pepper, tomato, garden pea, artichoke, asparagus, scorzonera, cucumber, sweet corn, and salsify.

The ability to cumulate nitrates in various cultivars of some species may vary considerably. Nitrate distribution in different parts of plants is not identical. Parts of the plant involving nutrient transport usually contain more NO_3^- than assimilative and generative organs. The highest concentrations are to be found in leaf veins, petioles, stalks, and stems, the lowest ones in leaf blades and fruits. In peel and layers near to the surface of the fruit, the nitrate content is higher.[75-77]

In fruits, nitrates are mostly present only in negligible quantities, but slightly higher concentrations may be found in bananas, strawberries, and melons, which are sometimes classified as vegetables. Small quantities of nitrates are present in wines.

The nitrate content of cereal grains as well as grains of other crops and weeds is usually largely below the limits of hygienic risk.

In spices, an increased nitrate accumulation has been found in sweet marjoram and ginger.

Occurrence in Foodstuffs of Animal Origin

Increased nitrate content is a nonphysiological constituent in animals in contrast to plants, where nitrates are a natural nutrient. For that reason and under normal circumstances, NO_3^- concentrations in raw materials of animal origin (meat and milk) are very low. Nitrates and nitrites can nevertheless enter final products during manufacture. They are used in the meat industry together with salt in curing mixtures in the meat for further processing, especially smoking.

Residual NO_3^- and NO_2^- concentrations in meat products are controlled by legislation. Sometimes these levels may be exceeded, not because of any error in the manufacturing process, but by a high nitrate content in the water or spices[10] used. The use of nitrites is also authorized in some countries for preparing some specially fermented fish products, whereas it is prohibited in the preparation of meatballs, meat fricassees, meat stuffings, and similar products from minced or chopped meat. For that purpose, even using nitrates is forbidden. Certain convenience foods which are usually baked can lead to a possible danger of nitrosamine formation. The same risk is, nevertheless, possible also in some meat stuffings and fillings contained in some combined meat-vegetable oven-ready food (for instance, kale and cabbage rolls), even when no nitrates or nitrites have been used during their preparation. The presence of secondary amines in meat together with nitrates and nitrites in vegetables (in unsuitably stored products), combined with cooking in the kitchen may give rise to conditions for nitrosamine formation (page 229). At any rate, it is recommended that vegetables with a low nitrate content be used for the production of meat-vegetable oven-ready meals; alternatively, compounds like ascorbic acid can be added to inhibit the formation of nitrosamines[79] (page 231).

In the production of hard sliced cheese, potassium nitrate is used to prevent consecutive swelling due to gases arising from some the activities of some bacteria, as for instance, *Clostridium tyrobutyricum*. In some countries, however, their use in the dairy industry is forbidden.

Milk reconstituted at home in the kitchen from dried milk products may contain excessive levels of nitrate derived from the main water supply, and this may be of special importance for children. A baby consuming, in proportion to its weight, five times more water than an adult, may suffer more from this than by being fed standard vegetable meals. The nitrate concentration in milk may be influenced by the nitrate content in the fodder of dairy cows.[80-81]

CHANGES DURING PROCESSING AND STORAGE

Storage

The method of harvesting as well as postharvest treatment and transport of vegetables and potatoes may significantly influence their biological value. Products damaged during the harvest, mechanically impaired and tainted, facilitate an increase in the activity of microorganisms, which can lead to reduction of nitrate to nitrite.[82] Poor transport and anaerobic storage conditions at an unsuitable temperature induce a greater risk, mainly in leaf vegetables. Processing factories should be situated as close as possible to farms to reduce the possibility of vegetable deterioration during transport.[83]

During storage of plant products, nitrate is reduced to nitrite by intramolecular respiration and, at a higher temperature, by microorganism activity, whereas this does not occur in freshly harvested plant material. Hildebrandt[84] studied spinach under different storage conditions. At 5°C the nitrate content in whole leaves remained practically unchanged during 15 days, and the nitrite content increased only slightly from the 5th day of the experiment. At 22°C, the nitrate content decreased after 7 d from 1,720 mg NO_3^-.kg^{-1} to 1,120 mg, and the nitrite concentration increased from an initial 8 mg NO_2^-.kg^{-1} up to 423 mg. In homogenized samples at 5°C, the nitrate content decreased during 15 d from 1,780 mg.kg^{-1} to 1,240 mg, and the nitrite content increased from the initial trace quantity up to 415 mg.kg^{-1}. At 22°C, the nitrate content reached zero after 4 d and the nitrite content increased in the same time from a trace quantity to 1,620 mg NO_2^-.kg^{-1}. At –18°C, there were no changes in NO_3^- and NO_2^- content in whole leaves which is the same for the homogenized leaves, even after 90 d of storage. Similar results were obtained in other vegetables like white and red cabbage, kale, endive, leek, and rhubarb.[85]

A similar study of nitrate and nitrite dynamics in carrots during storage was done by Barthová et al.[86] It was shown that blanching (5 min at 95°C) inactivated the enzymes and bacteria so that the NO_3^- reduction to NO_2^- was negligible in comparison with fresh matter. No significant changes were noticed during storage at 5°C after 48 h, and at 25°C there was, after 10 to 12 h, a significant nitrate reduction to nitrite that was later reduced to lower oxidation states (Tables 6 and 7).

Gislason et al.[87] studied the storage of five potato varieties grown in five localities at three fertilizing levels. In all experiments, the nitrate content decreased after a 6-month storage at 5°C. On average, the reduction was approximately 12% after 90 d of storage and 20% after 180 d of storage.

Gumargalieva et al.[88] showed that with several potato varieties a linear decrease of NO_3^- content occurs during storage.

Culinary and Industrial Processing

Current culinary and industrial processing of vegetables and potatoes are able to reduce markedly even high nitrate levels in the raw material. Cleaning and washing are of a great importance. Potatoes, for instance, may in this way lose some 30% of initial nitrate content and with further cooking a further 60%.[89,90]

In the production of sterile vegetable and potato products besides peeling and blanching, the method of sterilizing, as well as the nitrate contribution from any added preservative must be considered. (Table 8). Changes of nitrate and nitrite content in potato during different culinary processing is described by Cieslik[91] (Table 9).

Reduction of nitrate concentrations in vegetables and potatoes during their wet thermal processing has been studied in many countries. It has been concluded that boiling in water can reduce the initial nitrate content by as much as 70 to 80% according to the vegetable species, method of pretreatment, volume of water used and length and temperature of cooking.

According to Przybylowski and Sajko, the content of nitrates and nitrites in some milk and vegetable baby foods during 2 weeks' storage does not change; after 3 months storage a small decrease was detected.[92]

On the basis of large studies on spinach, a nomograph (Figure 5) has been plotted which allows one to estimate relatively precisely the leaching of nitrates by water (temperature between 70 and 130°C) and a leaching period from 0.5 to 16 min. These levels can also be used for other leaf vegetables, when appropriately modified.[93,94] Studies on spinach blanching at 85 to 90°C have shown that nitrate leaching is greatest during the first 3 minutes.[95] A detailed study has been done with spinach samples differing in the initial nitrate content, with the aim of determining the changes occurring during thermal sterilizing and freezing. The average residual NO_3^- content was 83% after sterilizing and 61% after freezing, compared to the nitrate content in the raw vegetable.[96-101]

Table 6 Nitrate and Nitrite Content in Carrot Stored at 5°C

	Nitrate ($mg.kg^{-1}$ in fresh matter)			Nitrite ($mg.kg^{-1}$ in fresh matter)		
Sample	**Initial**	**After 24 h**	**After 48 h**	**Initial**	**After 24 h**	**After 48 h**
Fresh	430	420	390	0.7	0.7	1.0
Purée	360	340	320	0.5	0.6	1.1
Juice	420	400	380	0.6	0.6	1.7
Blanched	360	350	330	0.5	0.5	0.7

From Barthová, Z., Madarič, A., and Görner, F., *Čs. Hyg.*, 29, 478, 1984. With permission.

Table 7 Nitrate and Nitrite Content in Carrot Stored at 25°C

	Nitrate ($mg.kg^{-1}$ in fresh matter)			Nitrite ($mg.kg^{-1}$ in fresh matter)		
Sample	**Initial**	**After 16 h**	**After 24 h**	**Initial**	**After 16 h**	**After 24 h**
Fresh	430	280	68	0.7	100	78
Purée	360	250	42	0.5	130	54
Juice	420	200	30	0.6	160	63
Blanched	360	290	130	0.5	17	11

From Barthová, Z., Madarič, A. and Görner, F., *Čs. Hyg.*, 29, 478, 1984. With permission.

Table 8 Effect of Boiling in Water on Nitrate Content of Some Vegetables (mg $Nitrate.kg^{-1}$ in Fresh Matter)

	Time of boiling	Nitrate content		
Species	**(min)**	**Raw sample**	**After boiling**	**In extract**
Kohlrabi	25	1,576	244	1,357
Celeriac	25	81	26	54
Carrot	20	192	45	140
Potatoes	20	134	30	109
Lettuce	10	2,280	413	1,816
Sauerkraut	25	269	41	224

Table 9 Changes of Nitrate and Nitrite Contents in Potatoes During Culinary Processing

	Decrease (%)	
Process	**Nitrate**	**Nitrite**
Potatoes		
Cooked unpeeled	16	60
Cooked peeled, whole	47	65
Cooked peeled, sliced	71	42
Cooked and stored in refrigerator until next day and warmed in oil	45	54
Peeled and pressure cooked	2	36
French-fried at 180°C	32	70
Unpeeled baked in slices at 300°C	20	50
Peeled and microwave baked	8	43
Peeled and microwave cooked	30	50

Note: Content of nitrate and nitrite in raw potatoes was 225 $mg.kg^{-1}$ and 3.71 $mg.kg^{-1}$, respectively.

From Cieslik, E., *Przem. Spoz.*, 46, 266, 1992. With permission.

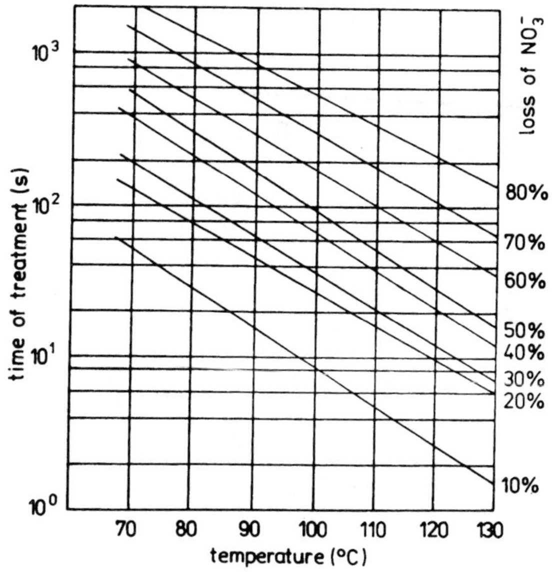

Figure 5 Nomograph to determine alternations of nitrate content in spinach during thermal treatment in water. From Paulus, K., *J. Food Sci.,* 44, 1169, 1979. With permission.

Vegetable products, especially when prepared from species with a high ability to accumulate nitrites, should be eaten as soon as possible after preparation. This is also true for frozen and pasteurized products.[102] After opening the tin, microorganisms able to reduce nitrates to nitrites may get into the product. Nitrites are formed by bacterial reduction not only at room temperature but also in the refrigerator. In samples where nonhygienic food preservation was modeled by inoculating with *Escherichia coli*, the nitrite content was much higher than in the control.[103] In Germany, a process aimed at reducing the nitrate content of food has been studied.[104] It is based on using pure cultures or mixtures of bacteria able to reduce nitrate without formation of undesirable metabolites and without causing deleterious effects on nutritional and sensory qualities of the products. These denitrification bacteria are, for instance, *Pseudomonas stutzeri, Pseudomonas denitrificans, Bacillus licheniformis*, and *Paracoccus denitrificans*. Experiments with the last-named microorganism were conducted with a view of reducing NO_3^- content in vegetable juice on the same principle as used in the treatment of drinking water.[104]

The presence of ascorbic acid, fiber, and possibly also tocopherols may compensate for increased nitrate levels in vegetables. Confirmation that vegetables contain protective factors against undesirable reactions may be substantiated, because no direct risks to human health have been reported, with the exception of infant methemoglobinemia due to an increased vegetable consumption. This applies even for such population groups in which consumption is considerably above the average, as for instance for vegetarians.

Equally in food of animal origin, ascorbic acid and tocopherols may serve as inhibitors of nitrosation processes. Products in which curing salts have been used should not be further processed at high temperature, such as, for instance, bacon or fried smoked meats.[105]

Dietary nitrate stress in the population may be reduced by using agricultural practices which are as natural as possible for the locality and variety. This may be done by controlling the agricultural processes, especially the use of fertilizers, postharvest processing, and storage. The food industry can also help by choosing suitable raw materials and by modifying manufacturing processes for plant and animal products. Finally, the consumer himself should be kept informed about the distribution of nitrates in different parts of the plant and about optimal cooking methods.

REFERENCES

1. Fergusson, J. E., *The Heavy Elements. Chemistry, Environmental Impact and Health Effects,* Pergamon Press, Oxford, 1988.
2. Nriagu, J. O., Food contamination with cadmium in the environment, in *Food Contamination from Environmental Sources,* Nriagu, J. O. and Simmons, M. S., Eds., John Wiley, New York, 1990.
3. Flegal, A. R., Smith, D. R., and Elias, R. W., Lead contamination in food, in *Food Contamination from Environmental Sources,* Nriagu, J. O. and Simmons, M. S., Eds., John Wiley, New York, 1990.
4. Friberg, L. and Elinder, C. G., Cadmium toxicity in humans, in *Essential and Toxic Trace Elements in Human Health and Disease*, Prasad, A. S., Ed., A. R. Liss,, New York, 1988, 559.
5. Skerfving, S., Toxicology of inorganic lead, in *Essential and Toxic Trace Elements in Human Health and Disease*, Prasad, A. S., Ed., A. R. Liss, New York, 1988, 611.
6. FAO/WHO, Sixteenth Rep. Joint FAO/WHO Expert Committee on Food Additives, WHO Tech. Rep. Ser. No. 505, World Health Organization, Geneva, 1972.
7. Jorhem, L., Mattson, P., and Slorach, S., Lead, cadmium, zinc and certain other metals in foods on the Swedish market, *Var Foda*, 36, Suppl. 3, 1984.
8. Slorach, S., Gustafsson, I. B., Jorhem, L., and Mattsson, P., Intake of lead, cadmium and certain other metals via a typical Swedish weekly diet, *Var Foda*, 35, Suppl. 1, 1983.
9. Ruick, G., Ergebnisse eines Monitoring-Programmes zur Emittlung der Aufnahme von Kupfer, Blei, Cadmium, Zink und Nickel mit Lebensmitteln, *Z. Lebensm. Unters. Forsch.*, 192, 249, 1991.
10. Sherlock, J. C., Lead in food and the diet, *Environ. Geochem. Health*, 9, 43, 1987.
11. Wolnik, K. A., Fricke, F. L., Capar, S. G., Braude, G. L., Meyer, M. W., Satzger, R. D. and Bonnin, E., Elements in major raw agricultural crops in the United States. I. Cadmium and lead in lettuce, peanuts, potatoes, soybeans, sweet corn and wheat, *J. Agric. Food Chem.*, 31, 1240, 1983.
12. Wolnik, K. A., Fricke, F. L., Capar, S. G., Meyer, M. W., Satzger, R. D., Bonnin, E., and Gaston, C. M., Elements in major raw agricultural crops in the United States. III. Cadmium, lead, and eleven other elements in carrots, field corn, onions, rice, spinach and tomatoes, *J. Agric. Food Chem.*, 33, 807, 1985.
13. Capar, S. G., Survey of lead and cadmium in adult canned foods eaten by young children, *J. Assoc. Off. Anal. Chem.*, 3, 257, 1990.
14. Jelinek, C. F., Levels of lead in the United States food supply, *J. Assoc. Off. Anal. Chem.*, 65, 942, 1982.
15. Seeger, R., Cadmium in Pilzen, *Z. Lebensm. Unters. Forsch.*, 166, 23, 1978.
16. Vetter, J., Vergleichende Untersuchung des Mineralstoffgehaltes der Gattungen *Agaricus* (Champingnon) und *Pleurotus* (Austernseitling), *Z. Lebensm. Unters. Forsch.*, 189, 346, 1989.
17. Kloke, A., Sauerbeck, D. R., and Vetter, H., The contamination of plants and soils with heavy metals and the transport of metals in terrestrial food chains, in *Changing Metal Cycles and Human Health,* Nriagu, J. O., Ed., Springer Verlag, Berlin, 1984.
18. Zurera, G., Estrada, B., Rincon, F., and Pozo, R., Lead and cadmium contamination levels in edible vegetables, *Bull. Environ. Contam. Toxicol.*, 38, 805, 1987.
19. Gutenmann, W. H., Bache, C. A., McCahan, J. B., and Lisk, D. J., Heavy metals and chlorinated hydrocarbons in marine fish products, *Nutr. Rep. Int.*, 38, 1157, 1988.
20. Tam, S. Y. K. and Mok, C. S., Metallic contamination in oyster and other seafood in Hong Kong, *Food Addit. Contam.*, 8, 333, 1991.
21. Narres, H. D., Valenta, P., and Nürnberg, H. W., Die voltammetrische Bestimmung von Swermetallen in Fleisch und inneren Organen von Schlachtrindern, *Z. Lebensm. Unters. Forsch.*, 179, 440, 1984.
22. Schelenz, R., Boppel, B., Zacharias, R., and Fischer, E.,Veränderung der Gehalte von Blei, Cadmium und Quecksilber in Gemüsen bei der haushaltsüblichen Zubereitung, *BFE - Ber.*, 1979/1.
23. Braude, G. L., Nash, A. M., Wolf, W. J., Carr, R. L., and Chaney, R. L., Cadmium and lead content of soybean products, *J. Food Sci.*, 45, 1187, 1980.

24. Kaiser, G. and Tölg, G., Mercury, in *Handbook of Environmental Chemistry,* Vol. 3, Part A, *Anthropogenic Compounds,* Hutzinger, O., Ed., Springer Verlag, Berlin, 1980.
25. Cibulka, J., *Pohyb olova, kadmia a rtuti v biosféřě (The Movement of Lead, Cadmium and Mercury in the Biosphere),* Academia, Prague, 1991.
26. Jensen, S. and Jernelov, A., Biological methylation of mercury in aquatic organisms, *Nature*, 223, 753, 1969.
27. FAO/WHO, Sixteenth Rep. Joint FAO/WHO Expert Committee on Food Additives, WHO Tech. Rep. Ser. No. 505, WHO, Geneva, 1972.
28. Gartrell, M. J., Craun, J. C., Podrebarac, D. S., and Gunderson, E. L., Pesticides, selected elements, and other chemicals in adult total diet samples, October 1980–March 1982, *J. Assoc. Off. Anal. Chem.*, 69, 146, 1986.
29. Van Dokkum, W., De Vos, R. H., Muys, Th., and Wesstra, J. A., Minerals and trace elements in total diets in The Netherlands, *Br. J. Nutr.*, 61, 7, 1989.
30. Palušová, O., Ursínyová, M. and Uhnák, J., Mercury levels in the components of the environment and diets, *Sci. Total Environ.*, 101, 79, 1991.
31. Hernandez Garcia, M. T., Martinez Para, M. C., and Masoud, T. A., Variacion en la cantidad de mercurio en muestras de pescado sometidas a diversos procesos culinarios, *Anal. Bromatol.*, 40, 291, 1988.
32. Nriagu, J. O. and Azcue, J. M., Food contamination with arsenic in the environmental, in *Food Contamination from Environmental Sources*, Nriagu, J. O. and Simrmons, M. S., Eds., J. Wiley, New York, 1990.
33. Vaessen, H. A. H. G. and van Ooik A., Speciation of arsenic in Dutch total diets: methodology and results, *Z. Lebensm. Unters. Forsch.*, 189, 232, 1989.
34. Schelenz, R., Veränderung des Gehaltes von Arsen in Gemüsen bei der haushaltsüblichen Zubereitung, *BFE - Ber.* 1980/3.
35. Greger, J. L., Aluminum content of the American diet, *Food Technol.*, 39, 73, 1985.
36. Sherlock, J. C. and Smart, G. A., Thallium in food and the diet, *Food Addit. Contam.*, 3, 363, 1986.
37. Combs, G. F., Jr., Selenium in foods, *Adv. Food Res.*, 32, 85, 1988.
38. Shamberger, R. J., *Biochemistry of Selenium*, Plenum Press, New York, 1983.
39. Higgs, D. J., Morris, V. C., and Levander, O. A., Effect of cooking on selenium content of foods, *J. Agric. Food Chem.*, 20, 678, 1972.
40. Maga, J. A., Phytate: its chemistry, occurrence, food interactions, nutritional significance and methods of analysis, *J. Agric. Food Chem.*, 30, 1, 1982.
41. Tomlinson, R. V. and Ballou, C. E., Myoinositol phosphate intermediates in dephosphorylation of phytic acid by phytase, *Biochemistry*, 1, 166, 1962.
42. Lolas, G. M., Palamidis, N., and Markakis, P., The phytic acid-total phosphorus relation in barley, oats, soybeans and wheat, *Cereal Chem.*, 53, 867, 1976.
43. O'Dell, B. L., de Boland, A. R., and Koirtyohann, S. R., Distribution of phytate and nutritionally important elements among the morphological components of cereal grains, *J. Agric. Food Chem.*, 20, 718, 1972.
44. de Boland, A. R., Garner, G. B., and O'Dell, B. L., Identification and properties of phytate in cereal grains and oilseed products, *J. Agric. Food Chem.*, 23, 1186, 1975.
45. Lolas, G. M. and Markakis, P., Phytic acid and other phosphorus compounds of beans (*Phaseolus vulgaris*). *J. Agric. Food Chem.*, 23, 13, 1975.
46. Uppstrom, B. and Svensson, R., Determination of phytic acid in rapeseed meal, *J. Sci. Food Agric.*, 31, 651, 1980.
47. Okubo, K., Waldrop, A. B., Iacobucci, G. A., and Meyers, D. V., Preparation of low-phytate soybean protein isolate and concentrate by ultrafiltration, *Cereal Chem.*, 52, 263, 1975.
48. de Rham, O. and Jost, T., Phytate-protein interaction in soybean extracts and low-phytate soy protein products, *J. Food Sci.*, 44, 596, 1979.
49. Szuhaj, B. F. and List, G. R., *Lecithins*, American Oil Chemists' Society, Champaign, IL, 1985.
50. Winters, D. D., Handel, A. P., and Lohrberg, J. D., Phytic acid content of crude degumed and retail soybean oils and its effect on stability, *J. Food Sci.*, 49, 1113, 1984.
51. McKenzie, J. M., Content of phytate and minerals in instant coffee, coffee beans and coffee beverage, *Nutr. Rep. Int.*, 29, 387, 1984.

52. Clydesdale, F. M. and Camire, A. L., Effect of pH and heat on the binding of iron, calcium, magnesium and zinc and the loss of phytic acid in soy flour, *J. Food Sci.*, 48, 272, 1983.
53. Hafez, Y. S., Mohammed, A. J., Perera, P. A., Singh, G., and Hussein, A. S., Effects of microwave heating and gamma irradiation on phytate and phospholipid contents of soybean (*Glycine max*. L.), *J. Food Sci.*, 54, 958, 1989.
54. Toma, R. B. and Tabekhia, M. M., Changes in mineral elements and phytic acid contents during cooking of three California rice varieties, *J. Food Sci.*, 44, 619, 1979.
55. Reinhold, J. G., Phytate concentrations of leavened and unleavened Iranian breads, *Ecol. Food Nutr.*, 1, 187, 1972.
56. Sing, P. P., Kothari, L. K., Sharma, D. C., and Saxena, S. N., Nutritional value of foods in relation to their oxalic acid content, *Am. J. Clin. Nutr.*, 25, 1147, 1972.
57. Faboya, O. O., The interaction between oxalic acid and divalent ions — Mg^{2+}, Zn^{2+} and Ca^{2+} — in aqueous medium, *Food Chem.*, 38, 179, 1990.
58. Libert, B. and Franceschi, V. R., Oxalate in crop plants, *J. Agric. Food Chem.*, 35, 926, 1987.
59. Najjar, M. F., Ben Amor, M. A., Oueslati, A., Chemli, R., Garnaoui, N., Boukef, K., and Zouaghi, H., Dietary oxalate and risk of lithiasis in Tunisia, *Lyon Pharm.*, 38, 291, 1987.
60. Narziss, L., Reicheneder, E., and Iwan, H. J., Possibilities of influencing of oxalate content of beer with special consideration of wheat malts and beer, *Monatsschr. Brauwiss.*, 39, 4, 1986.
61. Lagemann, M., Graef, V., and Anders, D., Determination of oxalic acid content of cocoa and cocoa products by the oxalate decarboxylase method, *Dtsch. Lebensm. Rundsch.*, 81, 140, 1985.
62. Treptow, H., Rhubarb (*Rheum sp.*) and its use, *Ernährung*, 9, 179, 1985.
63. Allison, R. M., Soluble oxalates, ascorbic and other constituents of rhubarb, *J. Sci. Food Agric.*, 17, 554, 1966.
64. Sachde, A. G., Al-Bakir, A. Y., Aziz, M. A. A., and Faris, J. A., Oxalic acid content of some common Iraqi vegetables, *Iraqi J. Agric. Sci. "Zanco"*, 2, 33, 1984.
65. Kitchen, J. W., Burns, E. E., and Perry B. A., Calcium oxalate content of spinach (*Spinacia oleracea* L.), *Proc. Am. Soc. Hortic. Sci.*, 84, 441, 1964.
66. Velíšek, J., unpublished data, 1993.
67. Gad, S. S., Esmat el-Zalaki, M., Mohamed, M. S., and Mohasseb, S. Z., Oxalate content of some leafy vegetables and dry legumes consumed widely in Egypt, *Food Chem.*, 8, 169, 1982.
68. Hiatt, W. R. and Owades, J. L., Oxalic acid removal in beer production, *U.S. Patent*, 4,652,452, 1987.
69. Moehler, K. and Scheerer, C., Bilanz der Bildung von Pökelfarbstoff in Muskelfleisch und Bilanzvergleich zwischen Fleischerzeugnissen des Handels und Modelversuchen mit Muskelfleisch und Nitrit, *Z. Lebensm. Unters. Forsch.*, 168, 381, 1979.
70. Spiegelhalder, B., Nitrosamine und Nitrosaminvorläufer in pflanzlichen Lebensmitteln, in *5th Joint Congr., X. CIQ XVIII, Deutsche Geselschaft für Qualitätforsahung Plant Foods and Human Health*, Kiel, 1982, 343.
71. Preussmann, R., Nitrite and Nitrate in der Nahrung und im Wasser, *Bibl. Nutr. Dieta*, 41, 66, 1988.
72. Causeret, J., Nitrates, nitrites, nitrosamines: apports alimentaires et sante, *Annu. Fals. Exp. Chim.*, 77, 133, 1984.
73. Selenka, F. and Brand-Grimm, D., Nitrat und Nitrit in menschlicher Nahrung. Bestimmung der täglichen Aufnahme und deren Schwankungsbreite, *Zentralbl. Bakteriol. Hyg. I. Abt., Orig. B*, 162, 449, 1976.
74. Prugar, J., Vaněk, V., Sokolov, O. A., and Semenov, V. M., Nitrates in plants, in *Nitrogen Cycles in the Present Agriculture*, Bielek, P. and Kudeyarov, V. N., Eds., Soil Fertility Research Institute, Príroda, Bratislava, 1991, 127.
75. Prugar, J., Kluever, M., and Prugarová, A., Sorteneinflüsse auf die Akkumulation von Nitrat in verschiedenen Gemüsearten und Kartoffeln, I, *Ernährung*, 14, 740, 1990.
76. Prugar, J., Kluever, M., and Prugarová, A., Sorteneinflüsse auf die Akkumulation von Nitrat in verschiedenen Gemüsearten und Kartoffeln, II, *Ernährung*, 15, 86, 1991.
77. Prugar. J. and Prugarová, A., Distribution des Nitrats in Gemüse und Kartoffeln, *Ernährung*, 15, 142, 1991.
78. Gerhardt, U. and Windmueller, R., Beeinflussung des Nitratgehalts in Fleischwaren durch Verarbeitung von Gewürzen, *Fleischerei*, 33, 1, 1982.
79. Lange, H. J., Nitratgehalte in Kohlrouladen, *Fleischwirtschaft*, 65, 1051, 1985.

80. Remond, D., La teneur du lait de vache en nitrate, *Le lait*, 55, 547, 1975.
81. Görner, F., Hluchan, E., Szokolay, A., and Antalíkova, E., Dusičnany a dusitany v mliečnych produktoch (Nitrates and nitrites in milk products), *Čs. Hyg.*, 23, 86, 1978.
82. Ahrens, E. and El Saidy, S., Einige Bedingungen der Nitritbildung bei der Lagerung von Blattgemüse, *Landw. Forsch.*, 35, 647, 1982, Sonderheft 38.
83. Benoit, F. and Ceustermans, N., Phytotechnie et nitrates en culture maraichere, *Rev. Agric.*, 41, 23, 1988.
84. Hildebrandt, E.-A., Zur Problematik der Nitrosamine in der Pflanzenernährung, Ph.D. dissertation, Justus Liebig-Universität, Giessen, 1976.
85. Schuster, B. E. and Lee K., Nitrate and nitrite methods of analysis and levels in raw carrots and in selected vegetables and grain products, *J. Food Sci.*, 52, 1632, 1987.
86. Barthová, Z., Madarič, A., and Görner, F., Redukcia dusičnanov v rastlinných materialoch (Reduction of nitrate in plant materials), *Čs. Hyg.*, 29, 478, 1984.
87. Gislason, J., Dahle, H. K., Baerug, R., Roer, L., and Ronson, K., *Potato Res.*, 27, 331, 1984.
88. Gumargalieva, K. Z., Kalinina, I. G., and Kuchumov, N. N., Changes in nitrate content of potatoes during storage, *Pishch. Prom.*, 1, 61, 1989.
89. Bergthaller, W. and Ocker, H. D., Einfluss der Verarbeitung und der küchentechnischen Zubereitung auf den Nitratgehalt von Kartoffelerzeugnissen, *Landw. Forsch.*, 41, 288, 1984.
90. Bergthaller, W., Putz, B., and Ocker, H. D., Der Einfluss der Verarbeitung auf die Nitratkonzentration in den Produkten der Kartoffelverarbeitung, *Kartoffelbau*, 37, 337, 1986.
91. Cieslik, E., Changes of nitrate and nitrite contents during potatoes cooking, *Przem. Spoz.*, 46, 266, 1992.
92. Przybylowski, P. and Sajko, W., Changes of nitrate and nitrite contents during baby food preservation, *Przem. Spoz.*, 46, 264, 1992.
93. Paulus K., Nomographs to determine alternations of essential components in leafy products during thermal treatment in water, *J. Food Sci.*, 44, 1169, 1979.
94. Fricker, A., Einfluss der Verarbeitung auf den Nitratgehalt pflanzlicher Lebensmittel, *Landw. Forsch.*, 41, 45, 1985.
95. Moehler, K., Landwirtschaftliche und technologische Möglichkeiten zur Verringerung des Nitrat- und Nitritgehaltes in Lebensmitteln, *Mittl. Komm. Wasserforsch. DFG*, III, 220, 1984.
96. Schijvens, E. P., Zandschulp, G. van de, and Kok, J. C., De invloed van steriliseren en diepvriezen op het nitraat-en drogestofgehalte von spinazie, *Voedingsmiddelen Tech.*, 20, 32, 1987.
97. Siciliano, J., Krulick, S., Heisler, E. G., Schwartz, J. H., and White, J. W., Nitrate and nitrite content of some fresh and processed market vegetables, *J. Agric. Food Chem.*, 23, 461, 1975.
98. Sistrunk, W. A., Kale greens quality, vitamin retention and nitrate content as affected by preparation, processing and storage, *J. Food Sci.*, 45, 679, 1980.
99. Sistrunk, W. A. and Bradly, G. A., Quality and nutritional value of canned turnip greens as influenced by processing technique, *Ark. Farm Res.*, 24, 5, 1975.
100. Sistrunk, W. A. and Cash, J, N., Spinach quality attributes and nitrate-nitrite levels as related to processing and storage, *J. Am. Soc. Hortic. Sci.*, 100, 307, 1975.
101. Sistrunk, W. A., Mahon, M. K., and Freemann, D. K., Relationship of processing methodology to quality attributes and nutritional value of canned spinach, *Hortic. Sci.*, 12, 59, 1977.
102. Eerola, M., Varo, P., and Koivistoinen, P., Nitrate and nitrite in spinach as affected by application of different levels of nitrogen fertilizer, blanching, and storage after thawing of frozen product, *Acta Agric. Scand.*, 24, 268, 1974.
103. Hlavsová, D., Tuček, J., and Turek, B., Hygienický význam redukce dusičnanů v zelenině (Hygienic relevance of nitrate reduction in vegetables), *Čs. Hyg.*,15, 264, 1970.
104. Mayer-Miebach, E., Rathjen A., and Kerner, M., Biologische Nitratentfernung aus Lebensmitteln unter Verwendung des *Bacteriums paracoccus denitrificans*, *Ber. Bundesforschungsanst. Ernähr.*, Karlsruhe, BFE-R-89-01, 129, 1989.
105. Hofmann, K., Einfluss der Verarbeitung auf den Nitratgehalt der Nahrung: Tierische Produkte, *Landw. Forsch.*, 37, 50, 1985, Sonderheft 41.

Section II
TOXIC AND ANTINUTRITIVE COMPOUNDS FORMED DURING FOOD PROCESSING AND STORAGE

Raw material of plant and animal origin and food are rather complicated heterogeneic materials, consisting of many substances of which some are very reactive.

During storage and food processing many reactions take plase and some toxic antinutritive compounds are also formed. The chapter covers toxic compounds arising from action of microorganism (bacterial toxins and mycotoxins), toxic compounds formed under the influence of physical factors and by chemical reactions (toxic compounds arising from proteins, carbohydrates, and lipids), and toxic compounds arising by interaction of food constituents with food additives (nitroso compounds and ethyl carbamate).

Chapter 3

Toxic Compounds Arising by Action of Microorganisms

Alexander Príbela and Terézia Šinková

Part A

Bacterial Toxins

CHARACTERIZATION OF BACTERIAL TOXINS

Microbial toxicosis often represents a serious public health hazard classified mostly as food poisonings. It is evident that bacterial toxicosis has increased both in developing countries and in developed ones. Microorganisms are widely distributed, but toxigenic bacteria are responsible for the induction of these diseases.

Predominantly, Gram-negative bacteria of genera *Escherichia, Salmonella, Shigella, Enterobacter, Klebsiella, Vibrio, Pseudomonas, Yersinia, Aeromonas, Plesiomonas,* some Gram-positive bacteria of *Staphylococcus, Clostridium, Streptococcus, Bacillus,* and some others are the source of bacterial toxins.

There are differences in production of bacterial toxins by individual microorganisms. Factors affecting production are conditions of cultivation (growth medium, temperature, pH, presence of oxygen) as well as the genus and species of bacteria. Details about bacterial toxins are discussed in various monographs.[1,2]

In particular, the activity of enterotoxins, neurotoxins, and some other toxins is important in food processing. Chemical structure, biological properties, and frequency of occurrence of some types of bacterial toxins such as botulotoxins and choleratoxins in some foods have been investigated fairly well. On the other hand, there is a lack of basic knowledge of the structure and biological properties of many other toxins. However, the relation between chemical structure and biological activity of toxins is essential in the prediction of bacterial pathogenity and prevention of bacterial toxicosis.[3]

Bacterial toxins are secondary bacterial metabolites. Their classification as endotoxins and exotoxins depends on the location in the microbial cell and the time of their release into the medium. Nevertheless, all of bacterial toxins can act as enterotoxins with harmful effects in the intestinal tract.

Endotoxins are the building compounds of the coating outer wall of Gram-negative bacteria released from dead cells under specific conditions, e.g., autolysis. They are defined as extremely thermoresistant compounds, surviving even a temperature of 126°C for 7 h or 146°C for 30 min.[4] Nevertheless, some exotoxins released from dead cells and some thermoresistant exotoxins have been observed. Endotoxin structure has been acknowledged as a macromolecular complex of lipopolysaccharides.[1,4,5]

Many diseases are caused by endotoxins — especially leucopenia, lethality, antigenicity, hypotension, pyrogenicity, hypoglycemia, aggregation of thrombocytes, hyperlipemia, tumor necrosis, stimulation of cyclic adenosine-3,5-monophosphate production, and

0-8493-4623-1/95/$0.00+$.50

induction of prostaglandin synthesis. A typical consequence of the endotoxin activity in a macroorganism is enterotoxin stress. Bioactivity of endotoxins depends mainly on sensitizing and retardant factors.

Exotoxins are bacterial poisons produced by multiplying microorganisms and excreted into the medium. Consequently, some of them will be transported to the individual body organs. The exotoxins remain in food even after the bacterial cells have died. They are proteins which are often enzymatically active.[3,6]

With the exception of choleratoxin and botulotoxin, the modes of action of the bacterial toxins have not been explained sufficiently. Frequently a number of reaction mechanisms operate simultaneously.

BACTERIAL TOXINS OF IMPORTANT MICROORGANISMS

TOXINS OF *CLOSTRIDIUM* SPECIES

Botulotoxins produced by *Clostridium botulinum* are considered the most dangerous bacterial toxins. Some antigenic types of them are known: A, B,Cα,Cβ D, E, F, and G. Especially types A, B, and E, and in particular also type F, are poisonous to humans. Types C and D are poisonous to poultry, cattle, and sheep. Type B is most prevalent in Europe, while type A tends to have a higher distribution in America. Type E occurs in seafood (fish, shell fish). Botulotoxins are produced under anaerobic conditions (cans, sausages). Optimum for *Cl. botulinum* production is a pH from 4.8 to 8.5 and a temperature of 30°C. The toxins can be produced at lower temperatures as well.

It is known that the protein structure of clostridial toxins are composed of 19 amino acids. The relative molecular weight of the types A and B is 900,000 to 1,000,000 Da. Poisoning of humans by a botulotoxin occurs 5 to 72 h after ingestion of the toxin, depending on the amount. Neurotoxins are responsible for headaches, weariness, discomfort, nausea, paralysis of eyes, larynx, and tongue nerves, and salivation. Death results from paralysis of the respiratory organs within 3 to 6 d. Botulotoxin poisoning of animals appears to be similar.[3,7,8]

Of the other producers of enterotoxins *Cl. perfrigens* is known mainly through its types A, C, and D. Type C is especially dangerous since it causes enteritis necroticans accompanied by high mortality, whereas type A causes only slight gastroenteritis. *Cl. perfrigens* produces few spores in foodstuffs and the enterotoxins production is therefore not significant. Nevertheless, it is able to produce intestinal spores.[3] *Cl. difficile* produces enterotoxins A, B, and toxic proteins C_1, C_2, and C_3. Comparing the last ones with toxins A and B, their chemical, biological, and antigen properties are different.[9] The response of human monocytes to the action of toxins A and B of *Cl. difficile* has been studied.[10]

TOXINS OF *ESCHERICHIA COLI* SPECIES

E. coli produces two types of toxins. Thermolabile toxin (LT) is a high molecular oligomer compound (relative molecular weight 180,000 to 200,000 Da) and contains two peptide subunits, A and B. Bioactivity of the thermolabile toxin is caused by binding specifity of subunit B and by enzymatic activity of subunit A as well. The enterotoxic activity of subunit A and the one of the choleragen are the same. The thermolabile enterotoxin of *E. coli* activates adenylatecyclase (EC 4.6.1.1).[11,12]

The thermoresistant enterotoxin (ST) is a low molecular weight, dialyzable compound (relative molecular weight 4,400 Da). The toxin activates guanylatecyclase (EC 4.6.1.2) and, in particular, this is the characteristic property which distinguishes its activity from the ones of choleragen and LT toxin.[13]

Similar types of enterotoxins are produced by species *Klebsiella pneumoniae*[14] and *Enterobacter cloacae.*[15]

TOXINS OF *SALMONELLA* SPECIES

Salmonella produce a number of toxins, of which enterotoxins are dangerous for human health. The relative molecular weight of the thermolabile toxin (S-LT) is about 90,000 Da, and its character is similar to choleragene. The thermoresistant enterotoxin (S-ST) will even resist a temperature of 70°C in either basic or acid media. It is also stable at a temperature of –20°C.[16,17] The species *S. typhimurium, S. enteritis, S. agona,* and *S. dublin* produce enterotoxins very extensively.[17-19] *Salmonella* produce endotoxin and cytotoxins (verotoxins) as well. The latter ones are involved in exterior cell membranes.[20]

TOXINS OF *STAPHYLOCOCCUS* SPECIES

There are seven serologically distinct types of enterotoxins, known as A, B, C_1, C_2, D, E, and F, produced mostly by *Staphylococcus aureus*. They represent proteins which are soluble in water (relative molecular weight 30,000 to 35,000 Da). Their heat stabilities are different. Enterotoxins B and C are relatively thermoresistant. They withstand heating at 90°C for 30 min. They even tolerate a medium of 10% NaCl, whereas toxin A can easily be inactivated. Enterotoxins B and C resist low temperatures. The toxicity of enterotoxin B is high. Toxicosis occurs with as little as 20 to 25 μg (total ingested amount) of enterotoxin B.[3,21,22]

TOXINS OF *BACILLUS* SPECIES

Bacillus cereus is one of the most dangerous toxin producers in foodstuffs, leading to the formation of some enterotoxins and cytolytic toxins. Food poisoning caused by diarrhea and emetic enterotoxins has been demonstrated. The diarrhea toxin, a labile protein (relative molecular weight about 50,000 Da, IP 4,9), causes disease of the lower intestinal tract, similar to that caused by *Cl. perfrigens.* A toxic protein fraction containing three detectable antigens was obtained.[23] The emetic enterotoxin, of relative molecular weight ranging from 5,000 to 15,000 Da is probably not a protein. It is thermoresistant and resists changes of pH. It causes mainly symptoms of the upper intestinal tract similar to the staphylococcal one.[24] In addition, *B. cereus* produces a number of cytolytic toxins.[25]

TOXINS OF *VIBRIO* SPECIES

Enterotoxins of genus *Vibrio,* chiefly those of *Vibrio cholerae,* have been studied in detail. Choleratoxin (relative molecular weight 84,000 Da) contains two units A and B linked noncovalently, and it has been named choleragen. The isolated units are not bioactive. Choleragen stimulates adenylatecyclase (EC 4.6.1.1) in liver cells, fat cells, leucocytes, and erythrocytes.[26,27] Enterotoxin produced by *V. parahaemolyticus* acts similarly. This bacterial type also produces hemolysine that is thermoresistant.[28]

OTHER BACTERIAL TOXINS

Toxins are produced by a number of other bacteria as well. Their occurrence and the consequences of their action are rare. Shigella enterotoxins, produced mainly by the species *Shigella dysenteriae 1* and *Shigella flexneri 2A* (relative molecular weight 50,000 to 70,000 Da), are cytotoxic to HeLa cells and lethal to rats. Their antigens are similar. They are inactivated at 90°C in 30 min.[29]

The molecule of shigatoxin is interesting since it is a bearer of three activities — neurotoxic, enterotoxic, and cytotoxic. The occurence of *Aeromonas hydrophila* enterotoxins and *A. sobria* in meat extracts at low temperatures has been observed.[30] The structure of enterotoxin A, produced by *Pseudomonas aeruginosa,*[31] *Enterobacter cloacae,*[15] and by some other bacteria has been described.

PREVENTION OF BACTERIAL TOXINS FORMATION AND POSSIBLE WAYS OF DETOXIFICATION

Particular attention has been paid to botulotoxin prevention.[10,21,22] A number of papers refer to the existence of some factors that lower the *Cl. botulinum* multiplication risk and consequently, the toxin production, mainly as far as the types A, B, and E are concerned. The factors involve water activity (a_w), NaCl content, spore germination temperature, pH, and some inhibitors such as nitrites, antimicrobial agents, and others.[21,22] A relation between a_w in pasta and toxin production by *Cl. botulinum* was observed.[32] No toxin was found at a_w 0.93 to 0.95 and 30°C in noodles after 10 weeks; therefore the a_w value in fresh pasta was acknowledged as the basic factor preventing botulotoxin production by *Cl. botulinum.* The vegetative cells and spores of the types A and B of *Cl. botulinum* were inhibited by *Cl. sporogenes* in chicken meat in which the degree of botulotoxin production depends on the relative concentrations of the spores of both microorganisms. Optimum results were obtained at a ratio of 10:1000 and 1000:1000, respectively.[8]

The effect of smoking and storage on toxin formation in vacuum-packed trout fillets was studied.[33] The samples were deliberately contaminated with spores of *Cl. botulinum*, type E. Germination and toxin production were not inhibited at 5 to 8°C, and the spores survived even hot smoke (60°C). The experiments suggested a possibility of preserving vacuum-packed smoked trout fillets safety by storage at temperatures below 5°C (optimum temperature is 3°C). Bacterial toxin prevention consists of careful sanitation and following optimum technical conditions (e.g., raw materials handling).

The content of endotoxins that have a special place in foodstuffs varies from 1 to 10, 000 $ng.g^{-1}$ in drinking water, from 10 to 50,000 $ng.g^{-1}$ in milk products, and from 180 to 10,000 $ng.g^{-1}$ in forcemeat.[4] Despite various activities, the endotoxins will bring only a low risk for health. Experimental results have not assigned their clinical effects, even at their high levels in diets.[4]

Food detoxification is more complicated than prevention. The feasibility of detoxification is limited by toxin properties and technological processes that do not lower the nutritious, technological, and organoleptic properties of the food product. Thermolabile toxins such as botulotoxins are inactivated at 80°C in 10 min, or at 100°C in a few seconds,[3,7,8] including the thermolabile toxin produced by *E. coli*,[11,12] enterotoxin B produced by *Staphylococcus aureus*,[3] and the thermolabile toxin produced by the *Salmonella* genus.[16,17] The shigella enterotoxins are inactivated by heating at 90°C in 30 min.[29] On the other hand, the thermostabile toxins cannot be destroyed completely, not even by extensive heating. Consequently, toxin prevention seems to be more advantageous than their suppression.

Part B

Mycotoxins

CHARACTERIZATION OF MYCOTOXINS

Food products, being organic substances containing essential nutrients, are suitable substrates for mold growth. Secondary metabolites — mycotoxins — are frequently produced by different varieties of fungus. They are contained in spores of the fungus thallus, or secreted in the substrate they grow on. Mycotoxins can pass their toxic properties into food either directly or indirectly through an animal whose organism is not able to detoxify the substance or that changes it into another harmless compound. Nevertheless, it is possible to consume mold-contaminated products without any hazard or influence on taste and appearance. The hazard becomes serious when mycocarcinogens such as aflatoxins are involved. Inhalation of aflatoxins can also impair human health.[34,35]

Food regularly contains a number of microbe species producing various mycotoxins with different potency. Some of the mycotoxins can predominate over others, and some of them may diminish the toxic potency of the others; and the final result combines the effects of the individual mycotoxins. From the toxicological viewpoint, it is the mycotoxin, not the mold, which is essential in the final evaluation. Furthermore, the presence of mold does not necessarily indicate the presence of a specific mycotoxin. Unfortunately, some metabolites from common molds, already identified and chemically characterized, have not yet been toxicologically evaluated.[36]

Mycotoxins can be produced by fungi grown on living plants, infested stored food products, and infested decaying organic matter. There are a wide range of suitable substrates for growing toxigenic fungi. Moisture is the most critical environmental factor influencing mold growth and toxin production. It is followed by temperature and time of storage.[37,38]

Toxic metabolites produced by three genera of molds — *Aspergillus, Fusarium,* and *Penicillium* — are of primary concern in commercial food safety. They can be commonly found in stored cereal grains and oilseeds and may cause various forms of specific human and animal mycotoxinoses.[34,35]

Numerous studies demonstrate that certain mycotoxins are extremely toxic to animals, and toxic effects in humans are also possible. Knowledge of action mechanisms, detoxification mechanisms, and absorption and transport are expected to explain a correlation between animal and human effects.[36]

The most important factors responsible for the biological activity of mycotoxins are physico-chemical properties, chemical structure and steric arrangement of the molecules, and the presence of bioactive moieties in the molecules. Statistical methods relating structure and activity have been used in mycotoxicology on a small scale.[38]

AFLATOXINS

Aflatoxins are produced by molds of the genus *Aspergillus* (*A. flavus, A. parasiticus, A. niger, A. wentii, A. glaucus, A. ruber, A. ochraceus, A. versicolor, A. oryzae*). In particular, *A. flavus,* a widely distributed species found in soil and many foodstuffs, produces very toxic and highly carcinogenic metabolites.[35,37-40]

Growth and aflatoxin production can be restricted by low or high temperatures and low a_w.[38] The growth and aflatoxin production of *A. flavus* in wheat and barley occurs over temperature and water activity (a_w) ranges of 10 to 42.5°C and 0.80 to 0.975, respectively. There is no single optimum temperature, but the optimum is between 25 and 35°C when the a_w is higher than 0.90. The limiting a_w for mold growth at 26 and 30°C is 0.73, 0.69, and 0.75 in maize, soybeans and pinto beans, respectively. The limiting a_w for aflatoxin production at the same temperature is in the range 0.85 to 0.89. Differences in the rate of occurrence of aflatoxin in various commodities might be due to morphological and environmental factors.[41] Aflatoxin accumulation generally increases with incubation time, although this is much less pronounced at optimal a_w.[42]

Some *Aspergillus* species can inhibit others for the biosynthesis of aflatoxin (e.g., *A. niger* or *A. tamarii,* when grown as mixed cultures with toxigenic *A. flavus*, inhibit the biosynthesis of aflatoxin by *A. flavus*). The composition of the media plays an important role in enhancement or reduction in aflatoxins but it does not need to influence the growth of fungi at the same time.[43,44] It is known that nitrogen regulates the biosynthesis of secondary metabolites in a variety of microorganisms.[45]

Structures and molecular weights of the most important aflatoxins are given in Figure 1. Among four major aflatoxins, aflatoxin B_1 has the greatest acute toxicity, followed by G_1, B_2, and G_2. The acute toxicity of aflatoxins and their conversion products to animals cannot be generalized, because it differs from species to species.

Aflatoxin B_1 is the most potent hepatocarcinogen, but tumors of other organs caused by it were also observed.[47,48] Although direct evidence of aflatoxinosis in humans is not available, it is assumed from the symptoms of poisonings caused by consuming mold-contaminated foodstuffs. The symptoms include: edema of legs, abdominal pain, palpable liver, liver necrosis, fibrosis, slightly fatty liver, and other symptoms, some of them known as Reye's syndrome, characterized by vomiting, hypoglycemia, convulsions, hyperammonemia, and coma.[49,50]

Toxicity and carcinogenity of aflatoxins are significantly affected by the molecular structure. The extent of their biological effects depends on the rates of the various pathways that metabolize the toxin. The cyclopentanone ring attached to the coumarin gives the molecule a greater toxic potency in B_1 compared to the lactone in G_2. Furthermore, conversion of the ketone to a hydroxyl function, as in aflatoxicol, reduces the toxic activity.[46] Not having the dihydrofurofuran moiety, the compound becomes inactive. Reduction of this portion of the molecule reduces the activity (B_1 vs. B_2 and G_1 vs. G_2.[47]

Aflatoxins B_1, B_2, G_1, and G_2 can be isolated from nuts, oilseeds, cereals, and some other materials. Aflatoxins M_1 and M_2 are not only naturally occurring fungal metabolites, but can also be found in milk as common metabolic products of aflatoxin B_1 and B_2 biotransformed by cytosolic and microsomal enzymes. They are as toxic as or slighly less toxic than the parent compounds. The conversion of aflatoxin B_1 in feed to aflatoxin M_1 in milk varies from 1 to 4%. Some other metabolites of aflatoxin B_1 were characterized as well: aflatoxin P_1, aflatoxin Q_1, and aflatoxin R_0 (aflatoxicol). As they are less mutagenic and carcinogenic than the parent toxin, the hydroxylation and demethylation reactions of aflatoxin B_1 are recognized as detoxification processes.[38]

Although the actual intake of aflatoxins seems to be small, aflatoxins, as important contaminants, have been involved in the Global Environment Monitoring System (GEMS) sponsored by the United Nations Environment Programme, that is a part of a national, regional, and international effort to provide assurance regarding a safe food supply. Food products for human use should contain the lowest levels of aflatoxins technically achievable within the need to maintain an adequate food supply. Current aflatoxin levels in the U.S. established by the Food and Drug Administration for human foods (except milk) are 20 $\mu g.kg^{-1}$, and for milk 0.5 $\mu g.kg^{-1}$.

OTHER IMPORTANT MYCOTOXINS

Some other mycotoxins, important from a commercial aspect, are shown in Figure 1. A number of other toxic compounds is also produced by various species of *Aspergillus, Penicillium, Fusarium,* and other genera. Many of them share similar conditions for growth, invade foodstuffs and feedstuffs, and represent potential poisons as well.

MYCOTOXINS IN COMMERCIAL FOODS AND FEEDS

The most serious problem of aflatoxins is that of M_1 aflatoxin in milk. Possible contamination of milk, milk products, and eggs with aflatoxins comes from feed ingredients and represents a hazard in terms of children who are exposed to them regularly. Consequently, it is necessary to control ingredients in the preparation of animal feeds.

Growth of molds requires contact with substrate. Natural vegetable products having outer tissues or layers are fairly well protected, but damage to these coverings causes easy access of mold spores to the internal tissues and nutrients. Other important factors for

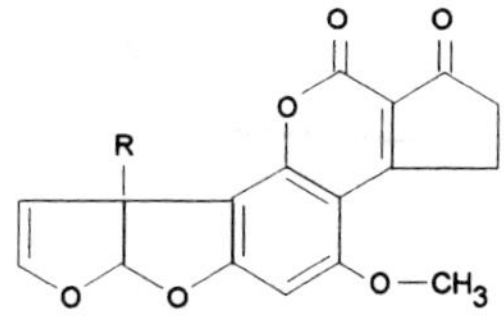

R = H, aflatoxin B_1
R = OH, aflatoxin M_1

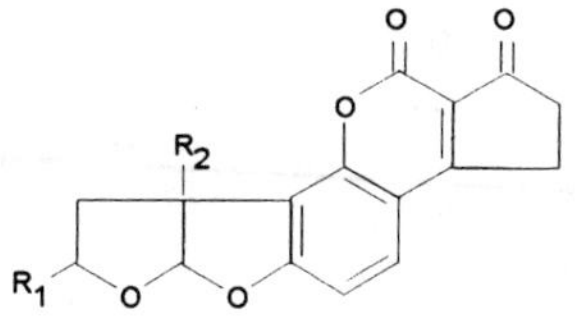

$R_1 = R_2 = H$, aflatoxin B_2
$R_1 = H, R_2 = OH$, aflatoxin M_2

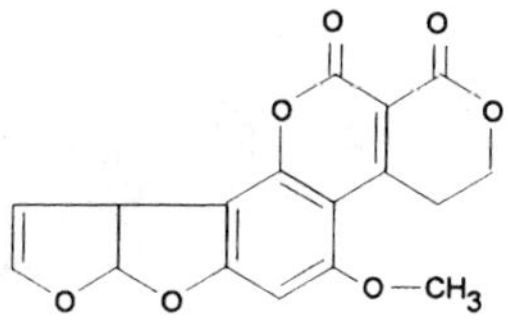

aflatoxin G_1

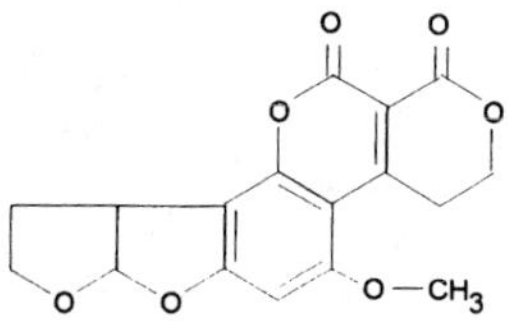

aflatoxin G_2

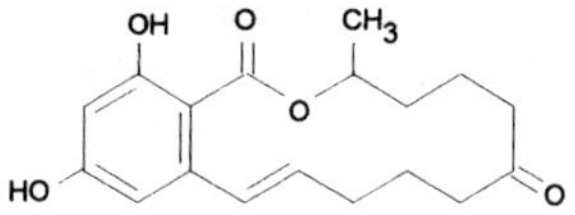

zearalenone

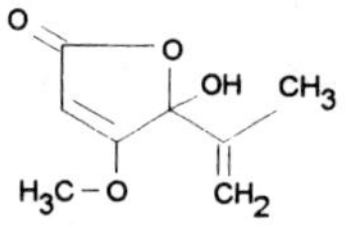

penicillic acid

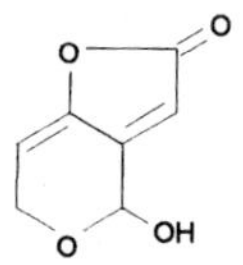

patulin

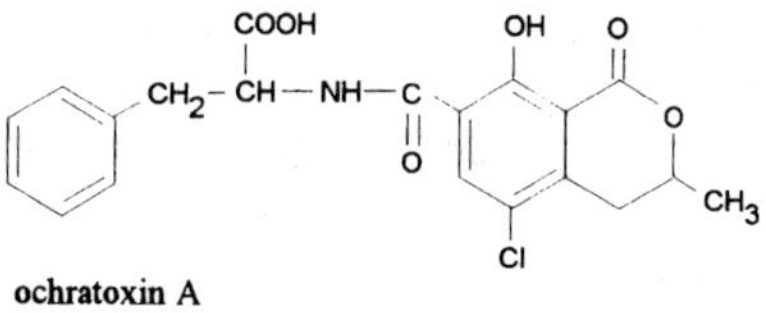

ochratoxin A

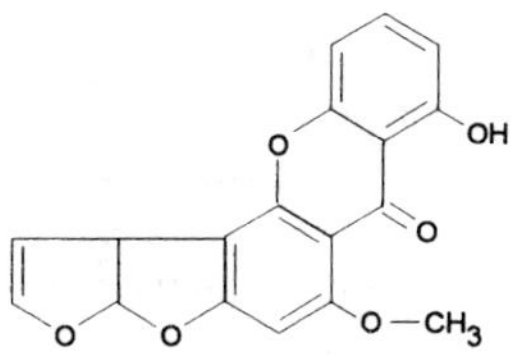

sterigmatocystin

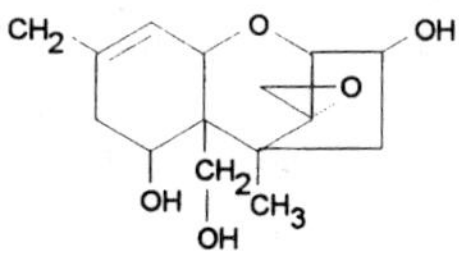

deoxynivalenol

Figure 1 Structure of some important mycotoxins.

mold growth and mycotoxin production are temperature, moisture, and time, because the maximum production occurs several days after germination. Availability of the nutrients needed for certain species growth, the presence of other microorganisms, and some chemicals in the environment also determine the conditions for mycotoxin production.

Although there are some species of *Penicillium* and *Fusarium* genera which grow on crops in the field rather than on stored products, it is mostly in stored products where mycotoxin production occurs. Needless to say, control of the conditions of storage and processing are essential to prevent potential health hazards of mycotoxin contamination of foodstuffs.[51]

Of the commercial grains, corn represents the material tending to have the highest mycotoxin contamination. The cereal grains are susceptible to contamination mostly with aflatoxins, zearalenone, penicillic acid, and ochratoxin. Since peanuts, almonds, walnuts, pistachios, and other nuts are good substrates for the aflatoxin-producing molds *Aspergillus flavus* and *A. parasiticus*, and the conidia of these fungi are ubiquitous in environments where nuts are grown and stored, it is of utmost importance to handle these commodities properly in order to protect them from becoming contaminated with aflatoxin. Environmental controls, such as low temperature and low moisture content, normal sorting and roasting of shelled nuts that inhibit outgrowth of the condidia, are effective measures to maintain good nut quality. Surface disinfection by direct chemical treatment of nuts for seed use and fumigation for the purpose of pest control are also successful. γ-Irradiation has been shown to be effective in reducing the natural mold contaminants of peanuts. However, some genera, mainly *Aspergillus* and *Penicillium,* are more resistant to irradiation compared to the other coexisting molds. Therefore, a combination of γ-irradiation and environmental control practices (proper drying, packaging, and storing at a low relative humidity) are recommended for reducing the natural microbial toxin producers.[52]

Dried fruits (figs, apricots, cherries, pears, and others) can be contaminated with aflatoxins and patulin. The latter toxin is often present in rotten apples and consequently in apple juice. Alcoholic fermentation degrades patulin completely. As aflatoxins and ochratoxin are partly resistant to fermentation, alcoholic beverages can be contaminated by these mycotoxins transferred from the raw materials (e.g., grapes and barley).

Neosartorya fischeri (producing fumitremorgins A and C and verrucuogen) is one of the most frequently isolated heat-resistant molds from fruit juices and other heat-processed fruit-based products. Its ascospores are exceptionally heat resistant compared to those of other molds, and the presence of the mold in processed fruit products may represent a public health concern.[53]

Meat products can be contaminated directly during their curing and aging. Sterigmatocystin, a known mycocarcinogen, was found in country-cured ham. Some other mycotoxins produced in meat products (e.g., patulin and penicillic acid) are supposed to be mostly destroyed by other components of products or to lose their activity by reaction with sulfhydryl groups in meat. Indirect contamination of meat and meat products comes from mycotoxin-contaminated feedstuffs. The original toxin may remain as such or in the form of a toxic metabolite.

Many other commercial commodities can contain aflatoxins (e.g., cassava, sweet potatoes, dried shrimp, fish, garlic, cottonseed, yucca, banana, black pepper), ochratoxin (e.g., coffee beans) and other mycotoxins, but their consumption is of less importance.

DETOXIFICATION OF FOODS CONTAMINATED BY MYCOTOXINS

Foodstuffs distributed to the population should not represent a potential health hazard; therefore detoxification of mycotoxin-contaminated products has been a continuing challenge for the food industry. A great deal of concern has been directed towards aflatoxins because of their potency and ubiquity. Most of the factors obtained from studies on aflatoxins can be applied to other mycotoxins.

The sensitivity of mycotoxins to physical or chemical treatment is affected by many factors, including moisture content, location of the toxin in the food, forms of the food, storage conditions, and interactions of the toxins with food components. It is important to understand these factors before a specific method can be recommended. In addition, the use of any applicable treatment conditions should not cause undesirable alteration of food quality.[54]

PHYSICAL METHODS

Stability of aflatoxins under various physical conditions has been studied. It is evident that higher temperatures and pressures can reduce the toxin levels. The relative heat stability of aflatoxins has been reported to be up to 270°C for B_1, 249°C for G_1, and 238°C for G_2.

The aflatoxin content of peanut oil heated at 160°C for 30 min and at 250°C for 10 min decreased by 20 and 4%, respectively. However, foods fried in oil contaminated with aflatoxins absorb aflatoxins at much higher levels than those calculated from the level of oil absorption by the foods.[56]

It was demonstrated that the aflatoxin content did not change at 100°C during heating of fruit juice and baking bread, nor was the toxin deoxynivalenol (produced by *Fusarium graminearum*) destroyed at 100°C during the cooking of noodles. (However, some toxin did leach into the cooking water.)[57]

When autoclaved at 120°C for 4 h, the aflatoxin content in peanut meal decreased from 7000 $\mu g.kg^{-1}$ to 370 $\mu g.kg^{-1}$.[55] A reduction in the level of aflatoxin during milk pasteurization and rice parboiling was observed.[58] The losses of aflatoxin B_1 in virgin olive oil (spiked with 100 ppb aflatoxin B_1) as a result of various physical treatments are shown in Table 1.[56]

When aflatoxin B_1 was exposed in the solvents ethanol, ethyl acetate, chloroform, and edible oils to radiation (solar, UV at 254 nm and 365 nm, and fluorescent light), only the combination of solar radiation and edible oils (coconut, corn, sesame, and soybean) degraded aflatoxin B_1 leaving no residual aflatoxin or new fluorescent compound. Nontoxicity of solar-irradiated coconut oil was established in tests on ducklings. No degradation of aflatoxin B_1 occurred in powdered copra meal as a result of solar radiation.[59]

γ-Irradiation was found suitable for the destruction of aflatoxins in solutions. The radiosensitivity of aflatoxins in increasing order is G_2, B_2, G_1, and B_1. Only about 5% of aflatoxin B_1 remains after irradiation of a standard solution (initial concentration 2.5 $mg.dm^{-3}$ at 5 kGy.[55]

The effect of γ-irradiation on the patulin content of apple juice concentrate was investigated. The radiation-induced reduction of the patulin content in relation to the absorbed dose followed an exponential relationship. The dose that reduced the patulin content to 50% of its initial value was 0.35 kGy. Disappearance of patulin from artificially contaminated apple juice concentrate (initial concentration 2 $\mu g.kg^{-1}$) was caused by doses greater than 2.5 kGy.[60,61]

Table 1 Losses of Aflatoxins B_1

Treatment	Loss of aflatoxin B_1 %
Storage in dark (25°C, 224 d)	<50
Heating (250°C, 10 min)	65
Exposure to sunlight (open air, 40 min)	95

The major aflatoxins can be completely destroyed during a typical hydrolyzed vegetable protein production process involving acidic hydrolysis of peanut meal at elevated pressure and temperature. Degradation products are nontoxic and nonmutagenic.[62]

Adsorbents, including bentonite and activated charcoal, can physically remove aflatoxins and patulin from liquid food such as apple juice. The adsorption capacity of powdered charcoal is approximately 10 times higher than that of a granulated one. An increase in the soluble solids content of a liquid, especially the sugar content, lowers the absorption efficiency.[38,63]

Sieving and dehulling were shown to be efficient in reducing the concentrations of deoxynivalenol (DON) and zearalenone (ZEN) in contaminated barley, wheat, corn, and rye. Coarsely ground barley, wheat, and corn containing 5 to 23 and 0.5 to 1.21 $mg.kg^{-1}$ DON and ZEN, respectively, were segregated into fractions by sieving. The largest particles (9-mesh barley, 9-mesh wheat, 16-mesh corn) contained 67 to 83% less toxin compared with the whole kernels. Removing the hull material from barley prior to sieving resulted in a further 16% reduction in the DON content of the 9-mesh fraction (from 73% reduction in intact barley to an 89% reduction in dehulled barley). Of the DON and ZEN, 40 to 100% was removed from the grain treated in a Scott-Strong dehuller. It was shown that both sieving and dehulling can represent useful procedures for reducing mycotoxin levels in contaminated grain, under certain circumstances.[64]

Low O_2 concentration and/or increased concentration of CO_2 or N_2 prevent mold development on grain and inhibit production of selected mycotoxins. The levels needed to inhibit mold growth are, however, much higher than those required for inhibition of mycotoxin production. For instance, patulin can be produced in apple juice at O_2 levels as low as 0.2%, but mold growth is completely inhibited by pure N_2 (less than 1 ppm O_2).[65,66]

An atmosphere enriched with high CO_2 levels allows inhibition of zearalenone production in high-moisture corn grains almost completely.[67] Reduction of aflatoxins can be observed after treating some foods with chlorine gas and ozone.[68]

BIOLOGICAL METHODS

It is known that mycotoxin production can be increased by mixed cultures in comparison with the pure ones,[69] whereas some microorganisms can reduce mycotoxin concentrations. In particular, metabolites of some lactobacillus species are effective in reducing aflatoxins, although the growth of microorganisms is not affected. Detoxification of aflatoxin B_1 by yogurt cultures was suggested.[70]

The effectiveness of some essential oils from spices on *Aspergillus parasiticus* growth and aflatoxin production was demonstrated. The concentration of thyme, cumin, clove, caraway, rosemary, and sage oils caused a 96% inhibition of total aflatoxin production at 0.2, 0.4, 0.4, 0.6, 2, and 2 $g.dm^{-3}$, respectively. There seems to be a relationship between the chemical structure of oils and their antifungal effect. The extent of inhibition could be attributed to the presence of an aromatic nucleus containing a polar functional group. A phenolic group can easily form hydrogen bonds with active sites of enzymes, resulting in inhibitory action. Besides the aromaticity of molecules, the inductive effect of the isopropyl group plays a part.[71]

The mycelial growth and toxin production by *A. parasiticus* were inhibited by a garlic concentration of 0.3 to 0.4%. When the fungus was grown on rice, the garlic concentration needed to inhibit of aflatoxin B_1 production was approximately 10 times higher (2.5%) than in broth (0.3%).[72]

The bitter glycoside of olives, oleuropein, was shown to be efficient in preventing aflatoxin production. Experimental results indicated that aflatoxin production can be reduced by 98% in the presence of 6 mg $oleuropein.ml^{-1}$ glucose + NH_4NO_3 broth (inoculated with 0.1 ml of suspension containing spores of *A. parasiticus*).[71,73]

Combination of salt and aqueous extracts of some vegetable leaves (*Azadirachta indica, Lawsonia alba, Pongamia glabra,* and *Tridax procumbers*) was suggested as a treatment for preventing aflatoxin contamination of peanuts during storage and transport.[74]

CHEMICAL METHODS

It is known that alkaline treatment causes a reduction in aflatoxins. During alkaline cooking of corn with lime (the process named nixtamalization), aflatoxins G_1 and G_2 are more susceptible than B_1 and B_2, and B_1 is more resistant than B_2.

A major product formed from reacting aflatoxin B_1 with ammonium hydroxide is aflatoxin D_1, which was found to be 130 times less mutagenic than aflatoxin B_1. The efficiency of detoxification by ammoniation was determined. Greater than 97% aflatoxin B_1 reduction in dried coconut meat was accomplished, depending on the ammonium hydroxide concentration and moisture content within 5 to 15 d.[75] The aflatoxin content of contaminated groundnut oil cakes was reduced considerably by pressurized application of ammonia, dropping from 1000 to 140 ppb at a gas pressure of 2 bar and to 60 ppb at 3 bar. The effectiveness of ammoniation increased proportionally with the application pressure. Ammoniation represents a practical solution to the problem of removing carcinogenicity from foodstuffs, and it seems to offer the best chance for aflatoxin inactivation on an industrial basis.[76] The parameters and application of aflatoxin decontamination by ammoniation are given in Table 2.[77]

Aflatoxin removal from peanut meals with aqueous ethanol and from naturally contaminated corn for making tortillas on a commercial scale is well known.[78,79]

Formaldehyde, being historically used as a milk preservative prior to refrigeration, has been shown to reduce levels of aflatoxins B_1, B_2, G_1 and G_2. The effect of formaldehyde on aflatoxin M_1 levels in raw and pasteurized milk stored in glass or plastic containers up to 4 weeks was studied. The results indicated that aflatoxin M_1 levels in milk preserved with 0.025 to 0.1% formaldehyde and stored at room temperature may be expected to decrease by 45 to 85% in a week. Because the negative effects of formaldehyde on aflatoxin M_1 in milk outweigh the benefits, formaldehyde should not be used as a preservative for aflatoxin M_1-contaminated milk.[80]

Mycotoxin production in the presence of some other chemicals has been investigated. Undissociated forms of acetic, benzoic, citric, lactic, propionic, and sorbic acids are able to inhibit aflatoxin production by aspergilli partially or completely.[81] Solutions of volatile

Table 2 Parameters and Application of Ammoniation/Aflatoxin Decontamination Procedures

	Process	
Parameter	**High pressure/ high temperature**	**Ambient temperature/ atmospheric pressure/**
Ammonia level	0.2–2%	1–5%
Pressure	35–50 psi	Atmospheric
Temperature	80–120°C	Ambient
Duration	20–60 min	14–21 d
Moisture	12–16%	12–16%
Commodities	Whole cottonseed	Whole cottonseed
	Cottonseed meal	Corn
	Corn	
	Peanut meal	
Applications	Feed mill	Farm

From Park, D., L., *Food Technol.*, 47(10), 92, 1993. With permission.

organic acids (acetic and propionic acid) have been suggested for the prevention of mold growth and attendant aflatoxin formation in corn stored in high moisture conditions. Comparing propionic and acetic acid at low concentration (0.25%), the former is more effective.[82]

Salts such as sodium chloride, potassium chloride, and sodium nitrate, at low concentrations can enhance aflatoxin production. At higher concentrations they become inhibitory, but marked inhibition requires amounts of the salts greater than are commonly used in foods.[81]

More than 75% degradation of aflatoxin B_1 was achieved after treatment of aflatoxin B_1 spiked corn meal, copra meal, and peanuts with 11 to 35 mg chlorine per gram material. The extension of the exposure period of meal (beyond 2.5 h) and peanuts (beyond 1 d) did not decrease the aflatoxin B_1 level. Mutagenicity of chlorine-treated materials was greatly reduced compared with untreated controls, and it correlated with the reduction in aflatoxin B_1 levels. New mutagenic compounds did not appear.[83]

Some other chemicals have been shown to be partly or completely effective: ammonium bicarbonate, sodium bicarbonate, H_2O_2, tartaric and ascorbic acids, 4-aminobenzoic acid, potassium sorbate, sodium benzoate, potassium benzoate, formaldehyde, SO_2, potassium sulfite, sodium bisulfite, potassium fluoride, barium hydroxide, phenolic antioxidants (especially BHA), methylxanthines (caffeine and theophylline), phosphates, and some insecticides and herbicides.[81,84-86] However, most of these cannot be added to foods to prevent aflatoxin formation because of their hazardous effect on human health. Any residues of processing aids in final food products have to be limited to an extent that does not represent a hazard at the expected levels of food consumption.

REFERENCES

1. Kadis, S. and Ciegler, A., *Microbial Toxins, Bacterial Protein Toxins*, Vol. I, IIA, IIB, III, *Bacterial Endotoxins,* Vol. IV-V, Academic Press, 1972.
2. Alouf, J. E. and Freer, J. H., *Sourcebook of Bacterial Protein Toxins*, Academic Press, London, 1991, 518.
3. Macholz, R. and Lewerenz, H. J., *Lebensmitteltoxikologie*, Akademie Verlag, Berlin, 1989, chap. 19.2.
4. Jülicher, B., Schütz, M., and Wiesner, H. U., Importance of endotoxins in foods — characterization and legal evaluation (in German), *Arch. Lebensmittelhyg.*, 40, 79, 1989.
5. Reitschel, T. E. and Brade, H., Bacterial endotoxins, *Sci. Am.*, 267, 27, 1992.
6. Gaman, P. M. and Sherrington, K. B., An introduction to microbiology, in *The Science of Food,* 2nd ed., Pergamon Press, Oxford, 1981, chap. 15.
7. Tompkin, B. R. and Christiansen, L. N., *Clostridium botulinum*, in *Food Microbiology, Public Health and Spoilage Aspects,* Defigueiredo, M. P. and Splittstoesser, D. F., Eds., AVI Publishing, Westport, CT, 1976, chap. 4.
8. Huhtanen, C. N., Inhibition of *Clostridium botulinum* toxin formation by *C. sporogenes* in culture media and in a meat system, *J. Food Protect.,* 54, 50, 1991.
9. Torres, J. F. and Lönnroth, I., Production, purification and characterization of *Clostridium difficile* toxic proteins different from toxin A and from toxin B, *Biochim. Biophys. Acta*, 998, 151, 1989.
10. Flegel, W. A., Müller, F., Däubener, W., Fischer, H. G., Hadding, U., and Northoff, H., Cytokine response by human monocytes to *Clostridium difficile* toxin A and toxin B, *Infect. Immunol.,* 59, 3659, 1991.
11. Fukuta, S., Magnani, J. L., Twiddy, E. M., Holmes, R. K., and Ginsburg, V., Comparison of the carbohydrate-binding specificities of cholera toxin and *Escherichia coli* heat-labile enterotoxins LTh-I, LT-IIa, and LT-IIb, *Infect. Immunol.,* 56, 1748, 1988.
12. Yoh, M., Narita, I., Honda, T., Miwatani., T., and Nishibuchi, M., Comparison of preservation methods for enterotoxigenic *Escherichia coli* producing heat-labile enterotoxin, *J. Clin. Microbiol.,* 29, 2326, 1991.

13. Chan, S. K. and Giannela, R. A., Amino acid-sequence of heat-stable enterotoxin produced by *Escherichia coli* pathogenic for men, *J. Biol. Chem.*, 256, 7744, 1981.
14. Klipstein, F. A. and Engert, R. F., Enterotoxigenic intestinal bacteria in tropical sprue, III. Preliminary characterization of *Klebsiella pneumoniae* enterotoxin, *J. Infect. Dis.*, 132, 200, 1975.
15. Klipstein, F. A. and Engert, R. F., Partial purification and properties of *Enterobacter cloacae* heat-stable enterotoxin, *Infect. Immunol.*, 13, 1307, 1976.
16. Sandefur, P. D. and Peterson, J. W., Isolation of skin permeability factors from culture filtrates of *Salmonella typhimurium, Infect. Immunol.*, 14, 671, 1976.
17. Koupal, L. R. and Deibel, R. H., Assay, characterization and localization of an enterotoxin produced by *Salmonella, Infect. Immunol.*, 11, 14, 1975.
18. Kuhn, H., Tschäpe, H., and Rische, H., Enterotoxigenicity among *Salmonellae*: prospective analysis for a surveillance program, *Zbl. Bakt. A.*, 240, 171, 1978.
19. Stinavage, P. S., Martin, L. E., and Spitznagel, J. K., A 59 kilodalton outermembrane protein of *Salmonella typhimurium* protects against oxidative intraleukocytic killing due to human neutrophils, *Mol. Microbiol.*, 4, 283, 1990.
20. Ashkenazi, S., Cleary, T. G., Murray, B. E., Wagner, A., and Pickering, L. K., Quantitative analysis and partial characterization of cytotoxin production by *Salmonella* strains, *Infect. Immunol.*, 56, 3089, 1988.
21. Sperber, W. H., Requirements of *Clostridium botulinum* for growth and toxin production, *Food Technol.*, 36, 89, 1980.
22. Christiansen, L. N., Factors influencing botulinal inhibition by nitrite, *Food Technol.*, 34, 237, 1980.
23. Thompson, N. E., Ketterhagen, M. J., Bergdoll, M. S., and Schantz, E. J., Isolation and some properties of an enterotoxin produced by *Bacillus cereus, Infect. Immunol.*, 43, 887, 1984.
24. Hughes, S., Bartholomew, B., Hardy, J. C., and Kramer, J. M., Potential application of a hep-2 cell assay in the investigation of *Bacillus cereus* emetic-syndrome, food poisoning, *FEMS Microb. Lett.*, 52, 7, 1988.
25. Gilmore, M. S., Cruz-Rodz, A. L., Leimeister-Wächter, M., Kreft, J., and Goebel, W., A *Bacillus cereus* cytolytic determinant, cereolysin-AB, which comprises the phospholipase C and sphingomyelinase genes nucleotide sequence and genetic linkage, *J. Bacteriol.*, 171, 744, 1989.
26. Sattler, J. and Wiegandt, H., Studies of the subunit structure of choleragen, *Eur. J. Biochem.*, 57, 309, 1975.
27. Van Heyningen, S., The subunits of cholera toxin. Structure, stechiometry and function, *J. Infect. Dis. Suppl.*, 133, 5, 1976.
28. Miwatani, T., Sakurai, J., Takeda, Y., and Shinoda, S., Studies on direct haemolysins of *V. parahaemolyticus*, in *Int. Symp. V. parahaemolyticus*, Saikon Publishing, Tokyo, 1974, 245.
29. O'Brien, A. D., Thompson, M. R., Gemski, P., Doctor, B. P., and Formal, S. B., Biological properties of *Shigella flexneri* 2A toxin and its serological relationship to *Shigella dysenteriae* 1 toxin, *Infect. Immunol.*, 15, 796, 1977.
30. Majeed, K. N. and MacRae, I. C., Experimental evidence for toxin production by *Aeromonas hydrophila* and *Aeromonas sobria* in a meat extract at low temperatures, *Int. J. Food Microbiol.*, 12, 181, 1991.
31. Klinger, K. W. and Shuster, C. W., A macromolecular structure produced by *Pseudomonas aeruginosa* is recognized by antibody to exotoxin A, *Infect. Immunol.*, 43, 912, 1984.
32. Glass, K. A. and Doyle, P. M., Relationship between water activity of fresh pasta and toxin production by proteolytic *Clostridium botulinum, J. Food Protect.*, 54, 162, 1991.
33. Dehof, E., Greuel, E., and Krämer, J., Tenacity of *Clostridium botulinum* type E in hot smoked vacuum-packed trout fillets (in German), *Archiv Lebensmittelhyg.*, 40, 27, 1989.
34. Joffe, A. Z., Toxin production in cereal fungi causing toxic alimentary aleukia in man, in *Mycotoxins in Foodstuffs,* Wogan, G. N., Ed., M. I. T. Press, Cambridge, MA, 1965.
35. Dvorackova, I., Aflatoxin inhalation and alveolar cell carcinoma, *Br. Med. J.*, 20, 691, 1976.
36. Concon, J. M., *Food Toxicology*, Part B, *Contaminants and Additives,* Marcel Dekker, New York, Basel, 1988.
37. Hesseltine, C. W., Conditions leading to mycotoxin contamination of food and feeds, in *Mycotoxins and Other Fungal Related Food Problems,* Rodricks, J. V., Ed., American Chemical Society, Washington, D. C., 1976.

38. Betina, V., *Mycotoxins. Chemical, Biological, and Environmental Aspects*, Elsevier, Amsterdam, 1989.
39. Kulik, M. M. and Holaday, C. E., Aflatoxin A: a metabolic product of several fungi, *Mycopathol. Mycol. Appl.*, 30, 137, 1966.
40. Van Walbeek, W., Scott, P. M., and Thatcher, F. S., Mycotoxins from foodborne fungi, *Can. J. Microbiol.*, 14, 131, 1968.
41. Trucksess, M. V., Stoloff, L., and Mislivec, P. B., Effect of temperature, water activity, and other toxigenic mold species on growth of *Aspergillus flavus* and aflatoxin production on corn, pinto beans and soybeans, *J. Food Protect.*, 51, 361, 1988.
42. Montani, M. L., Vaamonde, G., Resnik, S. L., and Buera, P., *Int. J. Food Microbiol.*, 6, 349, 1988.
43. Shanta, T., Rati, E. R., and Bhavani Shankar, T. N., Behavior of *Aspergillus flavus* in presence of *Aspergillus niger* during biosynthesis of aflatoxin B_1, *Antonie van Leeuwenhoek J. Microbiol. Serol.*, 58, 121, 1990.
44. Moss, M. O., Badii, F., and Clifford, M. N., Reduced aflatoxin production by *Aspergillus parasiticus* after growth on a caffeine-containing medium, *Lett. Appl. Microbiol.*, 10, 205, 1990.
45. Orvehed, M., Haeggblom, P., and Soederhaell, K., Nitrogen inhibition of mycotoxin production by *Alternaria alternata, Appl. Environ. Microbiol.*, 54, 2361, 1988.
46. Wogan, G. N., Edwards, G. S., and Newberne, P. M., Structure activity relationships in toxicity and carcinogenity of aflatoxins and analogs, *Cancer Res.*, 31, 1936, 1971.
47. Heathcote, J. G., Mycotoxins — production, isolation, separation, and purification, in *Mycotoxins, Chemical, Biological and Environmental Aspects,* Betina, V., Ed., Elsevier, Amsterdam, 1984, chap 7.
48. Heathcote, J. G. and Hibbert, J. R., *Aflatoxins: Chemical and Biological Aspects,* Elsevier, Amsterdam, 1978.
49. Serck-Hanssen, A., Aflatoxin-induced fatal hepatitis, a case report from Uganda, *Arch. Environ. Health,* 20, 729, 1970.
50. Robinson, P., Infantile cirrhosis of the liver in India. With special reference to probable aflatoxin etiology, *Clin. Pediatr.*, 6, 57, 1967.
51. Shapton, D. A. and Shapton, N. F., *Principles and Practices for the Safe Processing of Foods,* Butterworth-Heinemann, Oxford, 1991.
52. Chiou, R. Y. Y., Lin, C. M., and Shyu, S. L., Property characterization of peanut kernels subjected to gamma irradiation and its effect on the outgrowth and aflatoxin production by *Aspergillus parasiticus, J. Food Sci.*, 55, 210, 1990.
53. Nielsen, P. V., Beuchat, L. R., and Frisvald, G. C., Influence of atmospheric oxygen content on growth and fumitremorgin production by a heat-resistant mold *Neosartorya fischeri, J. Food Sci.*, 54, 679, 1989.
54. Samarajeewa, U., Sen, A. C., Cohen, M. D., and Wei, C. I., Detoxification of aflatoxins in foods and feeds by physical and chemical methods, *J. Food Protect.*, 53, 489, 1990.
55. Mutluer, B. and Erkoc, F. U., Effects of gamma irradiation on aflatoxins, *Z. Lebensm. Unters. Forsch.*, 185, 398, 1987.
56. Mahjoub, A. and Bullerman, L. B., Effects of storage time, sunlight, temperature, and frying on stability of aflatoxin B_1 in olive oil, *Lebensm. Wiss. Technol.*, 21, 29, 1988.
57. Nowicki, T. W., Gaba, D. G., Dexter, J. E., Matsuo, R., and Clear, R. M., Retention of the *Fusarium mycotoxin* deoxynivalenol in wheat during processing and cooking of spaghetti and noodles, *J. Cereal Sci.*, 8, 189, 1988.
58. Ogunsanwo, B. M., Faboya, O. O., Ikotun, T., and Idowu, R., Fate of aflatoxins in soybeans during the preparation of soyogi, *Nahrung*, 33, 485, 1989.
59. Samarajeewa, U., Solar degradation of aflatoxin B_1 in foods, *Proc. Jpn. Assoc. Mycotoxicol.*, 1, 91, 1988.
60. Zegota, H., Zegota, A., and Bachmann, S., Effect of irradiation and storage on patulin disappearance and some chemical constituents of apple juice concentrate, *Z. Lebensm. Unters. Forsch.*, 187, 321, 1988.
61. Zegota, H., Zegota, A., and Bachman, S., Effect of irradiation on the patulin content and chemical composition of apple juice concentrate, *Z. Lebensm. Unters. Forsch.*, 187, 235, 1988.

62. Dutton, M. F. and Williams, K., Detoxification of aflatoxin in peanut meal by acid hydrolysis, *Food Rev.*, 15(Suppl. 2), 70, 1988.
63. Van, J. A., Removal of patulin from apple juice by charcoal treatment, *Dissertation-Abstr. Int.*, 49, 3527, 1989.
64. Trenholm, H. L., Charmley, L. L., Prelusky, D. B., and Warner, R. M., Two physical methods for the decontamination of four cereals contaminated with deoxynivalenol and zearalenone, *J. Agric. Food Chem.*, 39, 356, 1991.
65. Paster, N. and Bullerman, L. B., Mould spoilage and mycotoxin formation in grains as controlled by physical means, *Int. J. Food Microbiol.*, 7, 257, 1988.
66. Orth, R., Wachstum und Toxinbildung von Patulin- und Sterigmatocystinbildenden Schimmelpilzen unter kontrollierter Atmosphäre, *Z. Lebensm. Unters. Forsch.*, 160, 359, 1976.
67. Paster, N., Blumenthal, Y. J., Barkai, G. R., and Menasherov, M., Production of zearalenone in vitro and in corn grains stored under modified atmospheres, *Int. J. Food Microbiol.*, 12, 157, 1991.
68. Maeba, H., Takamoto, Y., Kaminura, M., and Miura, T., Destruction and detoxification of aflatoxins with ozone, *J. Food Sci.*, 53, 667, 1988.
69. Luchese, R. H. and Harrigan, W. F., Growth of, and aflatoxin production by *Aspergillus parasiticus* when in the presence of either *Lactococcus lactis* or lactic acid and at different initial pH values, *J. Appl. Bacteriol.*, 69, 512, 1990.
70. Rasic, J. L., Skrinjar, M., and Markov, S., Detoxification of aflatoxin B_1 by yoghurt, lactic and acetic acids, *Food Biotechnol.*, 4, 608, 1990.
71. Farag, R. S., Daw, Z.Y., and Abo-Raya, S. H., Influence of some spice essential oils on *Aspergillus parasiticus* growth and production of aflatoxins in asynthetic medium, *J. Food Sci.*, 54, 74, 1989.
72. Patel, U. D., Govindarajan, P., and Dave, P. J., Inactivation of aflatoxin B_1 by using the synergistic effect of hydrogen peroxide and gamma-irradiation, *Appl. Environ. Microbiol.*, 55, 465, 1989.
73. Gourama, H. and Bullerman, L. B., Effects of oleuropein on growth and aflatoxin production by *Aspergillus parasiticus, Lebensm. Wiss. Technol.*, 20, 226, 1987.
74. Ghewande, M. P. and Nagaraj, G., Prevention of aflatoxin contamination through some commercial chemical products and plant extracts in groudnut, *Mycotoxin Res.*, 3, 19, 1987.
75. Mercado, C. J., Real, M. P., and Rosario, R. R., Chemical detoxification of aflatoxin-containing copra, *J. Food Sci.*, 56, 733, 1991.
76. Frayssinet, C. and Lafarge-Frayssinet, C., Effect of ammoniation on the carcinogenicity of aflatoxin-contaminated groundnut oil cakes: long-term feeding study in the rat, *Food Addit. Contamin.*, 7, 63, 1990.
77. Park, D. L., Controlling aflatoxin in food and feed, *Food Technol.*, 47(10), 92, 1993.
78. Arriola, M. C., Porres, E., Cabrera, S., Zepeda, M., and Rolz, C., Aflatoxin fate during alkaline cooking of corn for tortilla preparation, *J. Agric. Food Chem.*, 36, 530, 1988.
79. Abbas, H. K., Mirocha, C. J., Rosiles, R., and Carvajal, M., Effect of tortilla preparation process on aflatoxin B_1 and B_2 in corn, *Mycotoxin Res.*, 4, 33, 1988.
80. Heimbecher, S. K., Jorgensen, K. V., and Price, R. L., Interactive effects of duration of storage and addition of formaldehyde on levels of aflatoxin M_1 in milk, *J. Assoc. Off. Chem.*, 71, 285, 1988.
81. Rusul, G. and Marth, E. H., Food additives and plant components control growth and aflatoxin production by toxigenic aspergilli: a review, *Mycopathologia*, 101, 13, 1988.
82. Wilson, D. M., McMillian, W. W., and Widstrom, N. W., Field aflatoxin contamination of corn in south Georgia, *J. Am. Oil Chem. Soc.*, 50, 69, 1979.
83. Samarajeewa, U., Sen, A. C., Fernando, S. Y., Ahmed, E. M., and Wei, C. I., Inactivation of aflatoxin B_1 in corn meal, copra meal and peanuts by chlorine gas treatment, *Food Chem. Toxicol.*, 29, 41, 1991.
84. Montville, T. J. and Goldstein, P. K., Sodium bicarbonate inhibition of aflatoxigenesis in corn, *J. Food Protect.*, 52, 45, 1989.
85. El-Gazzar, F. E. and Marth, E. H., Role of hydrogen peroxide in the prevention of growth and aflatoxin production by *Aspergillus parasiticus, J. Food Protect.*, 51, 263, 1988.
86. Lee, E. G., Townsley, P. M., and Walden, C. C., Effect of bivalent metals on the production of aflatoxins in submerged cultures, *J. Food Sci.*, 31, 432, 1966.

Chapter 4

Toxic and Antinutritional Compounds Arising Under the Influence of Physical Factors and by Chemical Reactions

Part A

Toxic and Antinutritional Compounds Arising from Proteins

Jan Pánek, Jiří Davídek, and Zuzana Jehličková

Processing of natural foodstuffs can sometimes lead to the formation of a number of undesirable compounds. These compounds arise from various physical influences and chemical reactions. They may have a negative influence on the nutritional quality of the food. The formation of toxic compounds from proteins during cooking, industrial processing, and storage is mostly accompanied by a decrease of nutritional quality of the proteins. It usually leads to a decrease in digestibility of the proteins and, furthermore, to a decrease or even loss of availability of some reaction products of the amino acids.

Antinutritional and toxic compounds from proteins are formed during processing of proteins by reactions with other components of foodstuffs, e.g., carbohydrates (nonenzymatic browning reactions), lipids (binding of protein with oxidized lipids) or polyphenols (reactions similar to the enzymatic browning reactions). These compounds can, however, arise from single proteins, which are exposed to the influence of certain conditions (e.g., heating or alkali treatment). Reactions leading to the formation of antinutritional and toxic compounds from proteins and to the decrease in their nutritional quality are caused primarily by the presence of some very reactive essential and semiessential amino acids (lysine, methionine, cysteine or cystine, tryptophan), which often are the limiting amino acids in some foodstuffs. In this case, the formation of toxic compounds does not have to be the most significant, especially from the point of view of human nutrition. However, the accompanying loss of essential amino acids, which may lead to a significant decrease in nutritional quality of protein source, is of great importance.

NUTRITIONAL CHANGES IN FOOD PROTEINS

Proteins are necessary components of foodstuffs, because they are the main source of nitrogen and the only source of essential amino acids. For human nutrition, not only is the entire input of proteins important, but also their nutritional quality, which depends on their amino acid composition, digestibility of proteins, and physiological utilization of released amino acids. Physiological availability of amino acids varies and depends on protein source, processing treatment, and on the diet and health condition of the consumer.[1,2]

Food proteins are sometimes treated with heat and alkali during commercial and home processing. Many commercial foods contain proteins, such as sodium caseinate, textured

0-8493-4623-1/95/$0.00+$.50

soy protein, corn flour, wheat flour, etc., which have been previously exposed to alkali and/or heat treatment.

Alkali induces a number of changes in proteins. These include formation of cross-linked amino acids, such as lysinoalanine and related amino acids and racemization of amino acid residues.[2]

Heating causes large changes in the proteins of foodstuffs. By intensive heating, the bonds in amino acids can be shifted, and in this way digestibility can decrease. The intensity of changes in the protein, during heating, significantly depends on the water content. Heat treatment of protein preparations, which contain high amounts of water (e.g., during cooking or sterilization) results in substantially larger changes in amino acid composition than heat treatment under dry conditions.[3]

Heating protein preparations in the presence of water can lead to a large number of reactions of amino acids, which can decrease the nutritional quality of the protein by:

- Hydrolysis of peptide bonds of proteins
- Formation of low molecular fragments of proteins
- Oxidation of some functional groups of amino acids (e.g., oxidation of thiol to the disulfidic group)
- Oxidative deamination
- Decarboxylation to alkanals
- Racemization of L-amino acids to D-amino acids
- Cross-linking of amino acids

Serine, threonine, cysteine, and tryptophan are very unstable to heating, unlike neutral aliphatic amino acids like glutamic acid and proline, which are very stable.[1,3,4]

The above-mentioned reactions lead to decrease in nutritional quality of proteins, but need not lead to the formation of toxic compounds. Only racemization and cross-linking lead to the formation of these compounds.

D-AMINO ACIDS

Occurrence and Formation

D-amino acids (D-AA) can be rarely found in natural materials. Natural proteins contain solely L-amino acids.

D-AA are formed in protein preparations from natural L-amino acids during cooking and in industrial processes. Simultaneously, other atypical amino acids are formed, lysinoalanine being the most important of them.

In foodstuffs which were not exposed to intensive heating or unconventional treatment extensive racemization of L-amino acids does not occur, as shown in Tables 1 and 2. The only exception is D-aspartic acid since its content in untreated foodstuffs is relatively high.[4-6]

Table 2 shows that on intensive heating more racemization does not occur, and D-AA contents are approximately comparable to the control (Tables 1 and 2). Fermented milk products are an exception, because in them D-AA are present in higher amounts. From this point of view, D-alanine, D-aspartic acid, and D-glutamic acid reach the highest concentrations. In these products, microorganisms cause differences both in composition and content of D-AA. These microbial D-AA arise via biosynthesis, catalyzed with racemases and epimerases. A certain amount of D-AA can also occur during autolysis of microorganisms.[6]

Extensive racemization of all amino acids also appears in an alkaline medium at low temperatures. This alkaline medium is used for, e.g., destruction of some enzymes, microorganisms, and microbial toxins (page 177) and also for various technological

Table 1 D-Amino Acid Content in Raw Foods that have been Treated Under Very Mild Technological Conditions[4–6]

Food	D-Amino acid content (%)[a]								Ref.
	Ala	Val	Leu	Pro	Asp	Glu	Met	Phe	
White bread	2.4	0.9	3.2	0.9	5.6	2.8	2.3	2.3	5
Soy flour	2.5	1.0	1.4	2.3	4.4	3.1	—	2.8	5
Corn meal	2.3	1.3	2.5	1.5	5.2	3.4	2.4	1.5	5
Raw beef	3.2	1.6	3.1	2.0	6.2	4.9	2.4	2.8	5
Raw chicken	1.9	0.8	2.5	1.5	4.9	2.7	1.2	2.5	5
Raw cow milk	1.9	—	—	—	7.3	4.8	—	—	6
Pasteurized cow milk	1.8	—	—	—	7.3	5.1	—	—	6
Raw almond	0.0	0.0	3.0	—	2.6	—	—	1.1	4

[a] $\%\text{D-AA} = \dfrac{100.\text{D-AA}}{\Sigma\text{D-AA} + \text{L-AA}}$

Table 2 D-Amino Acid Content in Foods, that have been Treated in a Conventional Way[4–6]

Food	D-Amino acid content (%)[a]								Ref.
	Ala	Val	Leu	Pro	Asp	Glu	Met	Phe	
Toast (surface)	2.8	1.1	2.7	2.1	10.5	3.2	1.7	2.4	5
Extruded soy flour	2.7	0.8	2.7	1.6	7.6	3.9	—	2.4	5
Taco (shells)	3.2	1.5	3.8	1.0	5.8	3.8	1.1	—	5
Hamburger (surface)	2.8	1.5	3.2	1.8	5.5	2.4	2.9	2.7	5
Irradiated chicken	1.6	1.2	2.1	1.7	6.1	1.9	1.8	1.5	5
Kefir	37.4	5.6	22.6	—	17.6	4.9	—	—	6
Yogurt	61.3	—	—	—	20.9	12.4	—	—	6
Curdled milk	38.6	6.8	18.4	—	14.1	4.0	—	—	6
Fresh goat cheese	36.7	7.8	9.6	—	12.7	6.8	—	—	6
Peanut butter	3.1	1.2	2.2	1.5	4.9	3.7	2.0	2.7	5
Roasted almond	7.2	1.1	6.5	—	4.7	—	—	1.3	4

[a] $\%\text{D-AA} = \dfrac{100.\text{D-AA}}{\Sigma\text{D-AA} + \text{L-AA}}$

purposes, such as the production of protein concentrates and isolates, removing meat from bones (mechanically recovered meat), or for peeling fruit and vegetables. Aspartic acid and serine racemize most easily, while isoleucine, valine, threonine, and proline racemize very slowly. Free amino acids are about ten times more stable than those bonded in proteins. Racemization increases in the presence of glucose, where it accompanies nonenzymatic browning reactions and, further on, the presence of linoleic acid.[4,5]

Racemization begins with the removal of a proton from a free or peptide-bound amino acid. An optically inactive planar carbanion is formed as an intermediate, followed by reaction with a proton (H^+ ion), either a D-enantiomer or primary L-enantiomer being formed (Figure 1).

Nutritional and Physiological Aspects

Together with racemization, cross-linking of polypeptide chains occurs, which leads to the formation of a great number of xenobiotic amino acids, of which lysinoalanine is the best known. Both phenomena cause a decrease of digestibility of alkali-treated proteins. In these cases, digestibility decreases approximately by 10 to 20% in casein, by 40 to 70%

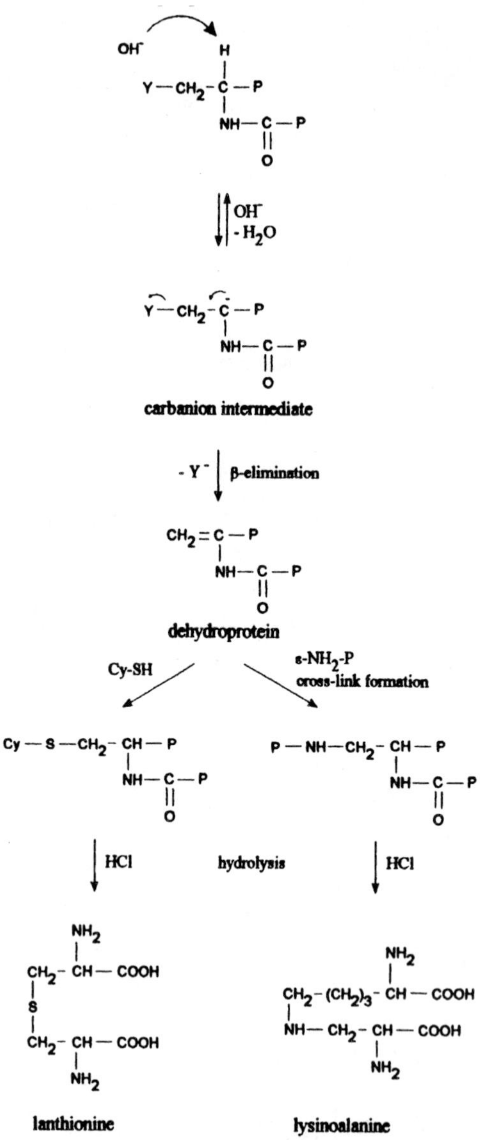

Figure 1 Possible mechanism for alkali-induced lysinoalanine and lanthionine formation and amino acid racemization in protein. Y = OH, OR, SH, SR, S^+R_2, S-SR, N^+R_3; P = protein side chain; Cy-SH = cysteine; ε-NH_2-P = ε-amino group of lysine bound in protein. Adapted from Friedman, M., Zahnley, J. C., and Masters, P. M., *J. Food Sci.*, 46, 127, 1981 and Velíšek, J. and Pokorný, J., *Potrav. Vědy*, 10, 59, 1992.

in soybean and wheat proteins. The decrease in the nutritional quality of the protein is caused by the decrease of digestibility and also by losses of amino acids, mainly of the essential ones. The loss of available lysine is the most significant. It is generally accepted that the degree of racemization and cross-linking corresponds to the decrease in digestibility.

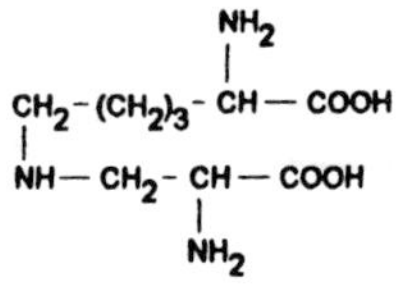

lysinoalanine
N^6-(2-amino-2-carboxyethyl)-lysine

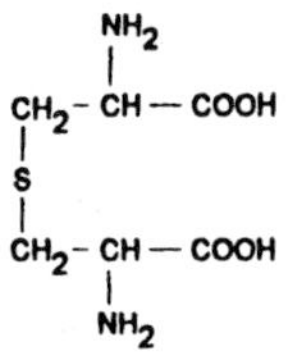

lanthionine
S-(2-amino-2carboxyethyl)-cysteine

Figure 2 Chemical structures of lysinoalanine and lanthionine.

It is accepted that in animal proteins more lysinoalanine (2 to 10 times) is formed, while the degree of racemization is higher in vegetable proteins.[7]

Absorption of amino acids in the intestinal tract is caused by various mechanisms, which are dependent on the structure of amino acids. L-Amino acids are absorbed through an active transport, while D-AA are absorbed passively, by diffusion. D-AA are less readily reabsorbed through the glomeruli of the kidneys. Acute toxicity of L- and D-enantiomers is comparable, only D-serine has higher toxicity, because it is nephrotoxic, like lysinoalanine.[2,4]

LYSINOALANINE, LANTHIONINE

Formation of Lysinoalanine (LAL) and Lanthionine (LAT)

Both compounds (Figure 2) usually range among so-called xenobiotic (unnatural, unusual, atypical) amino acids. A large number of these amino acids are known to be formed during alkali treatment of proteins, but in high concentration, only lysinoalanine and lanthionine are significant in foodstuffs and food sources. A survey of other atypical amino acids is given in another chapter (page 103).

The formation of LAL and LAT is schematically shown in Figure 1. LAL is formed mainly in an alkaline medium, even at low temperatures. At higher temperatures, LAL and LAT are formed even in a neutral and a low acidic medium. During alkali treatment, which is the most important from the point of view of possible LAL formation, the degree of formation depends on the treatment time, temperature, and the concentration of hydroxide ion. The formation of cross-linked amino acids is mostly accompanied by racemization of amino acids.

The reaction begins with β-elimination of the hydroxyl group of serine, *O*-phosphorylserine, or *O*-glycosylserine (Y = OH, OR) and/or the disulfide group of cystine (Y = S-SR). β-elimination of the hydroxyl group of threonine and its derivatives (Y = OH, OR) and the thiol group of cysteine (Y = SH), respectively, is also mentioned. The oxidation of the cysteine thiol group to cystine disulfide is required. The final product of β-elimination is the highly reactive dehydroalanine (DHA; 2-aminoacrylic acid), which is an intermediate in the formation of LAL, LAT, and other xenobiotic amino acids.

Temperature and pH have a large influence on the rate and degree of DHA formation. β-elimination is a base-catalyzed reaction, and that is why the increasing pH increases the reaction rate and shifts the reaction equilibrium towards the products.

At pH values higher than 9, there is also a very fast breakdown of disulfide groups, which is directly related to the rate of formation DHA and consequently with LAL and LAT formation. Temperature as well as pH has a very significant influence on DHA formation and consequent reactions. For example, during the heating of β-lactoglobulin A up to 97.5°C, DHA formation at pH 6.9 is very slow and a higher amount occurs after heating for 1 h, while at pH 9.8 it occurs after 5 to 10 min. On the other hand, during the heating of β-casein up to 120°C, DHA formation is very fast both at neutral and low acidic pH. Derivatization of function groups of amino acids has a strong influence on the β-elimination rate. Phosphorylated derivatives are considered to be most reactive. It is believed that enzymatic dephosphorylation decreases DHA formation to 10%.

DHA resulting from β-elimination is very reactive, and furthermore it can react with various amino compounds, e.g., amino acids, biogenic amines, etc. LAT arises from the reaction of DHA with cysteine, LAL from the reaction of DHA with lysine. At the same time, the course of these reactions is largely dependent on pH value. At neutral pH, the reaction is very slow, while at pH values higher than 9, it is relatively fast. The ε-amino group of lysine is much more reactive than other functional groups in amino acids. Therefore, LAL is formed in significantly higher concentrations in comparison with other products. For example, if we compare LAL with LAT, there is 2 to 100 times more LAL in most foodstuffs.[1,4,8-13]

Chemistry of Lysinoalanine

The stereochemistry of amino acids which are formed is relatively complicated. LAL contains two asymmetric centers and therefore four stereoisomers can exist. Theoretically, LL- and LD-LAL arise from L-lysine in equimolar ratio. When racemization of L-lysine to D-lysine takes place, DL-and DD-LAL are also formed. But in foodstuffs, only the LL- and LD-stereoisomers are present in significant concentrations. Both forms arise (Figure 1) in an approximately equal amount, but in acid medium, consecutive racemization of the LL- to the LD-form may occur. Racemization reaches its highest rate at pH values between 0 and 2, which is a value corresponding to the pH in the stomach. It is therefore very significant that the nephrotoxicity of the LD-form is about 10 times higher than that of the LL-form.[4,8]

Free LAL and LAT are partially unstable in alkaline medium and during longer heating at high temperatures. The breakdown of both amino acids increases with the increasing amount of water in the material. Figure 3 shows the influence of temperature and heating time of two enzymatic preparations on the formation of LAL and LAT.[3]

Occurrence of Lysinoalanine and Lanthionine

Xenobiotic amino acids such as LAL, LAT, and others usually occur in higher concentrations in various industrially treated and cooked foodstuffs, which contain a larger amount of vegetable and animal proteins that have been exposed to heat and/or alkali treatments (Table 3).

The LAL content in differently treated proteins largely depends on the concentration of the hydroxide ion, temperature and time of treatment. This dependence is shown in Figure 4.

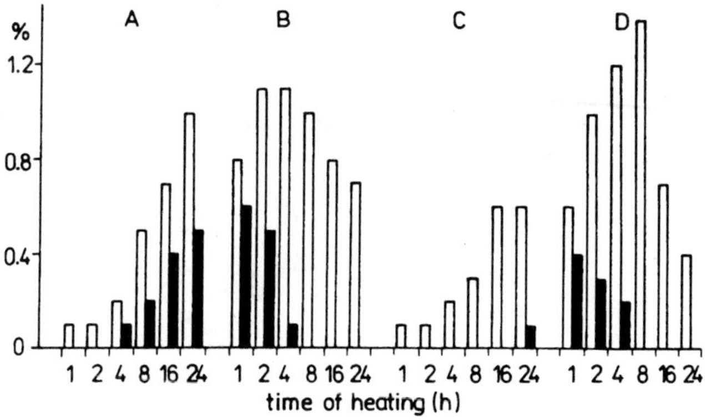

Figure 3 Dependence of lysinoalanine (LAL) and lanthionine (LAT) concentrations on the temperature and time of heating in enzymatic preparations. A = lysozyme (120°C); B = lysozyme (160°C); C = ribonuclease (120°C); D = ribonuclease (160°C). □ = LAL, ■ = LAT. Adapted from Scharf, U., and Weder, J.K.P., *Chem., Mikrobiol. Technol. Lebensm.*, 8, 71, 1983.

Table 3 Lysinoalanine (Lal) and Lanthionine (Lat) Content in Various Protein Preparations[4,7,9,10,14]

Protein source	LAL conc ($mg.g^{-1}$ protein)	LAT conc ($mg.g^{-1}$ protein)	Ref.
Defatted oilseed cakes			
Peanut	0.9	0.2	9
Soya	1.5	0.3	9
Sunflower	0.9	0.3	9
Rapeseed	1.5	0.1	9
Linseed	1.4	0.1	9
Textured broad been protein	0.3	0.1	9
Evaporated milk[a]	0.7[a]	—	7
α-Lactalbumin	0–83.4	—	7
β-Lactalbumin	0–28.1	—	7
Bovine serum albumine	0–64.7	—	7
Soy protein isolate	0.4–11.6	—	7,9,10
Wheat protein isolate	0.5–5.3	—	7,10
Hydrolyzed vegetable proteins	0.1–0.5	—	10
Alkali textured and spray-dried whey protein	0.2–30.0	—	9
Protein isolate from lobster shell	3.2	—	14
Casein isolate	0.6–16.2	—	4
Sour casein	0.1–0.2	—	4
Sodium caseinate	0.3–6.9	—	4,9
Calcium caseinate	0.4–1.0	—	4

[a] ΣLAL + LAT

Production of protein concentrates and isolates by alkali treatment has been known from antiquity. American Indians have long cooked corn in alkaline solution (lime water) for the production of masa and tortillas, which were traditional foods in Mexico. On the other hand, hominy is a traditional foodstuff for North American Indians and was prepared by cooking corn in water containing wood ash.

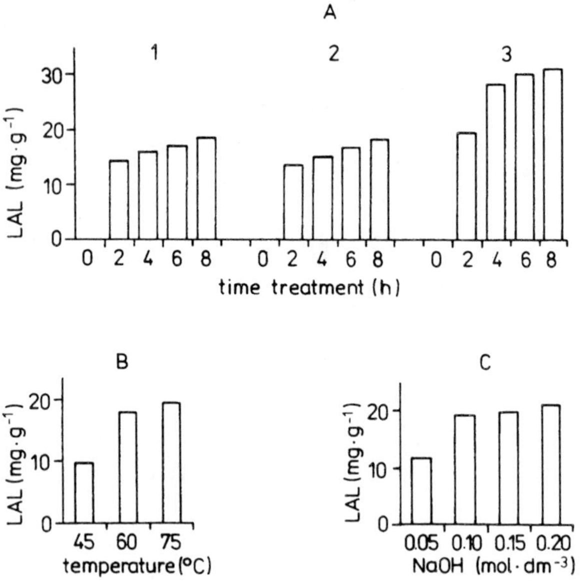

Figure 4 Lysinoalanine (LAL) concentration in alkali-treated protein materials. A, Dependence of LAL concentration on time treatment (0.1 mol.dm^{-3} NaOH, 75°C); 1 = canola meal, 2 = soybean protein isolate, 3 = casein. B, Dependence of LAL concentration on temperature treatment (0.1 mol.dm^{-3} NaOH, 3 h), canola meal. C, Dependence of LAL concentration on NaOH concentrations (3 h, 75°C), canola meal. Adapted from Pearce, K.N. and Friedman, M., *J. Agric. Food Chem.*, 36, 707, 1988.

Today products of this type in the North American countries are also prepared industrially, for example, dried masa flour, tortillas, corn chips, and canned hominy. Alkaline treatment of corn here results in losses of the amino acids arginine and cystine and formation of LAL. The losses are not too large — concentrations of LAL and LAT for the most part are not larger than 0.1% of the protein content in masa and tortillas, and 1.6% LAT and 0.3% LAL in hominy.[15]

Toxicological Aspects of Lysinoalanine and Lanthionine Formation

An evaluation of the formation of LAL and other xenobiotic amino acids must take into account two facts:

1. Toxicity of amino acids — only LAL toxicity has been studied in detail. Of all unusual amino acids, only LAL occurs in food proteins at high levels.
2. Lowering of the nutritional quality of proteins due to the formation of cross-linked bonds and by a decrease in the essential amino acids, mainly of available lysine.

The toxicity of LAL has been studied in detail. LAL has nephrotoxic effects and it can evoke an increase of nucleus and cytoplasm of the proximal renal tubule (nephrocytomegaly), cause microscopic lesions in kidney cells, and evoke an increase in the nucleoprotein content and consecutive disturbances of DNA synthesis and mitosis. The LD-stereoisomer has a relatively strong nephrotoxicity, while the other stereoisomers have significantly less influence (toxicity of the LD-isomer is about 10 times more than the LL-isomer). The toxicity of isomers is probably related to their affinity to Cu(II) and Zn(II) ions. With regard to the mechanism of toxicity, it is presumed that LAL operates as a trace metal chelator, because it is structurally similar to ethylenediaminetetraacetic acid (EDTA). Healthy kidney contains considerable amounts of copper and zinc bound in the metalloprotein metallothionein, which is located in tubular cells and is also extracellular in the tubules.

Because of its chelating ability, LAL can inactivate enzymes which contain metal ions, mainly Cu(II) and Zn(II) ions, the so-called metalloenzymes. Among them are, e.g., carboxypeptidase (peptidyl-L-amino acid hydrolase; EC 3.4.17.1), alcoholdehydrogenase (alcohol: NAD^+ oxidoreductase; EC 1.1.1.1) or polyphenoloxidase (*o*-diphenol: oxygen oxidoreductase; EC 1.10.3.1; tyrosinase). The LAL inhibition effect can be very significant, e.g., zinc-containing carboxypeptidase A can be higher than that of EDTA, but LAL toxicity can also inhibit other enzymes.

Kidney metalloenzymes contains copper in the cuprous (Cu[I]) state, which must be oxidized to the cupric state (Cu[II]) by hydrogen peroxide formed from catalase (hydrogen peroxide: hydrogen-peroxide oxidoreductase; EC 1.11.1.6). LAL and other similar amino acids inactivate metalloenzymic catalase. It is presumed that absorption, utilization, and uptake in urine has an influence on the occurrence and intensity of lesions. LAL has an influence on copper retention and redistribution and in this way also on the nutritional state of the organism in the copper area.

Other xenobiotic amino acids also have a very similar toxicity to LAL. They are present in significantly lower amounts, and therefore their toxicological importance is lower. Loss of enzymatic activity is higher not only with free LAL, but also with alkali-treated lysinoalanine-containing food proteins, such as casein, high lysine corn protein, lactalbumin, soy protein isolates, and wheat gluten, which contain various amounts of LAL, and even also by alkali-treated zein, which does not contain LAL.[8,10,11,15,17]

Use of Lanthionine

In human and veterinary medical practice, the group of synthetic antibiotics of the polypeptide type (so-called lanthibiotics), whose structure includes lanthionine bridges, are used. Apart from lanthionine, there are also other unusual amino acids, e.g., dehydroalanine, β-methyldehydroalanine, and β-methyllanthionine. Nisin, epidermin, and gallidermin are typical representatives of these antibiotics.[18-21]

OTHER XENOBIOTIC AMINO ACIDS

These amino acids, which are similarly formed in foods, also have similar physiological effects. But their formation is very limited, and concentrations are significantly lower than lysinoalanine and lanthionine.

Other xenobiotic amino acids and their stereoisomers can arise in the same way as LAL and LAT (Figure 1) by reactions of dehydroalanine or methyldehydroalanine with the secondary amino group of histidine, the hydroxy group of serine, threonine, or tyrosine, etc., and also by reaction with biogenic amines and ammonia.

The best known of these amino acids is ornithinoalanine, which is formed by reaction of dehydroalanine with ornithine, 3-[(2-phenylethyl)-amino]-DL-alanine (PEAA). The latter is formed by reaction of dehydroalanine with phenylethylamine, which is in turn a product of the decarboxylation of phenylalanine, DL-2,3-diaminopropanoic acid (DAPA; β-aminoalanine), formed by reaction of dehydroalanine with ammonia (Figure 5).[3,4,12,14,18,22]

NITROGENOUS COMPOUNDS ARISING FROM TRYPTOPHAN

Tryptophan is an essential amino acid which may be deficient in the diet of some members of the population. This is mainly due to the low content of tryptophan in cereals, which are practically the sole source of nutrition for a substantial part of the population,

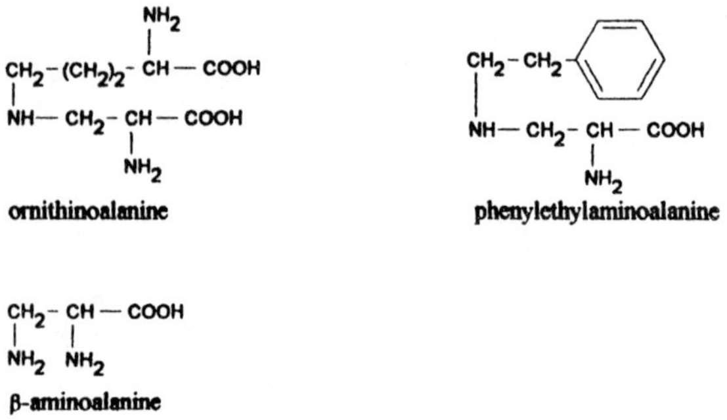

Figure 5 Chemical structures of other unusual amino acids.

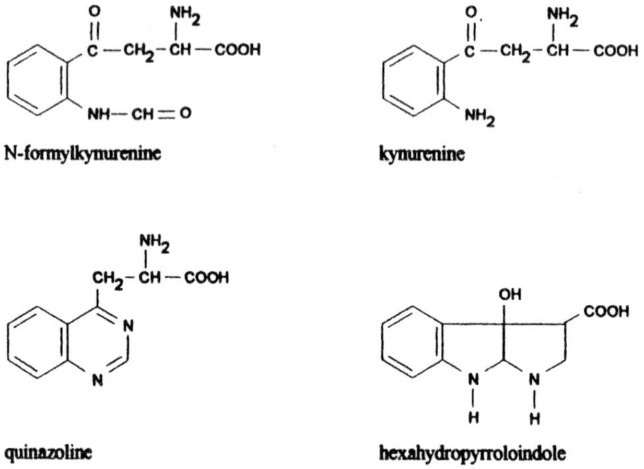

Figure 6 Some products of tryptophan reactions with ammonia.

and to its low stability during processing. The degree of tryptophan breakdown depends mainly on the presence of oxygen and on the temperature. In the presence of oxygen and at high temperature, the tryptophan hydroperoxidic radical is formed, which in the presence of ammonia reacts to form *N*-formylkynurenine and, consecutively, kynurenine or quinazoline or hexahydropyrroloindole (Figure 6).

Tryptophan can also condense with aldehydes, forming a 2-acyl-derivative, from which β-carboline is formed by cyclization and consecutive dehydrogenation. This compound, as well as its derivatives, are potentially carcinogenic. Tryptophan and tryptamine can react with carbonyl compounds via the Maillard reaction. At the same time partial dimerization can occur. The formation of (indolyl-methyl)-tetrahydrogen-β-carboline (Figure 7), as a condensation product of indolyl-3-pyruvic acid and tryptamine (products from oxidative deamination and decarboxylation of tryptophan, respectively) is an example.

The presence of products of lipid oxidation (hydroperoxides, cyclic peroxides, aldehydes, ketones) results in the breakdown of free and also protein-bound tryptophan.The diastereoisomers of dioxoindolyl-3-alanine, *N*-formylkynurenine, and kynurenine were identified as reaction products.

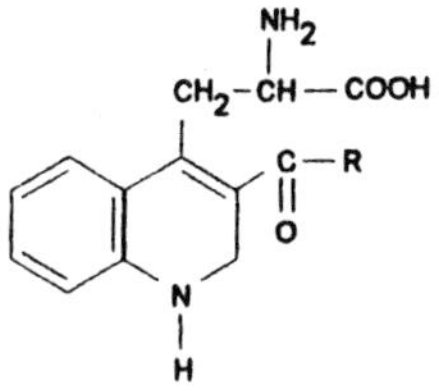

R = H, alkyl
2-acylderivative of tryptophan

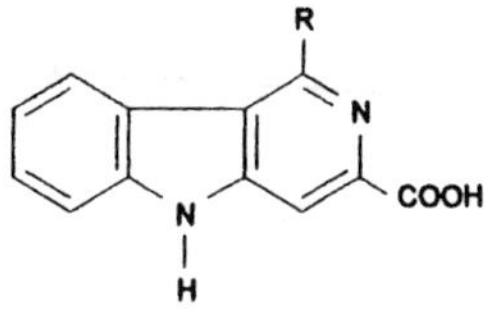

β-carbolin

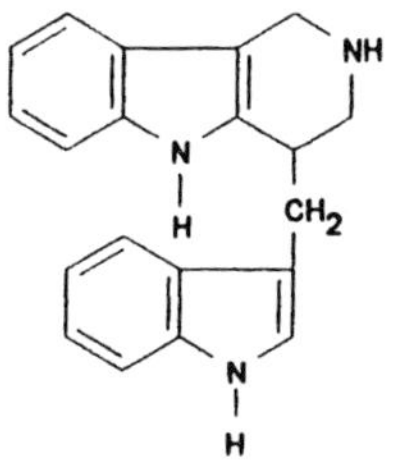

(indolylmethyl)-tetrahydrogen-β-carbolin

Figure 7 Some products of tryptophan reactions with aldehydes.

A decrease in bioavailability of tryptophan is a consequence of all these reactions. These compounds are found mainly in meat and meat products, heated milk, beer, and wine. The majority of the breakdown products of tryptophan are considered as potentially mutagenic and/or carcinogenic.[23]

REACTIONS OF PROTEINS WITH PLANT PHENOLS

Some plant polyphenols (phenolic acids, flavonoids, tannins) have various negative physiological effects and therefore belong to a group of natural toxic compounds (page 75). Orthodiphenols, phenolic acids, and caffeic and chlorogenic acids are easily oxidized by oxidoreductases, for example, by polyphenoloxidase (*o*-diphenol: oxygen oxidoreductase; EC 1.10.3.1; tyrosinase). Similarly, nonenzymatic oxidation can be catalyzed by heavy metal salts, mainly copper in the cuprous state (Cu[II]). Oxidation occurs very quickly in an alkaline medium, while in neutral and acidic media it is significantly slower. The primary products of oxidation are *o*-semiquinone radicals and *o*-quinones, which further react, forming dark polymeric products. These products are formed by reaction of *o*-quinones with primary *o*-diphenols, often in the presence of proteins, metals, and other compounds.

The production of protein concentrates by extraction of proteins from alkaline medium not only leads to the racemization of L-amino acids and the formation of lysinoalanine and similar compounds, but at the same time, the reactions of protein with phenolic compounds takes place. These reactions not only lead to disagreeable changes of color of protein preparations, but also to a decrease in nutritional quality of foodstuffs. Oxidized polyphenols easily react with the thiol group of cysteine, the ε-amino group of lysine, and the α-terminal amino group of protein-bound amino acids. Bound methionine and tryptophan are also very reactive. These reactions, which lead to a decrease of bioavailability of proteins, are very important, especially for proteins, in which lysine, methionine, and

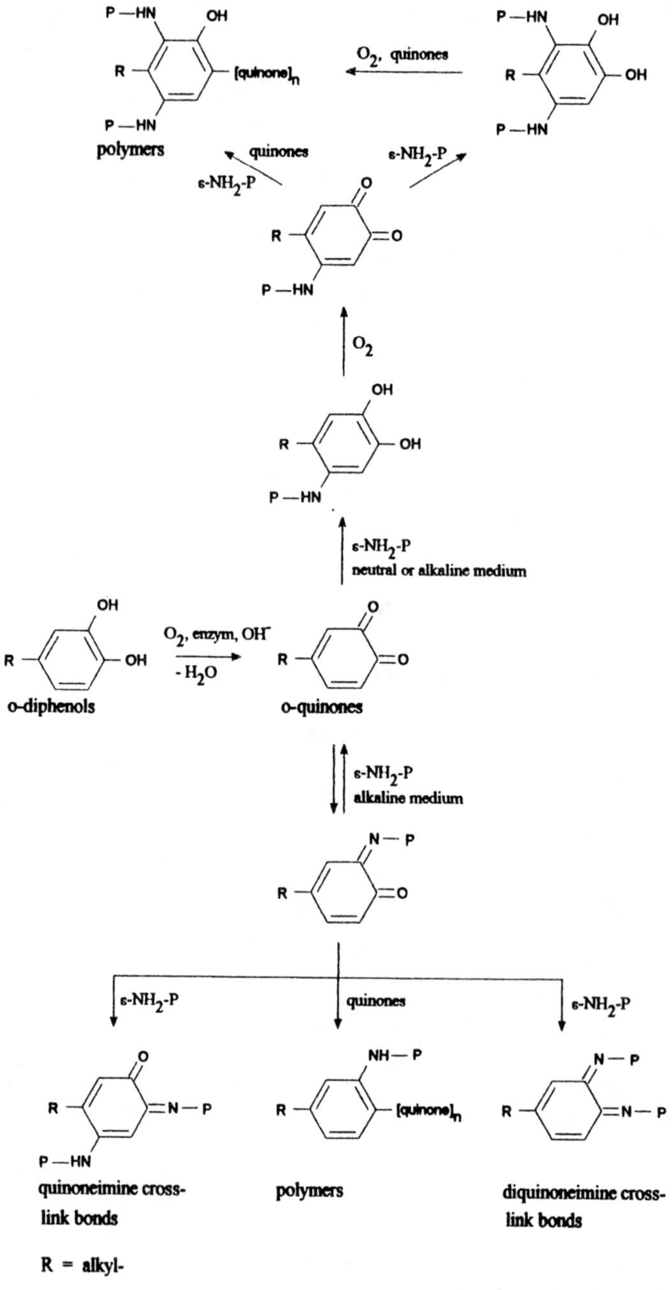

Figure 8 Possible mechanisms of lysine reactions with plant phenols. Adapted from Velíšek, J. and Pokorný, J., *Potrav. Vědy*, 10, 59, 1992 and Singleton, V. L., *Adv. Food Res.* 27, 149, 1981.

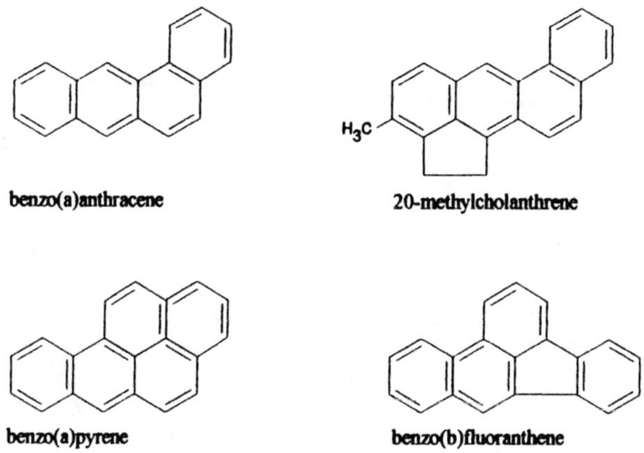

Figure 9 Some carcinogenic PAH.

tryptophan as essential amino acids are limiting amino acids. Methionine, cysteine, and tryptophan in addition are easily oxidized by quinones present, which can give rise to other secondary reactions, e.g., formation of lysinoalanine or tryptophan oxidation products. A side reaction is also the Strecker degradation of amino acids. The loss of essential amino acids is increased by various factors: in tryptophan, mainly by decreasing protein digestibility; in methionine, by its oxidation to methioninesulfoxide (which is less available than methionine); in lysine by its reaction with *o*-diphenols, mainly caffeic and chlorogenic acids, forming unavailable covalent compounds (Figure 8).

These reactions need not only have a negative physiological influence, since reactions of proteins with phenols can lead to their partial detoxification. For example, methionine can methylate break products of condensed tannins, mainly gallic acid and its derivatives. Similarly, cottonseed, as an important source of proteins in some regions, contains the toxic phenol gossypol, which by condensation of its aldehyde group with free amino groups in proteins, is largely detoxified during processing.

Catechins and other phenols can also react with proteins in the membrane cells, on collagen, in enzymes, etc. If phenols are bound on membranes of microorganisms and viruses, they increase their antimicrobial and antivirus effect.[4,24,25]

POLYCYCLIC AROMATIC HYDROCARBONS

Polycyclic aromatic hydrocarbons (PAH) are generated during incomplete combustion of organic matter, so their sources are numerous and differ greatly, including pollution and cotamination of air, water, and soil. Nowadays, they are ubiquitous in the environment and consequently they are present in foods. Moreover, they are formed in food in significant amounts during certain heat processes.

Chemistry

Polycyclic aromatic hydrocarbons can be defined as organic compounds containing two or more fused benzene rings, usually 3 to 7 (Figure 9). Conjugated π-electron systems of PAH determine their chemical stability. All PAH with exception of a few derivatives are solids and are the least volatile of all hydrocarbons. The high molecular weight of PAH and the absence of polar substituents groups make these compounds almost insoluble in water. There is a rough correlation between increasing molecular weight and decreasing solubility of PAH. When they react, they tend to retain their conjugated ring systems by forming derivatives by electrophilic substitution rather than addition. PAH chemistry has been comprehensively reviewed by Clar[26] and is discussed in various monographs.[27-29]

Toxicological aspects

Many PAH cause cancer in various animals species and it is suspected that they cause cancer in humans as well. The toxicological effects of PAH are structure dependent. These chemically relatively inert compounds are activated *in vivo*. Monooxygenates system of cytochrome P-450 (EC 1.14.14.1) and epoxide hydrolases (EC 3.3.2.3) participate in this activation process. For instance, benzo(*a*)pyrene (B(*a*)P) is metabolized to the transdihydrodiol-epoxide (7,8-dihydro-7,8-dihydroxybenzo(*a*)pyrene), which reacts with DNA and/or proteins by covalent binding. This form is probably an actual carcinogenic agent.[30]

Occurrence and Changes during Processing and Storage

PAH represent one of the most important classes of organic contaminants in food. Based on findings of many authors,[28,31-33] it can be concluded that human exposure to and risk from these compounds occurs via air, water, and food. The contamination of foods with PAH may also arise during processing and home cooking. Therefore, two main pathways can be roughly distinguished. The first one is the contamination resulting from environmental pollution (air, water, soil) and the second pathway, so-called secondary contamination or endogenous formation, is the contamination resulting mainly from smoking, roasting, grilling, broiling, and frying due to the pyrolysis of fats, proteins, sugars, and others.

PAH originating from the smoking of food seems to be probably the most important secondary source of contamination. Wigand and Jahr reported B(a)P content in commercial Bavarian smoked products.[34] A considerable number of samples, especially "black smoked" products, exceeded the value 1 $\mu g.kg^{-1}$, which was accepted as the safe limit for smoked products in Germany. B(a)P content in Frankfurter sausages, smoked in generators operating on various types of systems, i.e., smoke open-, closed-, friction open-, and steam systems, were determined. The highest level (0.7 $\mu g.kg^{-1}$), was found in sausages smoked in the closed system.[35] Smoke as well as smoke flavor contain various PAH, which during smoking are deposited on the surface of smoked products. Both the amount of PAH and their profile (presence of individual compounds) is dependent on the type of process, technology, and kind of processed food.

Since raw meat does not normally contain PAH, it is the smoking and other heat processes which are responsible for its formation. Occasionally the PAH levels in smoked products are relatively high. For instance, the B(a)P level in smoked beef reached up to 16.8 $\mu g.kg^{-1}$ (in the same unsmoked meat, no B(a)P was detected).[36]

The distribution of PAH in smoked meat is not homogeneous. About 60 to 70% of B(a)P is formed in the surface layer.[37,38] The degradation of B(a)P is influenced by its diffusion into the internal layer where it is stabilized due to the absence of light and oxygen.[39,40]

The incomplete combustion of charcoal can also contribute to the PAH content in meat. The surface area of treated products is an important parameter. Some authors[38] claim that a protective covering (e.g., cellophane, cotton fabric) reduces the PAH in smoked foods significantly. The skin of smoked fish and coverings of sausages seems to be a very effective barrier against PAH contamination.

Other culinary heating processes, such as grilling, roasting, and cooking also contribute to PAH secondary contamination of food. In the case of grilling, the heat is applied by radiation and the temperature may reach 350°C on the surface.[41] The precursors of

PAH can be proteins, lipids, and carbohydrates. For instance, starch heated at 370 to 390°C in the absence of air yields 0.7 μg.kg^{-1} B(a)P.[37]

The amount of PAH in heat-treated food is affected by a wide variety of factors. It seems that the presence of PAH in broiled meats is directly proportional to the temperature and duration of treatment. Most of the PAH are probably formed by pyrolysis of fats.[37,38] Decreasing fat content in beef also decreases the amount and profile of PAH.[42] The consumption of hamburgers which are cooked on a barbecue is very popular. With respect to the relatively high levels of PAH (from several hundreds to several tens of μg.kg^{-1}), such types of food contribute significantly to the total intake of PAH via nutrition.

In connection with smoking procedures, smoked cereal products should be mentioned, especially "talkhuna" or "talkhan". These local smoked cereal food are widely consumed in some Finnish and Russian localities.[43] They are prepared from smoked oats, barley, and peas. The average intake from this source is 430 μg per person per year.[44,45]

The first indication of possible formation of carcinogenic hydrocarbons during roasting of coffee was mentioned in 1938, and since then several reviews have been published.[38,46] The levels of PAH in normal roasted coffee beans range from 0.1 to 0.8 μg.kg^{-1} and increase with roasting temperature.[47] With respect to the form of coffee consumption, the PAH intake actually occurs only via the coffee brew and is very low due to its limited solubility.

In smoked tea leaves, type Lapsang Souchong, from 50 to 200 μg.kg^{-1} of B(a)P was found. However, tea prepared from 1 g tea leaves per 100 ml water, contaminated at a level of 180 μg.kg^{-1}, was less than 16 ng.dm^{-3} (WHO limit for drinking water is 0.01 μg.dm^{-3}).[48]

The presence of phenanthrene, fluoranthene, pyrene, benzo(*a*)pyrene, and benzo(*e*)pyrene was also detected in various kinds of whisky in very low concentrations (0.03 to 0.08 μg.dm^{-3}).[38]

The smoking, charcoal-broiling, grilling, and roasting, as has already been mentioned, are mainly responsible for secondary PAH contamination of meat, meat products, fish, coffee, tea, special kinds of cheese, and smoked cereal products. It is difficult to explain PAH formation during heating processing of food because very little is known about their formation in even simple models, and much less so in a complex matrix such as a foodstuff.

REFERENCES

1. Davídek, J., Janíček, G., and Pokorný, J., in *Chemie Potravin* (*Food Chemistry*), SNTL-ALFA, Prague, 1983, 15.
2. Friedman, M., Zahnley, J. C., and Masters, P. M., Relationship between *in vitro* digestibility of casein and its content of lysinoalanine and D-amino acids, *J. Food Sci.*, 46, 127, 1981.
3. Scharf, U. and Weder, J. K. P., Modelluntersuchungen zur Erhitzung von Lebensmittelproteinen — der Einfluss des Wassergehaltes auf die Aminosäurezusammensetzung von Lysozym und Ribonuclease nach der Erhitzung, *Chem. Mikrobiol. Technol. Lebensm.*, 8, 71, 1983.
4. Velíšek, J. and Pokorný, J., Antinutritional and toxic substances produced in foodstuffs by reaction of main nutrients, *Potrav. Vědy*, 10, 59, 1992.
5. Bunjapamai, S., Mahoney, R. R., and Fagerson, I. S., Determination of D-amino acids in some processed foods and effect of racemization on *in vitro* digestibility of casein, *J. Food Sci.*, 47, 1229, 1982.
6. Brückner, H. and Hausch, M., D-Amino acids in dairy products: detection, origin and nutritional aspects. I. Milk, fermented milk, fresh cheese and acid curd cheese, *Milchwissenschaft*, 45, 357, 1990.
7. Chung, S. Y., Swaisgood, H. E., and Catignani, G. L., Effects of alkali treatment and heat treatment in the presence of fructose on digestibility of food proteins as determined by an immobilized digestive enzyme assay (IDEA), *J. Agric. Food Chem.*, 34, 579, 1986.

8. Liardon, R., Friedman, M., and Philippossian, G., Racemization kinetics of free and protein-bound lysinoalanine (LAL) in strong acid media. Isomeric composition of bound LAL in processed proteins, *J. Agric. Food Chem.* 39, 531, 1991.
9. Aymard, C., Cuq, J. L., and Cheftel, J. C., Formation of lysino-alanine and lanthionine in various food proteins, heated at neutral or alkaline pH, *Food Chem.*, 3, 1, 1978.
10. Deng, Q. Y., Barefoot, R. R., Diosady, L. L., Rubin, L. J., and Tzeng, Y. M., Lysinoalanine concentrations in rapeseed protein meals and isolates, *Can. Inst. Food Sci. Technol. J.*, 23, 140, 1990.
11. Pearce, K. N. and Friedman, M., Binding of copper (II) and other metal ions by lysinoalanine and related compounds and its significance for food safety, *J. Agric. Food Chem.*, 36, 707, 1988.
12. Kleyn, D. H. and Klostermeyer, H., Dehydroalanin als Reaktionsprodukt bei der Erhitzung von β-Casein, *Z. Lebensm. Unters. Forsch.*, 170, 11, 1980.
13. Watanabe, K. and Klostermeyer, H., Bildung von Dehydroalanin, Lanthionin und Lysinoalanin beim Erhitzen von β-Lactoglobulin A, *Z. Lebensm. Unters. Forsch.*, 164, 77, 1977.
14. Oviedo, E., Garcia, I., and Henriques, R. D., Basic protein isolate from lobster shell, *Nahrung*, 29, 435, 1985.
15. Sanderson, J., Wall, J. S., Donaldson, G. L., and Cavins, J. F., Effect of alkaline processing of corn on its amino acids, *Cereal Chem.*, 55, 204, 1978.
16. Friedman, M., Grosjean, O. K., and Zahnley, J.C., Carboxypeptidase inhibition by alkali-treated food proteins, *J. Agric. Food Chem.*, 33, 208, 1985.
17. Friedman, M., Grosjean, O. K., and Zahnley, J.C., Inactivation of metalloenzymes by food constituents, *Food Chem. Toxicol.*, 24, 897, 1986.
18. Dodd, H. M., Horn, N., and Gasson, M. J., Analysis of the genetic determinant for production of the peptide antibiotic nisin, *J. Gen. Microbiol.*, 136, 555, 1990.
19. Hoerner, T., Zachner, H., Kellner, R., and Jung, G., Fermentation and isolation of epidermin, a lanthionine containing polypeptide antibiotic from *Staphylococcus epidermis, Appl. Microbiol. Biotechnol.*, 30, 219, 1989.
20. Hoerner, T., Ungermann, V., Zachner, H., Fiedler, H. P., Utz, R., Kellner, R., and Jung, G., Comparative studies on the fermentative production of lantibiotics by *staphylococci, Appl. Microbiol. Biotechnol.*, 32, 511, 1990.
21. Kaletta, C. and Entian, K. D., Nisin, a peptide antibiotics: cloning and sequencing of the nisA gene and posttranslational processing of its peptide product, *J. Bacteriol.*, 171, 1597, 1989.
22. Friedman, M. and Noma, A. T., Formation and analysis of (phenylethyl)-amino-alanine in food protein, *J. Agric. Food Chem.*, 34, 497, 1986.
23. Friedman, M. and Cuq, J. L., Chemistry, analysis, nutritional value, and toxicology of tryptophan in food. A review, *J. Agric. Food Chem.*, 36, 1079, 1988.
24. Singleton, V. L., Naturally occurring food toxicants: phenolic substances of plant origin common in foods, *Adv. Food Research*, 27, 149, 1981.
25. Smith, F. H., Effect of gossypol bound to cottonseed protein on growth of weanling rats, *J. Agric. Food Chem.*, 20, 803, 1972.
26. Clar, E., in *Polycyclic Aromatic Hydrocarbons*, Academic Press, New York, 1964, chap. 2.
27. Lee, M. L., Novotný, M., and Bartle, K. D., in *Analytical Chemistry of Polycyclic Aromatic Compounds*, Academic Press, London, 1981, chap.1.
28. Bjorseth, A. and Ramdahl, T., in *Handbook of Polycyclic Aromatic Hydrocarbons*, Marcel Dekker, New York, 1983, chap.1.
29. Vo-Dinh, T., in *Chemical Analysis of Polycyclic Aromatic Hydrocarbons*, John Wiley Sons, New York, 1989, chap. 2.
30. Farmer, P. B., Carcinogen adducts: use in diagnosis and risk assessment, *Clin. Chem.*, in press.
31. Suess, M. J., The environmental load and cycle of polycyclic aromatic hydrocarbons, *Sci. Total Environ.*, 6, 239, 1976.
32. Sloof, W. and Janus J. A., in Integrated Criteria Document PAHs, Rep. no. 758474011, RIVM, The Netherlands, 1989, chap. 3.
33. Sloof, W. and Janus, J. A., in Integrated Criteria Document PAHs: Effects of 10 Selected Compounds, Appendix to Rep. no. 758474011, RIVM, The Netherlands, 1989, chap. 2.
34. Wigand, W. and Jahr, D., Benzo(a)pyrene-Gehalt in gerauchter Fleisherzeugnisse, *Fleischwirtschaft*, 65, 915, 1985.

35. Mueller, I. M. and Wirth, F., Health and environmental protection in hot smoking of small cooked sausages, in *Proc. European Meeting of Meat Research Workers,* 30, 287, 1984.
36. Ogbadu, G. H. and Ogbadu, L. J., Levels of benzo(a)pyrene in some smoked ready-to-eat Nigerian foods, *Lebens. Wiss. Technol.,* 22, 313, 1989.
37. Lo, M. T. and Sandi, E., Polycyclic aromatic hydrocarbons (polynuclears) in foods, *Res. Rev.,* 69, 352, 1978.
38. Fazio, T., Polycyclic aromatic hydrocarbons, in *Food Constituents and Food Residues, Their Chromatographic Determination,* Lawrence, J. F., Ed., Marcel Dekker, New York, 1984, chap. 5.
39. Šimko, P., Gombita, M., and Karovičová, J., Determination and occurrence of benzo(a)pyrene in smoked meat products, *Nahrung,* 35, 103, 1991.
40. Šimko, P., Changes of benzo(a)pyrene in smoked fish during storage, *Food Chem.,* 40, 293, 1991.
41. Heimann, W., *Fundamentals of Food Chemistry,* Part II: *Behavior of Food During Preparation and Cooking,* AVI Publishing, New York, 1980.
42. Maga, J. A., Polycyclic aromatic hydrocarbons (PAH) composition of mesquite smoke and grilled beef, *J. Agric. Food Chem.,* 34, 249, 1986.
43. Karimov, M. A., Sarbekov, E. K., and Kostenko, L. D., Benzo(a)pyrene content in cereal products, *Vopr. Pytaniya,* 1, 57, 1988.
44. Tuominen, J. P., Pyysalo, H. S., and Sauri, M., Cereal products as source of polycyclic aromatic hydrocarbons, *J. Agric. Food Chem.,* 16, 118, 1988.
45. Tuominen, J. P., in *Determination of Polycyclic Aromatic Hydrocarbons by Gas Chromatography/ Mass Spectrometry and Method Development in Supercritical Fluid Chromatography,* Technical Research Centre of Finland (Valtion Teknillinenn Tutkimuskeskus), Espoo, 1990, chap.1.
46. Howard, J. W. and Fazio, T., Review of polycyclic aromatic hydrocarbons in foods, *J. Assoc. Off. Anal. Chem.,* 63, 1076, 1980.
47. Kruijf, N., Schouten, T., and Stegen, G. H. D., Rapid determination of benzo(*a*)pyrene in roasted coffee and coffee brew by HPLC with fluorescence detection, *J. Agric. Food Chem.,* 35, 545, 1987.
48. Joe, F. L. Jr., Salemme, J., and Fazio, T., Liquid chromatographic determination of trace residues of polynuclear hydrocarbons in smoked foods, *J. Assoc. Off. Anal. Chem.,* 67, 1076, 1984.

Part B

Toxic and Antinutritional Compounds Arising From Saccharides

Jan Velíšek

Saccharides, especially mono- and oligosaccharides participate in many reactions which occur during processing and storage of foods. Changes in saccharides may be either enzymatic or nonenzymatic and frequently proceed simultaneously. Nonenzymatic browning reactions belong to the most important reactions occurring in foods because they not only produce desirable flavors, tastes, aromas and colors but also give rise to off-flavors and off-tastes, undesirable discolorations, and serious deterioration of food quality from the nutritional point of view. Nonenzymatic browning involves a number of reactions of saccharides and other carbonyl compounds which occur either as natural constituents of foods or originate by breakdown of nutrients and other food components. The most frequently encountered, both as to frequency and possible consequences, is the Maillard reaction involving reducing sugars (and their derivatives, such as alduronic acids) and amino compounds (amino acids, both free and bound in proteins, amines, and ammonia or ammonium salts) and caramelizing reactions, which occur by heating saccharides at relatively high temperatures. The loss of nutritional quality is attributed to the destruction of essential amino acids and a decrease in digestibility of proteins. The production of antinutritional, inhibitory and toxic compounds including kidney-damaging compounds, growth inhibitors, mutagenic (DNA-damaging), clastogenic (chromosome-damaging), and carcinogenic compounds further reduces the nutritional value and the safety of foods. The Maillard reaction called glycosylation also occurs *in vivo* and contributes to some adverse processes related to diseases and aging. Antioxidant and antimutagenic effects of certain reaction products are positive aspects of nonenzymatic browning.

The chemical, nutritional, physiological, safety and other aspects of nonenzymatic browning reactions have been covered in several recent review articles and books.[1-14]

THE MAILLARD REACTION PRODUCTS

GLYCOSYLAMINES AND AMINODEOXYSUGARS

The first step in the Maillard reaction of a reducing sugar (nonreducing oligosaccharides and polysaccharides are first hydrolyzed to monosaccharides) with an amino compound (e.g., amino acid or protein) in solutions and foods, is the addition of the amine to the carbonyl function of sugar. The product looses one molecule of water, yielding an imine (Schiff base), an open-chain compound which undergoes cyclization to the corresponding *N*-substituted glycosylamine. Schiff bases and glycosylamines readily hydrolyze to the parent compounds, especially in acid media, and this is why this reaction step does not cause any change in the nutritive quality of foods. Under the influence of a suitable catalyst (chiefly hydroxonium or hydroxyl ions), glycosylamines isomerize (Amadori rearrangement) to 1-amino-1-deoxyketoses, also known as ketosamines, isoaldosamines, or Amadori products, which are the major forms of the so-called bound or unavailable amino acids in foods.

The toxic potential of these early Maillard reaction products is not clearly evident since it is difficult to discriminate the actual toxic effects from those due to dietary inadequacy resulting from the nutrient losses or blockage. The most important in respect to the nutritional quality of foods are reactions of D-glucose and other reducing sugars with the ε-amino group of lysine and with sulfur-containing amino acids (methionine and cysteine or cystine) bound in proteins which are accompanied by oxidation reactions of sulfur-containing amino acids and tryptophan (page 183). Relatively less important are reactions of reducing sugars with N-terminal amino acids and other amino acids of the protein peptide chain and reactions of sugars with free amino acids (creatine/creatinine is an exception). All these reactions lead to the formation of unavailable complexes, oxidation products, and other covalent compounds, enzyme-resistant cross-links between amino acids in protein side chains, which result in a decreased protein hydrolysis by proteolytic digestive enzymes and thus lead to the decrease of their nutritive quality (page 183).

DEGRADATION PRODUCTS

The reaction outlined above is, however, more complex. Glucose alone isomerizes and dehydrates via 1,2-enolization to more reactive α-dicarbonyl compounds such as 3-deoxy-D-glucosulose (3-deoxy-D-erythrohexosulose), 3,4-dideoxy-D-glucosulos-3-ene (3,4-dideoxy-D-glycero-2-hexosulos-3-ene), and finally to 5-hydroxymethyl-2-furancarboxaldehyde and other minor products. Via 2,3-enolization it isomerizes to aldoses and ketoses, splits to smaller more reactive fragments such as carbonyl, α-dicarbonyl, α-hydroxycarbonyl compounds, and reductones such as formaldehyde, glycolaldehyde, glyceraldehyde, and triosoreductone (hydroxymethylglyoxal). These compounds further isomerize, dehydrate and split to other reactive species such as methylglyoxal. Reactive di-D-glucosylamine arises as a minor product in the reaction of glucosylamine with the second molecule of glucose and rearranges to difructoseamine. A portion of D-glucosylamine may be split by the reverse-aldol condensation into a very reactive two-carbon fragment glycolaldehyde imine and D-erythrose, instead of being rearranged to the aminodeoxysugar. This cleavage is almost simultaneously followed by the bimolecular condensation of glycolaldehyde imine to *N,N'*-disubstituted dihydropyrazine, one-electron oxidation of which leads to the formation of a pyrazine radical and subsequently to pyrazinium salt. Very reactive glyoxal is formed as an oxidation product of glycolaldehyde.

Both fructosamine and difructosamine react further by several pathways including elimination, dehydration, aldol, and retroaldol condensation. This decomposition proceeds predominantly via 1,2-enolization in acid and neutral media and via 2,3-enolization in alkaline media and yields a large number of volatile and nonvolatile products, of which some are identical with the degradation products of sugars which arise in the absence of amino compounds and some are derived from the parent amino compounds. The reactive degradation products of sugars and aminodeoxysugars such as dicarbonyls and reductones also undergo a complex series of reactions with amino compounds responsible for the production of flavors and colors of the treated material. Of special importance is oxidative decarboxylation of amino acids called the Strecker degradation, which gives rise to aldehydes, aminoreductones, and heterocyclic compounds. The final products of many reactions are high-molecular weight melanoidins responsible for color changes of many foods on processing and storage.

A few other simple compounds formed during the Maillard reaction, such as some dicarbonyls and heterocycles, e.g., glyoxal, methylglyoxal, diacetyl (2,3-butanedione), D-glucosulose, 5-hydroxymethyl-2-furancarboxaldehyde and other furans, 2-methylthiazolidine, products of triose reductone reaction with amino acids, and products obtained from a maltol-ammonia reaction, were identified as mutagens.[15-20] These compounds showed a relatively weak effect of an order of magnitude lower than that of heterocyclic amines in bacteria (base pair in contrast to frameshift mutations as caused by heterocyclic amines). Furthermore the liver microsomal enzymes or catalases were able to abolish the mutagenic effect of these compounds, in contrast with heterocyclic amines which were activated by them. Examples of food products with weak mutagenicity and which underwent metabolic deactivation, being neither mutagenic nor carcinogenic in intact animals, are carbohydrate-rich food products such as bakery products, roasted coffee, cocoa, caramels, and to some extent also heated milk and meat products.

Mutagenic compounds also arise during the nitrosation of the Maillard reaction products. It has been shown that glycosylamines, Amadori compounds, α-carbolines arising from tryptophan and other *N*-heterocyclic compounds can be nitrosated yielding mutagenic products (page 229).

Very little is known about the reaction products of sugars with sulfur dioxide and bisulfites which are widely used to control and retard the development of nonenzymatic browning. In the case of some stable sulfur-containing compounds such as D-glucose-6-phosphate, D-glycero-D-ido-1,2,3,4,5,6-hexahydroxyhexylsulfonate, 4-sulfohexosulose (i.e., 3, 4-dideoxy-4-sulfo-D-glycero-hexosulose), and 3, 4-dideoxy-4-sulfo-2-D-hexosulose, their oxidation and benzilic acid type rearrangement products have been identified in foods treated with sulfur dioxide. Investigations carried out on 4-sulfohexosulose (Figure 1) demonstrated its low toxicity and the absence of mutagenicity.[21,22] Sulfites are, however, reported to induce asthmatic crises in 4 to 8% of exposed asthmatics.[23]

Certain Maillard reaction products and/or their fractions, such as carbonyl compounds and high-molecular weight melanoidins occurring during heat processing and storage of food, were reported to have strong antioxidant properties. These properties were exhibited in particular by the products of reactions in model systems containing D-glucose or D-xylose with histidine, lysine, arginine, and cysteine[24-30] and even by the reaction

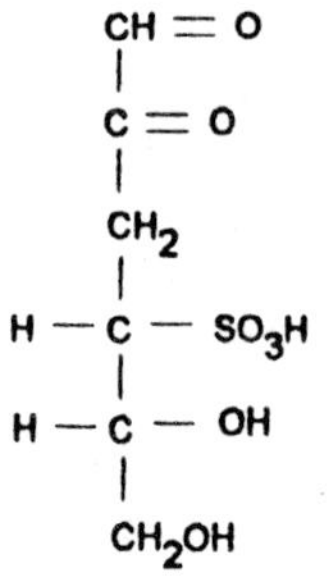

Figure 1 Structure of 3,4-dideoxy-4-sulfo-D-glycerohexosulose.

products of simpler systems such as glyoxal and glycine.[31,32] Some of the heated foods, such as heated milk, cereals, and meat, were shown to possess improved oxidative stability.[30] The hypothesis has therefore been put forward that Maillard reaction products might excert an anticarcinogenic activity by inactivating reactive oxygen species which are envolved in the process of cancer.[33] Feasible mechanisms are inhibition of nitrosamine formation by competition with electrophilic reaction of nitrite with secondary amines (page 231), direct scavenging of ultimate carcinogenic species, and antipromotor activity and modulation of monooxidase as a radical defence enzyme system. Results supporting this hypothesis were obtained with melanoidins and models which exerted antimutagenic and anticlastogenic effects.[33-35]

CARAMELIZATION PRODUCTS

In the solid state, sugars are relatively stable on moderate heating, but at temperatures exceeding 120°C they are pyrolyzed into a variety of products. If sugars are heated in controlled conditions together with acids, alkalies, sulfites, or ammonium salts, caramel colors of different flavor, color intensity, and other properties are obtained and widely used as color additives in foods.

In recent years, questions have arisen about the safety of caramel colors. Studies on long-term toxicity showed dose-related growth retardation and cecal enlargement for all the caramels produced by addition of accelerators. Hematological changes (a tendency to produce lymphocytopenia) were observed with ill-defined caramels, especially with positively charged caramels manufactured by the ammonia process.[36-38] Compounds responsible for toxic effects of caramels were 4-methylimidazole and 2-acetyl-4-(arabinotetrahydroxybutyl) imidazole, which are reaction products of carbonyl compounds with ammonia or ammonium ions (Figure 2). Both imidazoles occur in caramels at levels of several hundred $mg.kg^{-1}$.

Heat-Induced Mutagens

Studies conducted by the Japanese National Center in 1977 on cigarette smoke tar and smoke condensate from broiled fish and charred surfaces of broiled fish and meat proved a strong mutagenicity of these materials. This was partly ascribed to polycyclic aromatic hydrocarbons (page 195), but mainly to the basic fractions of the sample, which contained extremely potent frameshift mutagens, activated by microsomal enzymes (bacterial and/or *in vitro* mammalian cell test systems). These studies initiated and stimulated further extensive research on the chemistry, toxicity, and metabolism of a series of new toxic compounds which are formed as products of protein pyrolysis and nonenzymatic browning reactions.[10,14-16,33,39-45]

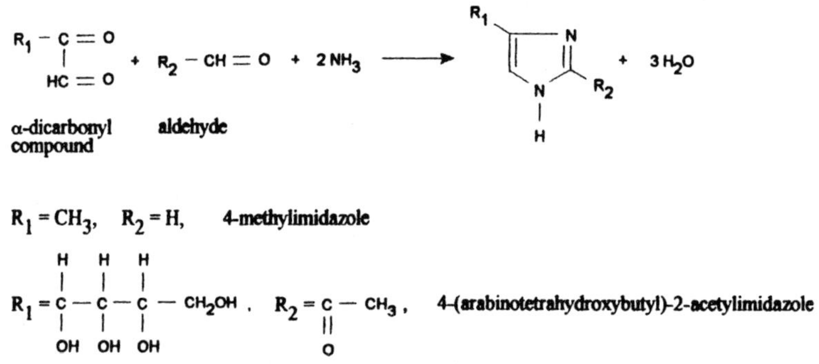

Figure 2 Formation of toxic imidazoles in caramel.

Mutagenic activity associated with the formation of browning products has been detected in all major protein-containing foods after heat treatment. Significant amounts of mutagens are found in beef, beef extracts, pork, ham, bacon, chicken, lamb, and eggs when fried or broiled. Seafood samples were more variable and generally showed a lower mutagenicity compared to meat and chicken. However, in some charcoal-broiled fish, mutagenicity has been observed at levels comparable to those found in red muscle meat. Products containing beef extracts (which are produced by intensive boiling) such as bouillon cubes, beef sauce concentrates, dried gravy mixes, dehydrated beef soups, and similar products have been shown to contain moderate amounts of mutagens. Milk, cheese, and certain organ meats like liver and kidney showed negligible mutagen formation under normal cooking conditions. The presence of mutagens has been demonstrated in a variety of canned meats and seafoods, but the levels found in canned foods were much lower than those found in fried or broiled food and showed a wide variation. The formation of mutagens is a complex function of cooking time and temperature, mode of cooking, and other variables. Time of cooking and temperature play an important role in the mutagen formation. For example, the mutagenicity increased by more than two orders of magnitude over the first 10 min of cooking, and mutagens were formed even at moderate temperatures. Below 150°C only very low levels of mutagenic activity were observed during pan frying of beef. With an increase in cooking temperature from 150 to 300°C, the mutagenicity increased ten to a hundred times. Both frying and broiling gave much higher levels of mutagenicity than other cooking methods like baking, stewing, and microwaving. The mutagenic activity increased with increased creatine and/or creatinine and glucose levels of the meat.[10,42] Concentrations of mutagens in cooked foods varied considerably, from a few to several hundred $mg.kg^{-1}$ of cooked material.

All the identified mutagenic compounds (with one exception, i.e., the pyrolytic product of lysine) were heterocyclic primary amines. They are classified into two types: the non-IQ type and the IQ (imidazoquinoline) type.

The non-IQ-type mutagens are mainly pyridoimidazoles and pyridoindoles (γ- and α-carbolines), first identified in amino acid and protein pyrolysates. Pyrolysis of tryptophan, glutamic acid, lysine, ornithine, and phenylalanine gave rise to a mutagenic activity stronger than that found for other amino acids. Strong mutagens also arose by pyrolysis of proteins such as casein, wheat gluten and soybean globulin (Figure 3). Among these compounds, two γ-carbolines (Trp-P-1, Trp-P-2) and two α-carbolines (AαC, MeAαC) showed the highest mutagenicity. These compounds were later identified in broiled fish and meat and beef extracts, but they do not seem to make a significant contribution to the overall mutagenicity and total mutagen level of foods.

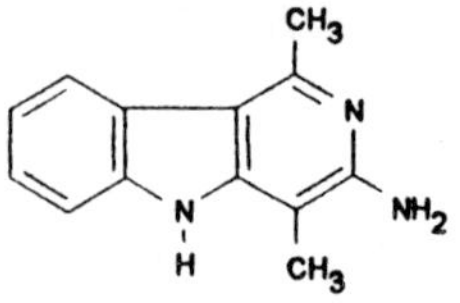

3-amino-1,4-dimethyl-5H-pyrido[4,3-b]indole (Trp-P-1)

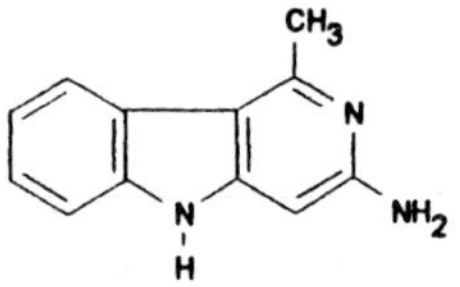

3-amino-1-methyl-5H-pyrido[4,3-b]indole (Trp-P-2)

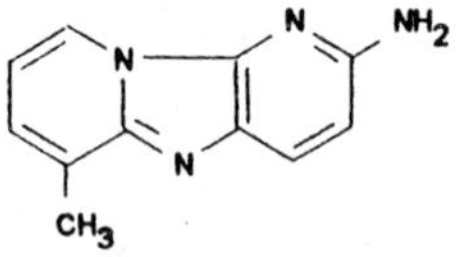

2-amino-6-methyldipyrido[1,2-a: 3',2'-d]imidazole (Glu-P-1)

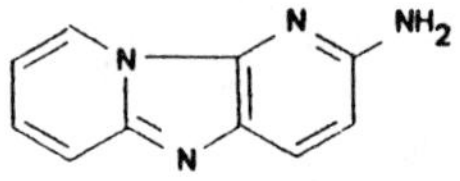

2-aminodipyrido[1,2-a: 3',2'-d]imidazole (Glu-P-2)

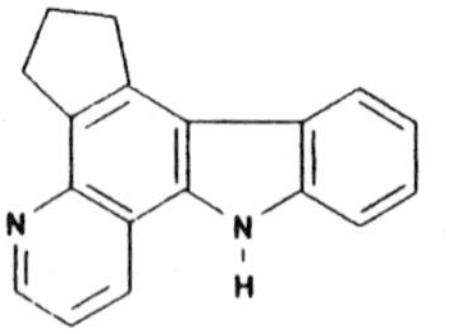

3,4-cyclopentenopyrido[3,2-a]carbazole (Lys-P-1)

Figure 3 Mutagens of non-IQ type identified in amino acid and protein pyrolysates and foods.

IQ-type mutagens, also called aminoimidazoazaarenes or high-temperature mutagens, are imidazoquinolines, imidazoquinoxalines, and imidazopyridines (Figure 4). Some other structures have recently been tentatively identified.[41] IQ-type mutagens were first identified in fried and broiled meat and fish and later in various cooked foods, the list of which was given above. They represent a dominating class of mutagens in foods of the Western diet cooked under normal domestic conditions.

Levels of the major mutagens arising in cooked meat and fish are listed in Table 1. In Figure 5, the increase of IQ compounds during heating of meat extract at 100°C is shown. Figure 6 demonstrates the influence of heating temperature on the formation of IQ compounds. Proportions in percent of mutagenicity due to non-IQ-type and IQ-type of amines in the basic fractions of various pyrolyzed materials were 3:88 in broiled sardine, 42:48 in broiled horse mackerel, 24:75 in fried beef, and 85:6 in cigarette smoke

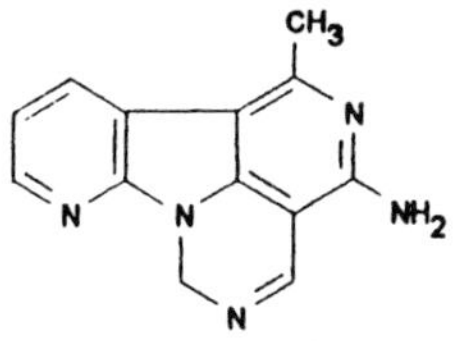

4-amino-6-methyl-1H-2,5,10,10b-tetraazafluoranthene (Orn-P-1)

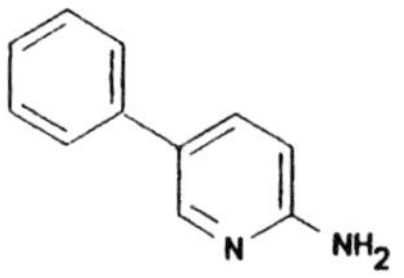

2-amino-5-phenylpyridine (Phe-P-1)

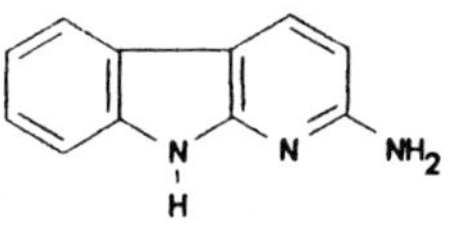

2-amino-9H-pyrido[2,3-b]indole (AαC)

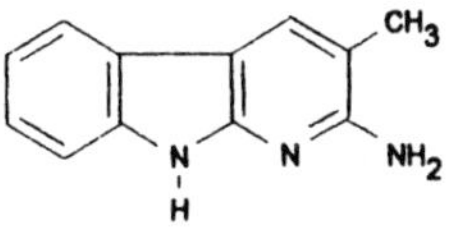

2-amino-3-methyl-9H-pyrido[2,3-b]indole (MeAαC)

Figure 3 (continued).

condensate.[42] 8-MeIQ$_x$ was often found at highest concentrations, and AαC was also frequently found at relatively high concentrations. Since MeIQ$_x$ is the main representative of the IQ compounds formed during the heating of foods, it can be used as an indicator compound for evaluating the extent of heating during processing. The specific mutagenicity of 8-MeIQ$_x$ is so high that it often accounts for 20 to 30% of the total mutagenicity in cooked foods. IQ and MeIQ possess an even higher mutagenicity. The mutagenic potential of AαC is about the same as that of IQ. Therefore, the risk of AαC would be higher than that of IQ, because the amount of AαC in foods is often higher than that of IQ. PhIP has low mutagenic activity, but its levels in cooked foods are often higher than those of other amines.

It seems that Maillard-type reactions are involved in the formation of mutagens. The precursors usually required for the formation of IQ-type mutagens are free amino acids and sometimes sugar, the imidazo part, common to all IQ-type mutagens originates from creatine via creatinine. A tentative route explaining the formation of the IQ compounds, starting from creatine and/or creatinine and the Maillard reaction products from glucose or other sugars and certain amino acids, is outlined in Figure 7. For example, IQ may be formed from creatinine, 2-methylpyridine, and formaldehyde or a related Schiff base formed from glycine through the Strecker degradation. The initial step may be a Mannich reaction or an aldol condensation. 4-MeIQ and 8-MeIQ$_x$ may analogously arise from creatinine, alanine, and 2-methylpyridine and creatinine, glycine, and 2,5-dimethylpyrazine, respectively.[42] Heating of model mixtures of creatinine, fructose, and alanine yielded

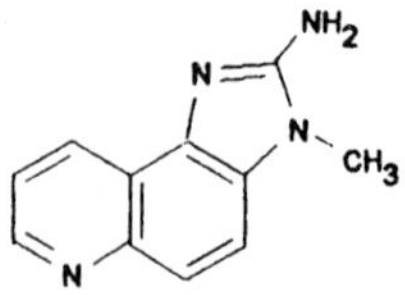

2-amino-3-methylimidazo[4,5-f]quinoline (IQ)

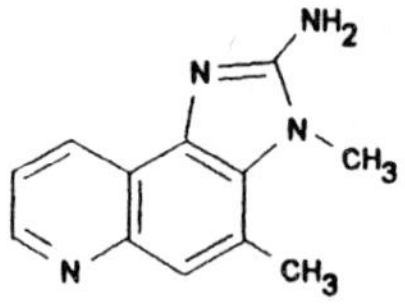

2-amino-3,4-dimethylimidazo[4,5-f]quinoline (4-MeIQ)

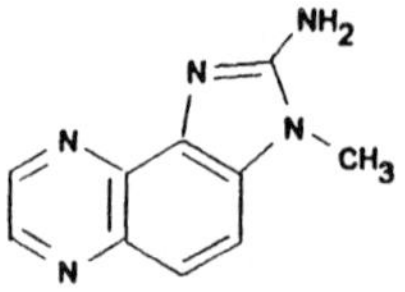

2-amino-3-methylimidazo[4,5-f]quinoxaline (IQ_x)

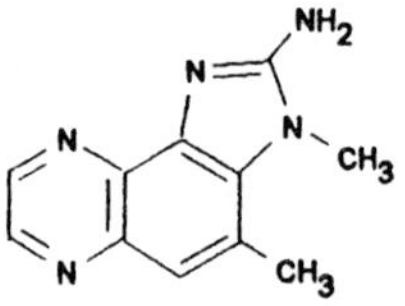

2-amino-3,4-dimethylimidazo[4,5-f]quinoxaline ($4\text{-}MeIQ_x$)

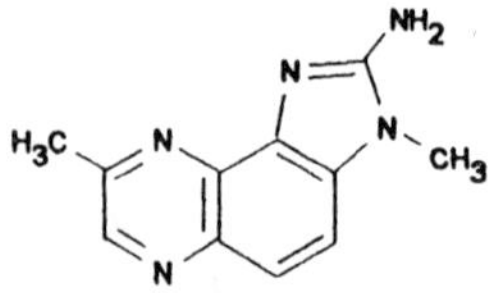

2-amino-3,8-dimethylimidazo[4,5-f]quinoxaline ($8\text{-}MeIQ_x$)

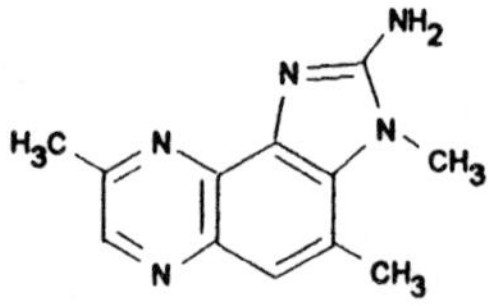

2-amino-3,4,8-trimethylimidazo[4,5-f]quinoxaline ($4,8\text{-}DiMeIQ_x$)

Figure 4 Mutagens of IQ type identified in foods.

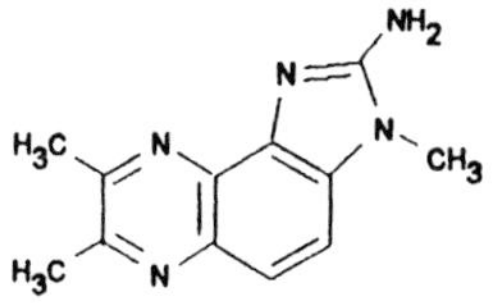

2-amino-3,7,8-trimethylimidazo[4,5-f]quinoxaline (7,8-DiMeIQ$_x$)

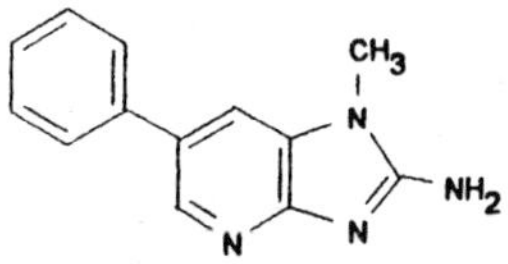

2-amino-1-methyl-6-phenylimidazo[4,5-b]pyridine (PhIP)

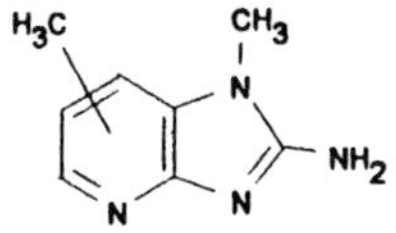

2-aminodimethylimidazopyridine (DMIP)

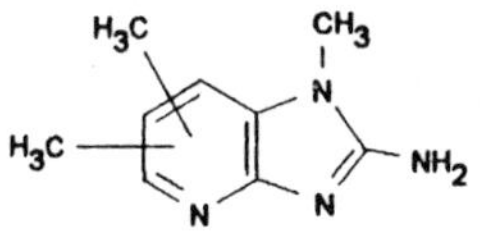

2-aminotrimethylimidazopyridine (TMIP)

Figure 4 (continued).

4,8-DIMeIQ$_x$ as the major mutagenic compound, whereas 4-MeIQ was a minor product.[43] Heating of creatine with proline gave rise to IQ.[44]

Some heterocyclic amines may well be carcinogenic to primates, including humans; some of them have other effects besides carcinogenicity. They may be related to development of degenerative changes of the cardiovascular system, brain, and pancreas.

Treatment with 2mM nitrite converts non-IQ-type heterocyclic amines to alcohols, but does not affect the amino group of IQ-type amines. This conversion is associated with the loss of mutagenicity. Treatment of IQ-type amines with more concentrated nitrite (50 m*M*) results in conversion of amino groups to nitro groups, and the resulting nitro compounds possess almost the same mutagenicity as the parent compounds. Treatment with hypochlorite results in loss of mutagenicity of both non-IQ-type and IQ-type amines. Heterocyclic amines of both types are readily soluble in many organic solvents and also in aqueous acidic solutions. They are quite stable and remain unchanged for at least 6 months when mixed with pellet diet and kept in dry conditions in a refrigerator. In aqueous solutions they are stable for 2 to 3 weeks when kept in a refrigerator. Their absorption from the gastrointestinal tract is efficient and rapid and a number of factors modifying their toxicity or even antimutagenic activity have been described. These include proteins, fiber, alcohol, vitamins, total fat, cholesterol, flavonoids, melanoidins (formed in the Maillard reaction), and other food constituents.[34,35,46-49] To minimize the

Table 1 Amounts of the Major Heterocyclic Amines (in $mg.kg^{-1}$) in Cooked Meat and Fish[10,15,40]

	Non-IQ-type mutagens					IQ-type mutagens					
Food	**Trp-P-1**	**Trp-P-2**	**Phe-P-1**	**AαC**	**MeAαC**	**IQ**	**4-MeIQ**	**8-MeIQ$_x$**	**4,8-DiMeIQ$_x$**	**PhIP**	**TMIP**
Broiled beef	0.21	0.25		1.20		0.19		2.11			
Broiled chicken	0.12	0.18		0.21				2.33	0.81		
Broiled mutton		0.15		2.50	0.19			1.01	0.67		
Fried ground beef											
At 200°C								1.3–2.4	0.5–1.2		
At 250°C						0.1	tr	1.00	0.50	15	0.50
Fried ground pork at 250°C						0.04	0.02	1.40	0.60	45	
Broiled sardine	13.3	13.1	8.6								

Note: tr = traces.

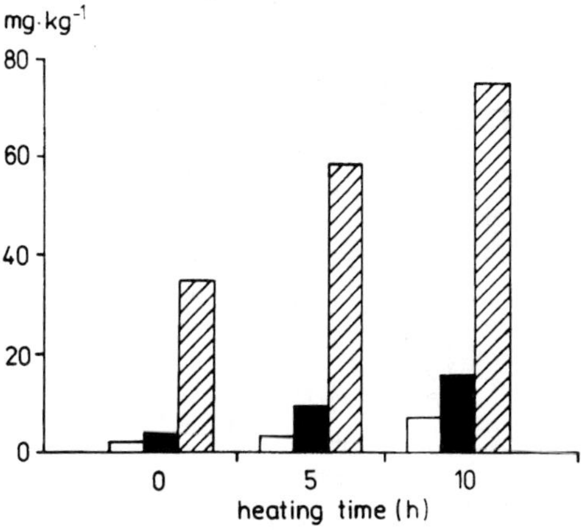

Figure 5 Formation of IQ-type mutagens in food grade meat extract at 100°C (related to dry weight, a_w = 0.42, water content 19.1%). □ = IQ, ■ = 4,8-DMIQ$_x$, ▨ = 8-MeIQ$_x$. (From Eichner, K., *Proc. Chemical Reactions in Foods II, VÚPP-STI, Prague,* 1992, 15. With permission.)

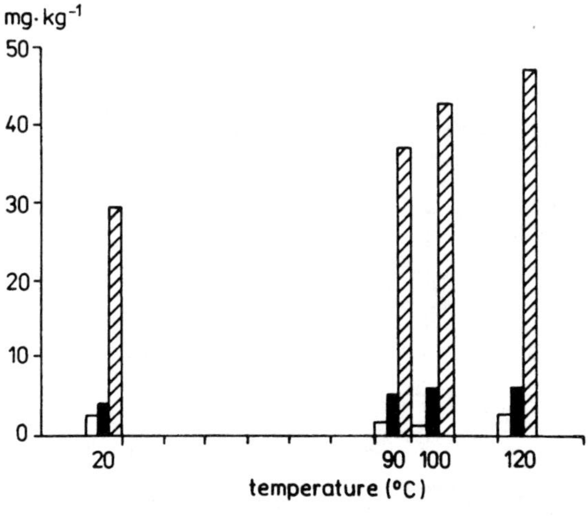

Figure 6 Formation of IQ-type mutagens in food grade meat extract at different temperatures (related to dry weight, a_w = 0.42, water content 19.1%). □ = IQ, ■ = 4,8-DMIQ$_x$, ▨ = 8-MeIQ$_x$ From Eichner, K., *Proc. Chemical Reactions in Foods II, VÚPP-STI, Prague,* 1992, 15. With permission.

risk of exposure to heterocyclic amines and other mutagens and carcinogens, it is recommended that exposure to smoke produced by broiling meat and fish and a high intake of food containing significant amounts of these compounds (broiled meat and fish and beef extracts) should be avoided. Higher temperatures must be avoided while drying meat extracts, and it is advisible to apply vacuum drying, especially at the low moisture level which favors the formation of IQ compounds.[45]

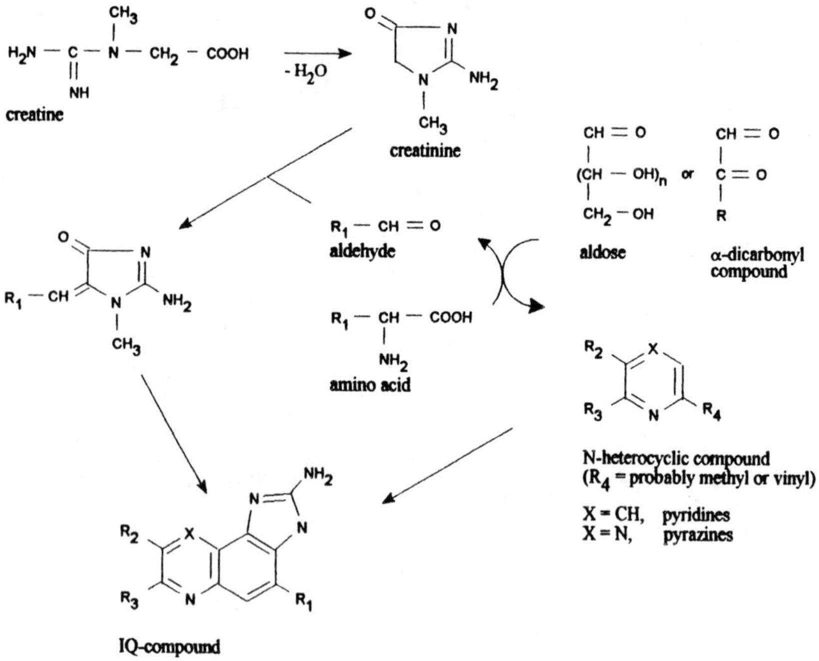

Figure 7 Formation of IQ-type mutagens.

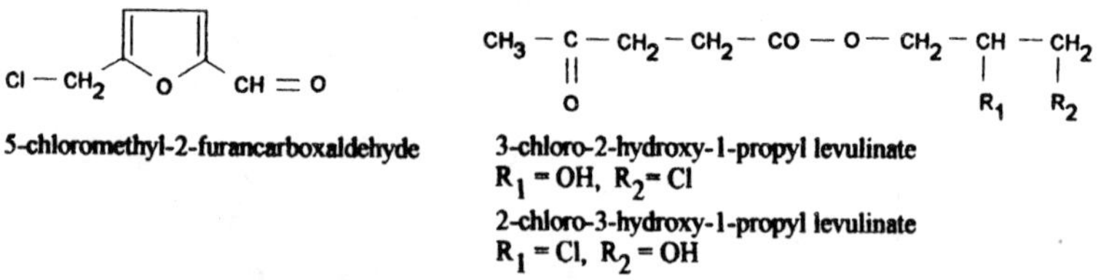

Figure 8 Chlorine-containing sugar degradation products.

CHLORINE-CONTAINING COMPOUNDS

Protein hydrolysates[50] produced by hydrochloric acid hydrolysis of proteinaceous materials and used as food seasonings contained 5-chloromethyl-2-furancarboxaldehyde at a level of 1.0 to 1.8 mg.kg^{-1}. This compound arose as a reaction product of hydrochloric acid with saccharides (Figure 8). Two other chlorine-containing compounds,[51] 3-chloro-2-hydroxy-1-propyl levulinate and 3-chloro-1-hydroxy-2-propyl levulinate have been found in hydrolysates at a level of 0.6 to 1.0 mg.kg^{-1}. These compounds arose as reaction products of levulinic acid (the major product of 5-hydroxymethyl-2-carboxfuraldehyde degradation in acid media) with 3-chloro-1,2-propanediol, which is the main contaminant of protein hydrolysates (page 221). All these chlorine-containing compounds arising from saccharides were destroyed by heating in alkaline medium.

REFERENCES

1. Eriksson, C., Ed., *Maillard Reactions in Food*, Pergamon Press, Oxford, 1981.
2. Waller, G. R. and Feather, M. S., Eds., *The Maillard Reaction in Foods and Nutrition*, American Chemical Society, Washington, D.C., 1983.
3. Danehy, J. P., Maillard reaction: nonenzymatic browning in food system with special reference to the development of flavor, *Adv. Food Res.*, 30, 77, 1985.
4. Baltes, W., Reaktionen vom Maillard-typ in Lebensmitteln, *Rev. Lebensmittelchem. Gericht. Chem.*, 40, 49, 1986.
5. Fujimaki, M., Namiki, M., and Kato, H., Eds., *Amino-Carbonyl Reactions in Food and Biological Systems*, Kodansha, Tokyo, 1986.
6. Quattrucci, E., Heat treatments and nutritional significance of Maillard reaction products, in *Nutritional and Toxicological Aspects of Food Processing*, Walker, R. and Quattrucci, E., Eds., Taylor & Francis, London, 1988, 113.
7. Namiki, M., Chemistry of Maillard reactions: recent studies on the browning reaction mechanism and the development of antioxidants and mutagens, *Adv. Food Res.*, 32, 115, 1988.
8. Monnier, V. M., Toward a Maillard reaction theory of aging, in *The Maillard Reaction in Aging, Diabetes and Nutrition*, Baynes, J. W. and Monnier, V. M., Eds., Liss, New York, 1989, 1.
9. O'Brien, J. and Morrissey, P. A., Nutritional and toxicological aspects of the Maillard browning reaction in foods, *Crit. Rev. Food Sci. Nutr.*, 28, 24, 1989.
10. Alexander, J., Becher, G. and Busk, L., Cooked food mutagens — a general overview, *Var Föda*, 2, 9, 1989.
11. Finot, P. A., Aeschbacher, H. U., Hurrell, R. F., and Liardon, R, Eds., *The Maillard Reaction in Food Processing, Human Nutrition and Physiology*, Birkhäuser Verlag, Basel, 1990.
12. Davídek, J., Velíšek, J. and Pokorný, J., Eds., *Chemical Changes during Food Processing*, Elsevier, 1990, 58.
13. Ames, J. M., Control of the Maillard reaction in food system, *Trends Food Sci. Technol.*, 1, 150, 1990.
14. Friedman, M., Prevention of adverse effects of food browning, in *Nutritional and Toxicological Consequences of Food Processing*, Friedman, M., Ed., Plenum Press, New York, 1991, 171.
15. Nagao, M., Sato, S., and Sugimura, T., Mutagens produced by heating foods, in *The Maillard Reaction in Foods and Nutrition*, Waller, G. R. and Feather, M. S., Eds., American Chemical Society, Washington, D.C., 1983, 521.
16. Omura, H., Jahan, N., Shinohara, K. and Murakami, H., Formation of mutagens by the Maillard reaction, in *The Maillard Reaction in Foods and Nutrition*, Waller, G. R. and Feather, M.S., Eds., American Chemical Society, Washington, D.C., 1983, 538.
17. Aeschbacher, H. U. and Würzner, H. P., An evaluation of instant and regular coffee in the Ames mutagenicity test, *Toxicol. Lett.*, 5, 139, 1980.
18. Shibamoto, T., Nishimura, O., and Mihara, S., Mutagenicity of products obtained from a maltol-ammonia browning model system, *J. Agric. Food Chem.*, 29, 643, 1981.
19. Kasai, H., Kumeno, K., Yamaizumi, Z., Nishimura, S., Nagao, M., Fujita, Y., Sugimura, T., Nukaya, H., and Kosuge, T., Mutagenicity of methylglyoxal in coffee, *Gana*, 73, 681, 1982.
20. Shinohara, K., Kim, E.-H., and Omura, H., Furans as the mutagens formed by amino-carbonyl reactions, in *Amino-Carbonyl Reactions in Food and Biological Systems*, Fujimaki, M., Namiki, M., and Kato, H., Eds., Kodansha, Tokyo, 1986, 281.
21. Walker, R., Mendoza-Garcia, M. A., Ioannides, C., and Quattrucci, E., Acute toxicity of 3-deoxy-4-sulphohexosulose in rats and mice and *in vitro* mutagenicity in the Ames test, *Food Chem. Toxicol.*, 21, 299, 1983.
22. Walker, R., Mendoza-Garcia, M. A., Quatrucci, E., and Falci, M., Short-term toxicity studies on 3-deoxy-4-sulphohexosulose (DSH) in rats and mice, *13th Int. Cong, Nutr,*, Brighton, U.K., 1985.
23. Fan, A. M. and Book, S. A., Sulfite hypersensitivity: a review of current issues, *J. Appl. Nutr.*, 39, 71, 1989.
24. Eichner, K., Antioxidative effect of Maillard reaction intermediates, in *Maillard Reactions in Food*, Eriksson, C., Ed., Pergamon Press, Oxford, 1981, 441.

25. Yamaguchi, N., Antioxidative activity of the oxidation products prepared from melanoidins, in *Amino-Carbonyl Reactions in Food and Biological Systems,* Fujimaki, M., Namiki, M., and Kato, H., Eds., Kodansha, Tokyo, 1986, 281.
26. Yamaguchi, N., Koyama, Y., and Fujimaki, M., Fractionation and antioxidative activity of browning reaction products between D-xylose and glycine, in *Maillard Reactions in Food,* Eriksson, C., Ed., Pergamon Press, Oxford, 1981, 429.
27. Eiserich, J. P., Macku, C., and Shibamoto, T., Volatile antioxidants formed from an L-cysteine/D-glucose Maillard model system, *J. Agric. Food Chem.,* 40, 1982, 1992.
28. Waller, G. R., Beckel, R. W., and Adeleye, B. O., Conditions for the synthesis of antioxidative arginine-xylose Maillard reaction products, in *The Maillard Reaction in Foods and Nutrition,* Waller, G. R. and Feather, M. S., Eds., American Chemical Society, Washington, D.C., 1983, 125.
29. Lingnert, H., Eriksson, C. E., and Waller, G. R., Characterization of antioxidative Maillard reaction products from histidine and glucose, in *The Maillard Reaction in Foods and Nutrition,* Waller, G. R. and Feather, M. S., Eds., American Chemical Society, Washington, D.C., 1983, 335.
30. Lingnert, H. and Hall, G., Formation of antioxidative Maillard reaction products during food processing, in *Amino-Carbonyl Reactions in Food and Biological Systems,* Fujimaki, M., Namiki, M., and Kato, H., Eds., Kodansha, Tokyo, 1986, 273.
31. Velíšek, J., Davídek, J., El-Zeany, B. A., Pokorný, J. and Janíček, G., Antioxidant activity of some brown pigments in L-ascorbic acid solutions, *Z. Lebensm. Unters. Forsch.,* 154, 151, 1974.
32. El-Zeany, B. A., Pokorný, J., Velíšek, J., Davídek, J. and Janíček, G., Antioxidant activity of some brown pigments in lipids, *Z. Lebensm. Unters. Forsch.,* 153, 316, 1973.
33. Aeschbacher, H. U., Anticarcinogenic effect of browning reaction products, in *The Maillard Reaction Products in Food Processing, Human Nutrition and Physiology,* Finot, P. A., Aeschbacher, H. U., Hurrell, R. F., and Liardon, R., Eds., Birkhäuser Verlag, Basel, Boston, Berlin, 1990, 335.
34. Lee, E., Chuyen, N. V., Hayase, F., and Kato, H., Absorption and distribution of [^{14}C] melanoidins in rats and the desmutagenicity of absorbed melanoidin against Trp-P-1, *Biosci. Biotech. Biochem.,* 56, 21, 1992.
35. Yen, G.-C. and Lii, J.-D., Influence of the reaction conditions on the antimutagenic effect of Maillard reaction products derived from xylose and lysine, *J. Agric. Food Chem.,* 40, 1034, 1992.
36. Evans, J. G., Butterworth, K. R., Gaunt, I. F., and Grasso, P., Long-term toxicity study in the rat of a caramel produced by the "half-open half-closed pan" ammonia process, *Food Cosmet. Toxicol.,* 15, 523, 1977.
37. Scheutwinkel-Reich, M. and von der Hude, W., Mutagenicity of caramel colors, *Z. Lebensm. Unters. Forsch.,* 181, 455, 1975.
38. Coulson, J., Miscellaneous naturally occurring colouring materials for foodstuffs, in *Developments in Food Colours-1,* Walford, J., Ed., Applied Science Publishers, London, 1980, 189.
39. Dolara, P. and Bianchini, F., Genotoxicity studies of cooked food, in *Nutritional and Toxicological Aspects of Food Processing,* Walker, R. and Quattrucci, E., Eds., Taylor & Francis, London, 1988, 125.
40. Sugimora, T., Wakabayashi, K., Nagao, M., and Ohgaki, H., Heterocyclic amines in cooked food, in *Food Toxicology: a Perspective on the Relative Risks,* Taylor, S. L. and Scanlan, R. A., Eds., Marcel Dekker, New York, 1989, 31.
41. Jägerstad, M. and Skog, K., Formation of meat mutagens, in *Nutritional and Toxicological Consequences of Food Processing,* Friedman, M., Ed., Plenum Press, New York, 1991, 83.
42. Jägerstad, M., Laser Reutersward, A., Öste, R., Grivas, S., Olsson, K., and Nyhammar, T., Creatinine and Maillard reaction products as precursors of mutagenic compounds formed in fried beef, in *The Maillard Reaction in Foods and Nutrition,* Waller, G. R. and Feather, M. S., Eds., American Chemical Society, Washington, D. C., 1983, 507.
43. Nyhammar, T., Grivas, S., Olsson, K., and Jägerstad, M., Isolation and identification of beef mutagens (IQ compounds) from heated model systems of creatinine, fructose and glycine or alanine, in *Amino-Carbonyl Reactions in Food and Biological Systems,* Fujimaki, M., Namiki, M., and Kato, H., Eds., Kodansha, Tokyo, 1986, 323.
44. Yoshida, D., Okamoto, H., Kushi, A., Fukuhara, Y., and Mizusaki, S., Mutagenicity of the heated products of nitrogenous compounds with the addition of glucose, in *Amino-Carbonyl Reactions in Food and Biological Systems,* Fujimaki, M., Namiki, M., and Kato, H., Eds., Kodansha, Tokyo, 1986, 335.

45. Eichner, K., Role and significance of the Maillard reaction during food processing, in *Proc. Chemical Reactions in Foods II,* Velíšek, J., Ed., VÚPP-STI, Prague, 1992, 15.
46. Kim, S. B., Hayase, F. and Kato, H., Desmutagenic effects of melanoidins against amino acid and protein pyrolysates, in *Amino-Carbonyl Reactions in Food and Biological Systems,* Fujimaki, M., Namiki, M., and Kato, H., Eds., Kodansha, Tokyo, 1986, 383.
47. Yoshida, S., Ye-Xiuyun, and Nishiumi, T., The binding ability of α-lactalbumin and β-lactoglobulin to mutagenic heterocyclic amines, *J. Dairy Sci.,* 74, 3741, 1991.
48. Lee, H., Jiaan, C.-Y., and Tsai, S.-J., Flavone inhibits mutagen formation during heating in a glycin/creatine/glucose model system, *Food Chem.,* 45, 235, 1992.
49. Yoshida, S. and Ye-Xiuyun, The binding ability of bovine milk caseins to mutagenic heterocyclic amines, *J. Dairy Sci.,* 75, 958, 1992.
50. Velíšek, J., Ledahudcová, K., Pudil, F., Davídek, J., and Kubelka, V., Chlorine-containing compounds derived from saccharides in protein hydrolysates, I. 5-Chloro-2-furanocarboxaldehyde, *Lebensm. Wiss. Technol.,* 26, 28, 1993.
51. Velíšek, J., Ledahudcová, K., Kassahun, B., Doležal, M., and Kubelka, V., Chlorine-containing compounds derived from saccharides in protein hydrolysates, II. Levulinic acid esters in soybean meal hydrolysates, *Lebensm. Wiss. Technol.,* 26, 430, 1993.

Part C

Toxic and Antinutritional Compounds Arising from Lipids

Jan Pokorný and Jan Velíšek

Lipids are generally oxidized or isomerized during food processing and storage. The products possess only low toxicity, at least in amounts generally consumed in the diet. Nevertheless, the nutritional value moderately decreases by various secondary reactions. In addition, some lipid oxidation products produce rancidity, which is objectionable to the consumer. Excessive amounts of natural (unchanged) lipids in the diet (as usually consumed in industrial countries) are far more dangerous than small amounts of oxidized lipids.

CHEMISTRY OF LIPID OXIDATION

Lipids may be oxidized following different mechanisms (Table 1), but autoxidation is the most important reaction under conditions occurring in food technology.

Most raw materials for food production, especially of plant origin, contain lipoxygenases (linoleate:oxygen oxidoreductase, EC 1.13.11.12), which catalyze the oxidation of linoleic and linolenic or related polyenoic fatty acids into the corresponding hydroperoxides.[1] The reaction is stereospecific and positional specific[2] and depends on the type and origin of the enzyme. Oxidation products inhibit seed germination.[3] The enzyme is easily deactivated by reaction products. Hydroperoxides are unstable and are cleaved by action of hydroperoxide lyases, which are usually present in the same material.[4] The enzyme-catalyzed oxidation is a free radical reaction, which is inhibited by phenolic antioxidants, but is activated by metal ions.

Singlet oxygen is produced by the action of light in the presence of photosensitizers,[5] such as chlorophyll pigments. Chlorophylls and, mainly, their degradation products, i.e., pheophytins, are present in traces in vegetable oils, and are active catalysts of oxidation on light,[6] while carotenoids inhibit oxidation by quenching singlet oxygen.[7] A molecule of singlet oxygen attacks the double bond of a polyenoic fatty acid, the final product being again a hydroperoxide.[5] The composition of isomeric hydroperoxides produced by singlet

Table 1 The Most Important Mechanisms of Lipid Oxidation

Mechanism of oxidation	Occurrence
Enzyme/catalyzed oxidation	Storage of raw material or raw food product
Oxidation by singlet oxygen	Storage in light
Autoxidation	Heating or storage
Oxidation by metal ions	Rare in foods
Oxidation by hydroperoxides	Mostly in storage of raw foods or prolonged storage of dry food products

oxygen is not identical with that of hydroperoxides produced by enzyme-catalyzed oxidation or autoxidation.

Autoxidation is caused by spontanous oxidation of unsaturated lipids by air oxygen. It is a free radical chain reaction consisting of three steps:[8] (1) chain initiation, (2) chain propagation, and (3) termination reactions. The reaction chain is usually initiated by a free radical produced by decomposition of a hydroperoxide or another labile molecule; however, it may be initiated by irradiation or heating. The lipid free radical is rapidly oxidized by air oxygen (or by oxygen dissolved in the medium) with the formation of a peroxy radical. The peroxy radical attacks a lipid molecule, forming another lipidic free radical and a molecule of hydroperoxide. This reaction continues until the chain is terminated by combination of two free radicals.

Hydroperoxides produced by these reactions have the hydroperoxy group attached on either carbon atom adjacent to a double bond system,[2] since free radicals produced as intermediates rearrange into a conjugated free radical. The positional isomerization is usually accompanied by *cis, trans*-isomerization so that the resulting hydroperoxides have either a *cis, trans*- or a *trans, trans*-configuration.

Autoxidation is catalyzed by transient heavy metal ions or complexes,[9] as they initiate the decomposition of hydroperoxides into free radicals. Iron and copper are the most important oxidation catalysts among metals encountered in fats and oils or other foods. Edible oils usually contain 0.05 to 0.5 $mg.kg^{-1}$ iron and 0.01 to 0.05 $mg.kg^{-1}$ copper, which reduce the stability on storage to 20 to 40%. Metals are deactivated by metal-chelating agents, such as phosphoric or citric acids, which are often added to oil during refining.[10-11] All other free radical-producing agents catalyze the lipid oxidation as well, but they are not important in foods.

Autoxidation is inhibited by antioxidants.[9,12] They are mainly polyphenolic substances, such as substituted pyrocatechols, pyrogallols, or hydroquinols, but a hydroxylic group may be methoxylated. Antioxidants react with free peroxy radicals with the formation of a hydroperoxide and a free radical of the antioxidant. The phenolic radical is less active, and cannot produce free radicals from lipids. They are slowly deactivated by combination with another peroxide or phenolic free radical.[9] At high concentration, however, phenolic free radicals slowly cause decomposition of lipid hydroperoxides (reverse reaction). The rate of this latter reaction is negligible at low concentrations of phenolics, common in foods. Nevertheless, the antioxidant activity moderately decreases with increasing concentration. At very high levels, the initiation reaction may even prevail. The concentration of tocopherols, which are among the most common phenolic antioxidants, is close to the optimum in edible oils,[13] so that further addition of tocopherols has no effect or may even decrease the stability.

Lipid hydroperoxides are very reactive substances. They decompose rapidly at higher temperatures and slowly at storage temperatures. Their most important reactions are shown in Table 2. Hydroperoxides are easily oxidized into dihydroperoxides or

Table 2 The Most Important Reactions of Lipid Hydroperoxides

Reaction type	Products
Autoxidation	Dihydroperoxides, hydroperoxydioxides
Reactions not affecting the carbon number	Carbonyl compounds, epoxides, hydroxyl derivatives
Polymerization reactions	Dimers and higher oligomers, cyclic products
Chain cleavage	Volatile aldehydes, ketones, alcohols, and hydrocarbons

combinations of hydroperoxides with dialkylperoxides (usually, six-member heterocycles) of various structures.[2] Diperoxides are very labile compounds, easily split into products of low molecular weight.

Another group of reaction products is formed by decomposition of the hydroperoxide group;[14] namely, by splitting off of water, a carbonyl derivative is formed (Figure 1), or by reaction of a hydroperoxide group with a double bond. Epoxides and hydroxyl groups are formed in this way. Hydroxyl derivatives can be produced by homolytic cleavage of a hydroperoxide group followed by abstracting a hydrogen atom. All these compounds are labile and can be further oxidized or changed in different ways.

Lipid oxidation products form various types of dimers,[14-16] where the two fatty acid chains are bound by a C-C link or an ether or a peroxide linkage. The former type prevails in frying fats, while the latter type occurs in oils oxidized in thin films at room temperature (such as in oil paintings). Dimers are the predominant type in food materials, but small amounts of trimers and traces of higher oligomers are detected as well. Fatty acid chains are sometimes bound by two bonds. Cyclic compounds are produced in this way. Two types of internal polymers are possible as well: (1) those produced by reaction between two different fatty acid chains of the same triacylglycerol molecule; and (2) those produced by reaction between two reactive groups of the same fatty acid chain; the molecular weight is not affected by these two reactions.

Decomposition by rearrangement and cleavage[17] is very important because volatile, sensory active substances are produced. They give rise to a rancid off-flavor, which is objectionable unless very weak. Typical cleavage products are volatile aldehydes and hydrocarbons (Figure 2), but nonvolatile substances are produced at the same time from the triacylglycerol remainder of the molecule. The molecule can be cleaved on either side of the hydroperoxide group so that a variety of homologous compounds are generally produced. The aldehyde reaction products can be further oxidized into carboxylic acids[18] (Figure 2). Unsaturated aldehydes are oxidized into volatile hydroperoxides, which are decomposed with the formation of malonaldehyde[19] (Figure 2).

Oxidized lipids contain several types of functional groups so that they can react with many food components. Typical examples are reactions with food proteins. Several functional groups of proteins can participate in the reactions (Table 3). Various reactions of oxidized polyunsaturated lipids with hide proteins are the basis of the chamois-leather tanning. The formation of multiple hydrogen bonds between oxidized lipids and proteins results in the formation of insoluble macromolecular complexes.[20] Lipids cannot be extracted from such complexes with common organic solvents, such as hexane or chloroform.[21] Hydroperoxides or free peroxy radical groups attack sulfur groups of amino acids bound in proteins.[22] Cysteine is oxidized into cystine and, still further, into sulfinic acid.[23] Methionine is oxidized into the respective sulfoxide or even sulfone.[24] Hydroperoxides react with amine groups, forming imines[25] (Figure 3). Many other reactions are possible. The final product is brown melanoidin, where the lipid moiety is bound to protein both by multiple hydrogen bonds and by covalent bonds. Melanoidins are not

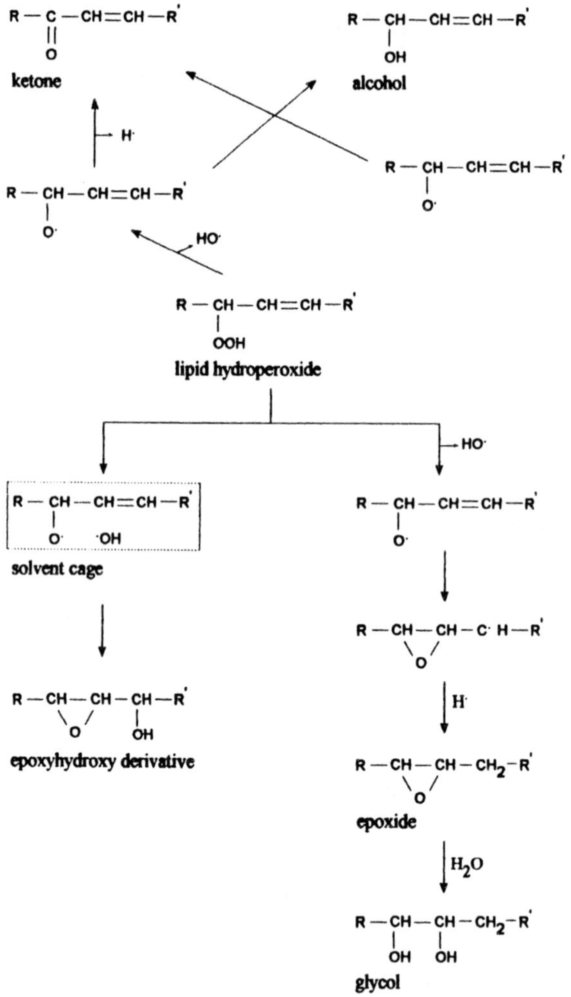

Figure 1 Reactions of lipid hydroperoxides not affecting the carbon number.

attacked by proteolytic digestive enzymes, or are attacked only with difficulty, which may cause excessive bile excretion.

STEROL OXIDATION

Sterols are minor components in all edible fats and oils. Cholesterol is the only sterol present in animal fats. Several phytosterols are found in vegetable oils. Sterols are relatively stable in pure preparations, but are oxidized rather easily when dissolved in fats or present in dry foods.

The mechanism of their oxidation is well known and has been reviewed.[24-27] Primary oxidation products are again free radicals and because the corresponding hydroperoxides are very unstable, they are rapidly transformed into the respective epoxides or diol derivatives and various other products. A list from various sources is given in Table 4. Both α and β derivatives are usually produced. They may be further oxidized to other

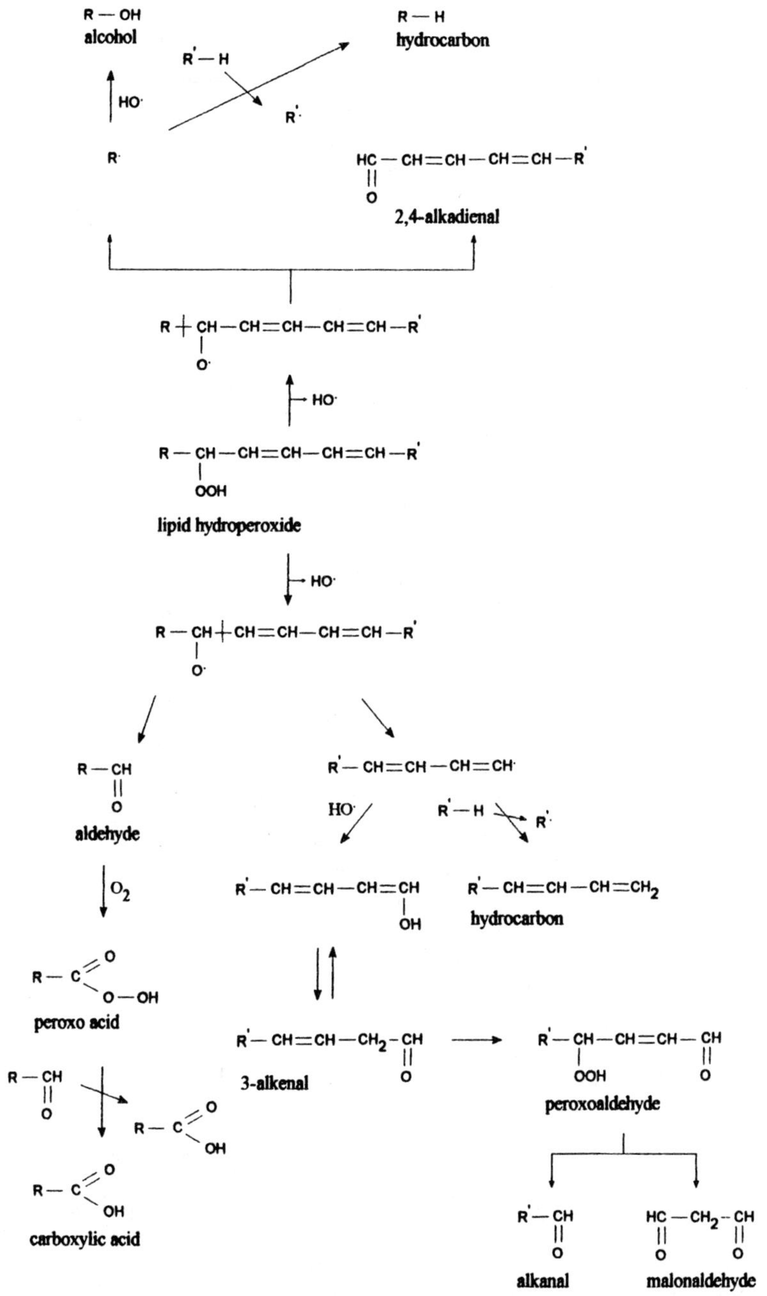

Figure 2 Formation of volatile products by rearrangement cleavage of lipid hydroperoxides.

products or react with proteins in an analogous manner to oxidized fatty acids.[28] The resulting insoluble complexes are similar to those produced from oxidized lipids. Under simulated gastric conditions, sterol oxidation products are converted into the respective chlorosubstituted derivatives.[29]

Table 3 Functional Groups Participating in Interactions Between Oxidized Lipids and Proteins

Functional group of lipid	Functional groups of proteins
Hydroperoxidic	Amine, thiol, sulfide, disulfide,
Epoxy (oxirane)	Hydroxyl, amine, carboxylic
Hydroxylic	Carboxylic, hydrogen bonds
Aldehydic	Amine, phenol, hydrogen bonds
Ketone	Amine

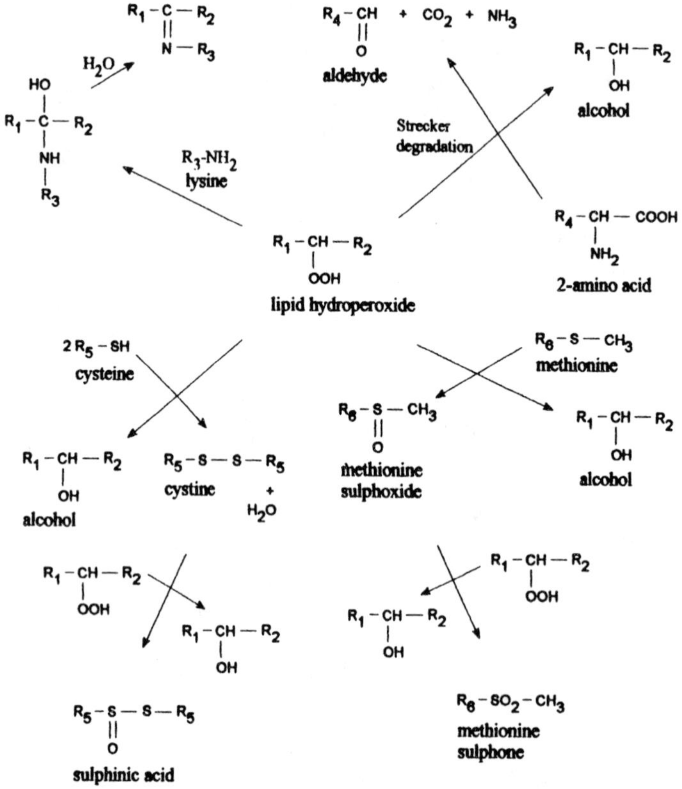

Figure 3 Reactions of hydroperoxides with basic and sulfur-containing amino acids.

Phytosterols react similarly to cholesterol, as they differ only in the structure of the side chain. Very little is known about the structure of oxidation products.

Sterols are dehydrated into hydrocarbons by heating to high temperatures or are dehydrated into disteryl ethers[30] and the corresponding hydrocarbons.[31] These products have been detected in refined edible oils, where they are produced during bleaching and deodorization.

Table 4 Typical Cholesterol Oxidation Products Detected in Foods

Oxidized product	Foods
5-Cholesten-3,7-diol	Processed meat, dried eggs, freeze-dried meat, heated tallow, stored butter
7-Oxocholesta-3,5-diene	Frying fat, dried pork, irradiated eggs, processed meat, fried bacon
3,5,6-Trihydroxy-5-cholestene	Heated fat, french fries, irradiated eggs, processed meat
5,6-Cholestan-5,6-epoxy-3-ol	Stored lard, bacon, french fries, dried eggs

Table 5 Major Isomerization Reactions of Lipids During Food Processing

Chemical process	Technological operation
Ester interchange (interesterification)	Deodorization, frying, hydrogenation
Double bond conjugation	Deodorization, frying, hydrogenation, oxidation
cis, trans-Isomerization	Hydrogenation, heating
Double bond shifting	Hydrogenation, extreme heat

ISOMERIZATION REACTIONS OF LIPIDS

The composition of fats and oils changes on heating even in the absence of oxygen. The most important reactions are summarized in Table 5. Three types of isomerization reactions may proceed in lipids during food processing. Fats and oils consist of triacylglycerols in which three acyls are bound to a molecule of glycerol. Their positions are not random, but each position in the triacylglycerol molecule is occupied by fatty acids of different composition. During the heating of lipids, especially in presence of water and acids, interesterification reactions take place, and acyls exchange their positions in the molecule of triacylglycerol[32] or between two or three different molecules. This ester interchange moderately affects the digestibility of fats and oils and, sometimes substantially, their stability against autoxidation.[33]

More serious reactions (from the nutritional standpoint) proceed during the heating of lipids to temperatures higher than 200°C, particularly in the presence of steam, acids, or some active clays. Fats and oils are deodorized during industrial refining under these conditions. Intermediary free radicals are formed, which rearrange into a conjugated double bond system. The positional isomerization is accompanied by *cis, trans*-isomerization.[34] Monoenoic fatty acids react more slowly after analogous mechanisms.

Similar reactions occur during industrial catalytic hydrogenation of vegetable or fish oils.[35] Unsaturated fatty acids are chemisorbed on the surface of nickel catalyst, where they are either hydrogenated or desorbed. During the desorption, double bonds may be shifted by one carbon atom in either direction, and/or may be *cis, trans*-isomerized. The majority of double bonds in hydrogenated fats are in the *trans*-configuration. Other types of isomers are produced during the hydrogenation. If linolenic (9, 12, 15-octadecatrienoic) acid is hydrogenated, three isomers may result, i. e., 9,12-; 9,15-; and 12,15-octadecadienoic acids, respectively. Similarly, two monoenoic acids are produced by hydrogenation of linoleic (9,12-octadecadienoic) acid, which can be present either as the *cis*- or the *trans*-isomer. Similar reactions proceed during the enzymatic hydrogenation in the rumen of ruminants; therefore, butter or beef tallow always contain isomeric unsaturated fatty acids.[36]

Table 6 Deterioration of Lipids during Food Processing

Technological operation	Extent of the reaction
Boiling	Almost no change
Roasting	Oxidation up to 3%, mainly in the surface layer
Frying	Oxidation up to 10%, polymerization
Drying	Oxidation up to 3%
Freezing, freeze-drying	Almost no change or oxidation up to 2 to 3%, respectively
Bleaching and deodorization	Isomerization up to 1 to 3%
Hydrogenation of oils	Isomerization up to 70%
Storage of edible oils	Oxidation up to 1%
Storage of raw food	Enzymic oxidation up to 1 to 2%
Storage of cooked food	Little change
Storage of dry food	Oxidation up to 10 to 20%
Storage of frozen food	Oxidation up to 5 to 10%

Table 7 Content of Oxysterols in Some Foods

Type of food	Oxysterol content (% total sterols)
Dried egg powder	5–49
Dried milk powder	1–19
Grated cheese	0.2–1.5
Stored lard	0.05–0.1
French fries (stored)	10–25
Heated oil (olive)	0.1–0.3
Butter (stored or heated)	0.1–2.5
Cooked meat, processed meat	0.3–0.8
Fried bacon	0.5

FORMATION OF OXIDATION AND ISOMERIZATION PRODUCTS OF LIPIDS DURING FOOD PROCESSING AND STORAGE

Deterioration reactions of lipids during food processing and storage cannot be avoided. Their extent is extremely variable, depending on the technology of food production (Table 6). Moderate isomerization occurs during fat and oil refining, particularly during the bleaching and deodorization. A high degree of isomerization results from side reactions during industrial hydrogenation.

Some technological operations cause only moderate oxidation in foods containing water, since the aqueous phase protects lipids against the access of oxygen. The only exception is deep-frying,[37] when frying oils are exposed to temperatures between 150 to 120°C for several hours. Oxidation products are polymerized under high temperature. The content of polar compounds and polymers may reach 20 to 25% and 10%, respectively.[38] Frying oils are not directly eaten, but they are adsorbed into the fried food and some oxidized products are bound to it by covalent bonds.

During drying, hydrated proteins lose water, so that the lipid layer remains unprotected, and it is exposed to oxygen; therefore, dry foods are easily oxidized on storage.[39] During heating, the material is dehydrated as well and lipids come in direct contact with oxygen and are slowly oxidized. If enzymes in the food material are not heat inactivated, lipoxygenases present in the tissues catalyze slow oxidation even in a hydrated medium. The oxidation soon reaches equilibrium, but the content of oxidation products is usually sufficient to produce rancidity.

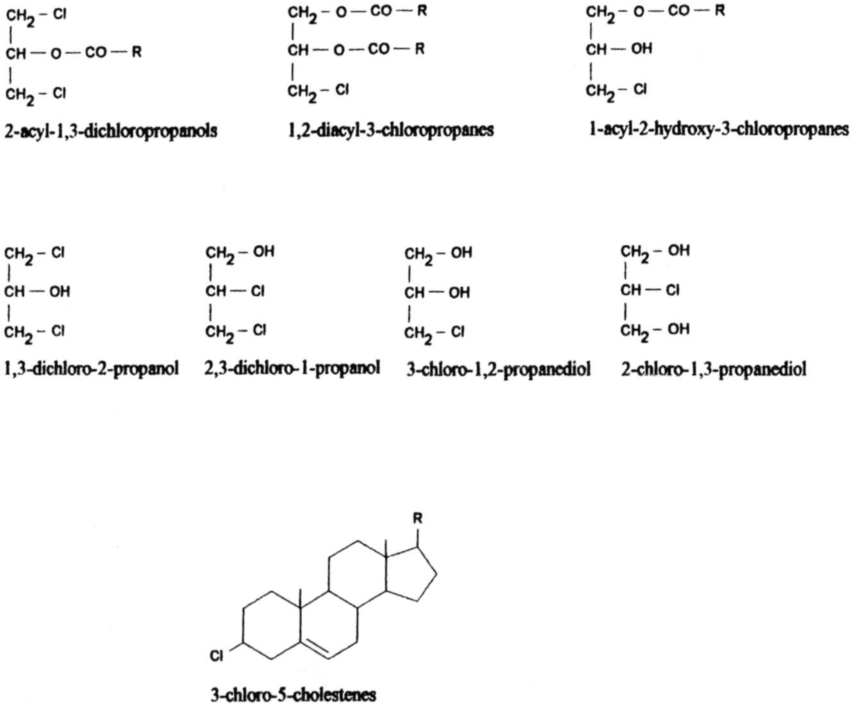

Figure 4 Structure of chlorine-containing compounds occurring in protein hydrolysates.

Cholesterol is oxidized very little (Table 7), except on frying or during the storage of dehydrated foods,[40] where the content of oxidation products can reach 3 to 7%. Sitosterol can be oxidized on heating as well.

FORMATION OF CHLORINE-CONTAINING PRODUCTS OF LIPIDS DURING FOOD PROCESSING AND STORAGE

Reaction of hydrochloric acid with residual lipids of oilseed meals and some other vegetable proteinaceous materials, such as wheat gluten, which are used for the production of hydrolyzed vegetable proteins, leads to the formation of a variety of chloropropanols,[41] their esters with higher fatty acids,[42] and chlorine-containing analogs of sterols,[43] (Figure 4). Glycerol monochlorohydrins, 3-chloro-1,2-propanediol and 2-chloro-1,3-propanediol, have been identified as the major protein hydrolysate contaminants, being present in concentrations amounting up to 1000 $mg.kg^{-1}$ and 100 $mg.kg^{-1}$, respectively. Glycerol dichlorohydrins, 1,3-dichloro-2-propanol and 2,3-dichloro-1-propanol, occur at the level of approximately 10 and 1 $mg.kg^{-1}$, respectively. Esters of chloropropanols with oleic, linoleic, palmitic, stearic, and other fatty acids have been found only in raw, unripe hydrolysates in trace amounts as well as chlorine-containing sterols, analogs of cholesterol, sitosterol, campesterol, and stigmasterol.[44]

HEALTH RISKS ARISING FROM THE LIPID DEGRADATION

The toxicity of oxidized lipids is low (Table 8), excepting volatile lipid hydroperoxides and cyclic dimers or monomeric cyclohexenoic products. Hydroperoxides are toxic only

Table 8 Toxicity of Oxidized Lipids

Compound or material tested	Toxic effect
Lipid hydroperoxide	Necrosis of lymphocytes, damage of thymus and spleen, decrease in leucocytes, inhibition of prostaglandin E synthesis, destruction of peroxidase and other enzymes, oxidation of phospholipids in membranes and in plasma
Hydroperoxyalkenals (mainly C5 to C9)	High acute toxicity, hepatotoxicity, mutagenicity, inhibition of succinate dehydrogenase, thiokinase, hemolysis
4-Hydroxy-2-nonenal	Cytotoxicity, destruction of lymphatic tissues, inhibition of glycine-6-phosphorylase
trans-5-Hydroxy-2-nonenal	Nephrotoxicity, hepatotoxicity
Hydroperoxides and secondary degradation products	Necrosis, fat accumulation, congestive hyperemia, damage to small intestine, liver, lungs, kidney
Rancid fats (oxidized at room temperature)	Inhibition of growth, hepatotoxicity, nephrotoxicity, damage of the skin permeability
Cyclohexene condensation products	Growth inhibition, death, damage of various organs
Heated fats (at frying conditions without food)	Histological changes in heart, liver, kidneys, seborrhea, diarrhea, polyuria, hair loss, edemas, atrophy, inflammation, destruction of alkaline phosphatase
Frying oils	Very low or no mutagenic effect, other damage of organs only in extreme cases, direct toxicity only exceptionally

in higher concentrations. The toxicity of oxidized lipids decreases in the following order: hydroperoxyalkenals[45] > hydroxyalkenals > alkenals > hydroperoxides > alkanals.[46]

Products of lipid oxidation and isomerization may be considered as antinutritional compounds (Table 9). Essential fatty acids, particularly linoleic and linolenic acids, are very oxylabile so that they are destroyed by oxidation and converted into neutral or nutritionally negative compounds.[47] In our laboratory, we have observed losses of 5 to 30% during the technological processing or storage. Tocopherols,[48] carotenes, and vitamin A[49] are oxidized into inactive compounds. We have found losses of 20 to 50% during storage of feed mixes at room temperature. Oxidized lipids react with proteins and decrease their digestibility, since the resulting complexes are only slowly and incompletely attacked by digestive enzymes; in mixtures of soybean oil and casein, the digestibility of protein decreased by 60% during a week of storage. At the same time, lysine[50] and other essential amino acids (cysteine, cystine, methionine, tryptophan) are converted into unavailable products.[51] Some vitamins of the B complex (especially thiamine and riboflavin) are destroyed by lipid hydroperoxides or free radicals arising from their decomposition; we have observed losses of 20 to 60% under normal storage conditions of dehydrated cereal, dairy, and meat products. Losses of vitamin C are very high as well,[52] sometimes up to 50 to 90%. The digestibility of oxidized lipids is lower than that of the original fats and oils; in particular, lipid oligomers are digested very poorly if at all.[53,54]

Isomerization reactions deactivate essential fatty acids as well, and *trans*-fatty acids have been found to be a risk factor in the development of cardiovascular diseases, when ingested in very high amounts.[55]

Table 9 Antinutritional Effect of Oxidized or Isomerized Lipids

Compound tested	Antinutritional effect
Isomerized fats, *trans* derivatives	Loss of activity as essential fatty acid; unfavorable effect on blood lipids (in excess doses)
Hydroperoxides	Destruction of essential fatty acids, tocopherols, carotenes, and vitamin A; destruction of lysine and sulfur containing amino acids
Aldehydes	Decrease of digestibility and nutritional value of protein; protein crosslinking
Heated oils	Destruction of liposoluble vitamins; destruction of ascorbic acid; destruction of essential amino acids and serine, cysteine, and proline; lower nutritional value of proteins; lower digestibility
Rancid oils	Muscular distrophy; slower growth, decrease of essential fatty acids in tissues; decomposition of carotenoids and tocopherols

During recent years, the content of polyenoic fatty acids has increased in the diet in most developed countries because of their beneficial effect on the development of atherosclerosis. However, they are easily oxidized *in vivo* when antioxidants such as ascorbic acid, tocophenols, selenium, polyphenolic substances, or thiol derivatives are not simultaneously consumed. Lipid free radicals and other free radicals are produced during the *in vivo* oxidation, which may cause severe damage of tissues, and initiate malignant tumor growth.[56,57] Oxidized lipids accelerate all stages of chronic heart diseases.[58] With proteins, they form insoluble deposits (lipofuscin) in the artery wall or in neural tissues.[59] These brown macromolecular compounds slowly accumulate with increasing age and, therefore, they are called age pigments.[60] Humans can absorb oxysterols, but they are rapidly transferred in the form of lipoproteins. Cholesterol oxides have angiotoxic, mutagenic, and carcinogenic properties.[61] Oxysterols (oxidation products of cholesterol) form similar insoluble products with plasma proteins as oxidized triacylglycerols. They are more dangerous than the original cholesterol in this respect. The role of oxidized lipids and oxysterols in the development of cardiovascular diseases has produced much concern among physiologists, and has become the subject of intensive research.

Chloropropanols and their esters with fatty acids have been shown to possess mutagenic activity.[62]

DETOXIFICATION OF FOODS FROM OXIDIZED AND ISOMERIZED LIPIDS AND OTHER RELATED COMPOUNDS

Food detoxification from oxidized or isomerized lipids would require complex technological treatments, involving extraction and fractionation, which are not possible on an industrial scale. The only exceptions are edible fats and oils, which may be treated by adsorbing clays to remove oxidation products.[63] Therefore, the prevention of these processes is the only possible protection in most foods.

Some suggestions for the protection of lipids during food processing and storage are summarized in Table 10. Several similar processes are used on an industrial scale. If the producer or the consumer do not prevent lipid oxidation, it is best to discard the food. Fortunately, foods become objectionable from the standpoint of their sensory value well before they become dangerous because of their content of oxidized products.

A very common and frequently used way of lipid protection is by the addition of inhibitors. A mixture of phenolic substances, synergists (mainly polyvalent organic acids), and chelating agents are added.[64] Several synthetic inhibitors have been permitted

Table 10 Protection of Lipids Against Deterioration Reactions

Operation	Protection of lipids
Refining of edible oils	Short-time low-temperature processes, nitrogen blanketing, use of stainless steel tanks
Hydrogenation of edible oils	Use of special catalysts and technological conditions, replacement by interesterification in vacuum, replacement by solid fat blends
Sterilization, boiling	Use of vacuum, short-time processing
Baking	Use of stabilized or hydrogenated fats
Roasting (coffee, nuts)	Use of steam or another inert gas
Frying in fat	Protection of oil by iron plates, use of steam, antioxidants
Storage generally	Using low temperature, darkness, inert gas
Storage of oils and fats	Use of antioxidants, protection against light
Storage of dried food	Use of inert gas, antioxidants in the packaging material
Storage of raw food	Blanching, steaming before storage
Refrigerated storage	Antioxidative coating
Frozen storage	Inhibitors
Storage of freeze-dried foods	Inert gas

for food use on the basis of sophisticated toxicological tests, but natural inhibitors have often been preferred more recently[65] due to superstition.[66]

Isomerized lipids possess no adverse flavor, so that humans are not protected against their consumption. The most important items are hydrogenated oils, which may be a risk factor in persons suffering from cardiovascular diseases. Technological processes are now available, which decrease the content of isomers in the hydrogenated product. It is possible to eliminate the hydrogenation entirely, replacing it by interesterification[32,67] or by combination of vegetable oils with solid fats.

The excessive consumption of natural fats and oils is a much greater risk for human health than modest or occasional consumption of oxidized or isomerized lipids, anyway.

Oxidized lipids are rarely present in foods at levels which would have any pronounced effect on human health. However, their constant intake in small amounts could contribute to many risk factors, influencing the development of cardiovascular diseases or carcinogenesis. Changes of lipids occurring during food processing or storage could have a moderate antinutritional effect. Losses of essential fatty acids, essential amino acids, liposoluble vitamins and some water-soluble vitamins are characteristic for these reactions.

Levels of chlorine-containing organic compounds in protein hydrolysates are, to a certain extent, influenced by the reaction conditions employed during the hydrolysis (temperature, time, hydrochloric acid concentration, etc.). Compounds already present can be destroyed by heating of hydrolysates in slightly alkaline media (Table 11). It was shown that under these conditions, 3-chloro-1,2-propanediol reacts with ammonia and amino acids under the formation of the corresponding 3-amino-1,2-propanediol, 2-amino-1,3-propanediol, *bis* (2,3-dihydroxypropyl)amine, *tris* (2,3-dihydroxypropyl)amine, and *N*-(2,3-dihydroxypropyl)amino acids[68-70] (Figure 5).

Table 11 Degradation of 3-Chloro-1,2-Propanediol and 2-Chloro-1,3-Propanediol in Soybean Meal Hydrolysate[a]

Temperature (°C)	pH	Time (h)	3-Chloro-1,2-propanediol ($mg.kg^{-1}$)	2-Chloro-1,3-propanediol ($mg.kg^{-1}$)
100	7.75	24	0	0.2
100	8.00	24	0	0.1
100	8.25	24	0	0.1
100	8.50	5.25	0	0.8
100	8.75	3.87	0	1.0
80	9.00	47.42	0	0.1
90	9.00	4.42	0	2.4
100	9.00	0.13	27.6	38.0
100	9.00	0.27	7.4	33.3
100	9.00	0.50	1.4	24.0
100	9.00	0.75	0.2	13.2
100	9.00	1.10	0	2.6

[a] Original concentration: 3-chloro-1,2-propanediol, 337 $mg.kg^{-1}$; 2-chloro-1,2-propanediol, 49 $mg.kg^{-1}$.

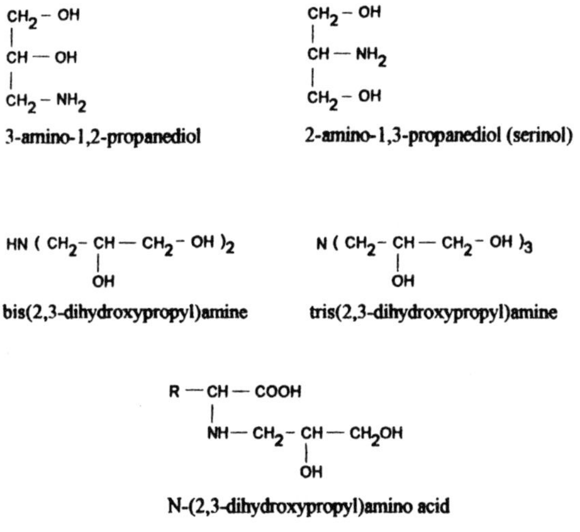

Figure 5 Structure of reaction products of 3-chloro-1,2-propanediol with amino compounds.

REFERENCES

1. Whitaker, J. R., Lipoxygenases, in *Oxidative Enzymes in Foods*, Robinson, D. S. and Eskin, N. A. M., Eds., Elsevier, London, 1991, chap. 5.
2. Chan, H. W.-S. and Coxon, D. T., Lipid hydroperoxides, in *Autoxidation of Unsaturated lipids*, Chan, H. W.-S., Ed., Academic Press, London, 1987, chap. 2.
3. Gardner, H. W., Dornbos, D. L., Jr., and Desjardins, A. E., Hexanal, *trans*-2-hexenal, and *trans*-2-nonenal inhibit soybean, *Glycine max*, seed germination, *J. Agric. Food Chem.*, 38, 1316, 1990.
4. Gardner, H. W., Weisleder, D., and Plattner, R. D., Hydroperoxide lyase and other hydroperoxide-metabolizing activity in tissues of soybean, *Glycine max*, *Plant Physiol.*, 97, 1059, 1991.
5. Bradley, D. G. and Min, D. B., Singlet oxygen oxidation in foods, *Crit. Rev. Food Sci. Nutr.*, 31, 211, 1992.

6. Endo, Y., Usuki, R., and Kaneda, T., Prooxidant activities of chlorophylls and their decomposition products on the photooxidation of methyl linoleate, *J. Am. Oil Chem. Soc.*, 61, 781, 1984.
7. Lee, E. C. and Min, D. B., Quenching mechanism of β-carotene on the chlorophyll sensitized photooxidation of soybean oil, *J. Food Sci.*, 53, 1894, 1988.
8. Chan, H. W.-S., The mechanism of autoxidation, in *Autoxidation of Unsaturated Lipids*, Chan, H. W.-S., Ed., Academic Press, London, 1987, chap. 1.
9. Pokorný, J., Major factors affecting the autoxidation of lipids, in *Autoxidation of Unsaturated Lipids*, Chan, H. W.-S., Ed., Academic Press, London, 1987, chap. 5.
10. Dijkstra, A. J., Degumming, refining, washing and drying fats and oils, in *Proc. World Conf. Oilseed Technol. Util.*, Applewhite, T. H., Ed., AOCS Press, Champaign, IL, 1993, 138.
11. Bernardini, M., Deodorization, in *Proc. World Conf. Oilseed Technol. Util.*, Applewhite, T. H., Ed., AOCS Press, Champaign, IL, 1993, 186.
12. Pospíšil, J., Antioxidants and related stabilizers, in *Oxidation Inhibition in Organic Materials*, Vol. 1, Pospíšil, J. and Klemchuk, P. P., Eds., CRC Press, Boca Raton, FL, 1990, chap. 3.
13. Mukai, K., Sawada, K., Kohno, Y., and Terao, J., Kinetic study of the prooxidant effect of tocopherol. Hydrogen abstraction from lipid hydroperoxides by tocopherol in solution, *Lipids*, 28, 747, 1993.
14. Gardner, H. W., Reactions of hydroperoxides: products of high molecular weight, in *Autoxidation of Unsaturated Lipids*, Chan, H. W.-S., Ed., Academic Press, London, 1987, chap. 3.
15. Neff, W. E., Frankel, E. N., and Fujimoto, K., Autoxidative dimerization of methyl linolenate and its monohydroperoxides, hydroperoxy epidioxides, and dihydroperoxides, *J. Am. Oil Chem. Soc.*, 6, 616, 1988.
16. Miyashita, K., Hara, N., Fujimoto, K., and Kaneda, T., Dimers formed in oxygenated methyl linoleate hydroperoxides, *Lipids*, 20, 578, 1985.
17. Grosch, W., Reactions of hydroperoxides: Products of low molecular weight, in *Autoxidation of Unsaturated Lipids*, Chan, H. W.-S., Ed., Academic Press, London, 1987, chap. 4.
18. Pokorný, J., Kmínek, M., Janitz, W., Novotná, E., and Davídek, J., Autoxidation of hexanal in presence of nonlipidic components, *Nahrung*, 29, 459, 1985.
19. Roubal, W. T., Free radicals, malonaldehyde, and protein damage in lipid protein systems, *Lipids*, 6, 62, 1971.
20. Gardner, H. W., Lipid hydroperoxide reactivity with proteins and amino acids, *J. Agric. Food Chem.*, 27, 220, 1979.
21. Pokorný, J., Über die Bildung von Komplexverbindungen bei der Reaktion oxydierter Lipide mit Eiweisstoffen, *Fette, Seifen, Anstrichm.*, 65, 278, 1963.
22. Gardner, H. W., Kleiman, R., Weisleder, D., and Inglett, G. E., Cysteine adds to lipid hydroperoxide, *Lipids*, 12, 655, 1977.
23. Yee, J. J. and Shipe, W. F., Effects of sulfhydryl compounds on lipid oxidation catalyzed by copper and heme, *J. Dairy Sci.*, 65, 1414, 1982.
24. Kobayashi, K., Murata, M., Matsudomi, N., and Kato, A., Damage to methionine and lysine in proteins involved with oxidation of lipids, *Nippon Eiyo Shokuryo Gakkaishi*, 36, 379, 1983.
25. Pokorný, J., Browning from lipid-protein interactions, *Proc. Food Nutr. Sci.*, 5, 421, 1981.
26. Beck, J.-P. and Crastes de Paulet, A., Activité biologiques des oxysterols, in *Activité biologiques des Oxysterols*, Inserm, Paris, 1988, chap. 1.
27. Maerker, G., Cholesterol autoxidation: current status, *J. Am. Oil Chem. Soc.*, 64, 388, 1987.
28. Nelson, G., Lipids and health focus on symposium, *INFORM*, 4, 1200, 1993.
29. Maerker, G., Nungesser, E. H., and Bunick, F. J., Reactions of cholesterol 5,6-epoxides with simulated gastric juice, *Lipids*, 23, 761, 1988.
30. Schulte, E. and Weber, N., Analysis of disteryl ethers, *Lipids*, 22, 1049, 1987.
31. Mariani, C., Gasparoli, A., Venturini, S., and Fedeli, S., Strutto vergine e strutto raffinato: loro differenziazione analytica, *Riv. Ital. Sost. Grasse*, 70, 275, 1993.
32. Rozendal, A., Interesterification and fractionation, in *Proc. World Conf. Oilseed Technol. Util.*, Applewhite, T. H., Ed., AOCS Press, Champaign, 1992, 180.
33. Lau, F. Y., Hammond, E. G., and Ross, P. F., Effect of randomization on the oxidation of corn oil, *J. Am. Oil Chem. Soc.*, 59, 407, 1982.
34. Billek, G., Veränderungen von Nahrungsfetten bei höheren Temperaturen, *Fat Sci. Technol.*, 94, 161, 1992.

35. Patterson, H. B. W., *Hydrogenation of Fats and Oils*, Elsevier, London, 1986.
36. Parodi, P. W., Distribution of isomeric octadecenoic fatty acids in milk fat, *J. Dairy Sci.*, 59, 1870, 1976.
37. Blumenthal, M. M., *Optimum Frying: Theory and Practice*, 2nd ed., Libra, Piscataway, NJ, 1987, 20.
38. Lumley, D., Polar compounds in heated oils, in *Frying of Food*, Varela, G., Bender, A. E., and Morton, I. D., Eds., VCH, Weinheim, 1988, 666.
39. Lingnert, H., Influence of food processing on lipid oxidation and flavor stability, in *Lipid Oxidation in Food*, St. Angelo, A. J., Ed., American Chemical Society, Washington, D.C., 1992, chap. 16.
40. Kim, S. K. and Nawar, W. W., Parameters influencing cholesterol oxidation, *Lipids*, 28, 917, 1993.
41. Velíšek, J., Davídek, J., Hajšlová, J., Kubelka, V., Janíček, G., and Mánková, B., Chlorohydrins in protein hydrolysates, *Z. Lebensm. Unters. Forsch.*, 167, 241, 1978.
42. Velíšek, J., Davídek, J., Kubelka, V., Janíček, G., Svobodová, Z., and Šimicová, Z., New chlorine-containing organic compounds in protein hydrolysates, *J. Agric. Food Chem.*, 28, 1142, 1980.
43. Velíšek, J., Davídek, J., and Kubelka, V., Formation of $\Delta^{3,5}$-diene and 3-chloro-Δ^5-ene analogs of sterols in protein hydrolysates, *J. Agric. Food Chem.*, 34, 660, 1986.
44. Velíšek, J. and Ledahudcová, K., Problems concerning organic chlorine compounds in protein hydrolysates, *Potrav. Vědy*, 11, 149, 1993.
45. Yoshioka, M. and Kaneda, T., Studies on the toxicity of autoxidized oils. III. The toxicity of hydroperoxyalkenals, *Yukagaku*, 23, 321, 1974.
46. Tovar, G. L. R. and Kaneda, T., Studies on the toxicity of the autoxidized oils. VI. Comparative toxicity of secondary oxidation products in autoxidized methyl linoleate, *Yukagaku*, 26, 169, 1977.
47. Esterbauer, H., Lipid peroxidation products: formation, chemical properties and biological activities, in *Free Radicals in Liver Injury*, Poli, G., Cheeseman, K. H., Dianzani, M. U., and Slater, T. F., Eds., IRL Press, Oxford, 1986, 29.
48. Kajimoto, G., Takaoka, M., Yoshida, H., and Shibahara, A., Decomposition of tocopherol by oxidative products of oils, and the production of red coloring materials, *Nippon Nogeikagaku Kaishi*, 63, 37, 1989.
49. Eschenbach, R. and Hartfiel, W., Einfluss von oxidierten Ölen sowie α-Tocopherol- und Antioxidantienzugaben auf das Wachstum und die Vitamin E- und A-Gehalte in Geweben von Masthuehnerkueken, *Fette, Seifen, Anstrichm.*, 87, 363, 1985.
50. Matoba, T., Yonezawa, D., Nair, B. M., and Kito, M., Damage of amino acid residues of proteins after reaction with oxidizing lipids: estimation by proteolytic enzymes, *J. Food Sci.*, 49, 1082, 1984.
51. Nielsen, H. K., Finot, P. A., and Hurrell, R. F., Reactions of proteins with oxidizing lipids. II. Influence on protein quality and on the bioavailability of lysine, methionine, cyst(e)ine, and tryptophan as measured by rat assays, *Br. J. Nutr.*, 53, 75, 1985.
52. Bauernfeind, J. C., Antioxidant function of L-ascorbic acid in food technology, *Int. J. Vitamin Nutr. Res. Suppl.*, 27, 307, 1985.
53. Combe, N., Intestinal absorption of heated fats, *Riv. Ital. Sost. Grasse*, 57, 226, 1980.
54. Marquez-Ruiz, C., Perez-Camino, M. C., and Dobarganes, M. C., Digestibility of fatty acid monomers, dimers, and polymers in the rat, *J. Am. Oil Chem. Soc.*, 69, 930, 1992.
55. Mensink, R. P. and Katan, M. B., Effect of dietary *trans* fatty acids on high-density and low-density lipoprotein cholesterol levels in healthy subjects, *N. England J. Med.*, 327, 439, 1990.
56. Duthie, G. G., Wahle, K. W. J., and James, W. P. T., Oxidants, antioxidants and cardiovascular disease, *Nutr. Res. Rev.*, 2, 51, 1989.
57. Duthie, G. G., Antioxidant hypothesis of cardiovascular disease, *Trends Food Sci. Technol.*, 2, 205, 1991.
58. Haumann, B. F., Health implication of lipid oxidation, *INFORM*, 4, 800, 1993.
59. Nagy, I. Z., *Lipofuscin: State of Art*, Akademiai Kiado, Budapest, 1988, chap. 1 through 5.
60. Fukuzumi, K., Relationship between lipoperoxide and aging, *Oleagineux*, 36, 251, 1981.
61. Pie, J. E., Spahis, K., and Seillan, C., Evaluation of oxidative degradation of cholesterol in food and food ingredients: identification and quantification of cholesterol oxides, *J. Agric. Food Chem.*, 38, 973, 1990.
62. Šilhánková, L., Šmíd, F., Černá, M., Davídek, J. and Velíšek, J., Mutagenicity of glycerol chlorohydrins and their esters of higher fatty acids present in protein hydrolysates, *Mutation Res.*, 103, 77, 1982.

63. Mancini-Filho, J., Smith, L. M., Creveling, R. K., and Al-Shaikh, H. F., Effects of selected chemical treatments on quality of fats used for deep frying, *J. Am. Oil Chem. Soc.*, 63, 1452, 1986.
64. Pokorný, J., Stabilization of food, in *Oxidation Inhibition in Organic Materials*, Vol. I, Pospíšil, J. and Klemchuk, P. P., Eds., CRC Press, Boca Raton, FL, 1990, chap. 11.
65. Loelliger, J., Natural antioxidants for the stabilization of foods, in *Flavor Chemistry*, Min, D. B. and Smouse, T., Eds., AOCS Press, Champaign, IL, 1989, 302.
66. Haumann, B. F., Antioxidant: firms seeking products they can label as "natural", *INFORM*, 1, 1002, 1990.
67. Seher, A., Hydrogenation and transesterification, in *Lipids*, Vol. 2, Paoletti, R., Jacini, G., and Porcellati, R., Eds., Raven Press, New York, 1976, 527.
68. Velíšek, J., Davídek, T., Davídek, J., and Hamburg, A., 3-Chloro-1,2-propanediol derived amino alcohol in protein hydrolysates, *J. Food Sci.*, 56, 136, 1991.
69. Velíšek, J., Davídek, T., Davídek, J. Kubelka, V., and Víden, I., 3-Chloro-1,2-propanediol derived amino acids in protein hydrolysates, *J. Food Sci.*, 56, 139, 1991.
70. Velíšek, J., Ledahudcová, K., Hajšlová, J., Pech, P., Kubelka, V., and Víden, I., New 3-chloro-1,2-propanediol derived dihydroxypropylamines in hydrolyzed vegetable proteins, *J. Agric. Food Chem.*, 40, 1389, 1992.

Chapter 5

Toxic Compounds Arising by Interaction of Food Constituents with Food Additives

Part A

Nitroso Compounds

Jiří Čulík and Vladimír Kellner

In 1956 nitrosamines were found to be carcinogenic in animals. Since that time considerable research attention has been paid to determine the levels of occurrence and formation of these substances in the environment and particularly in food.

CHEMISTRY OF NITROSATION

All nitroso compounds have the nitrosyl functional group –N≠ O in the molecule. The most widespread are *N*-nitroso compounds with the functional group –N–N≠ O. But O-, C-, and S-nitroso compounds are also known.

N-nitroso compounds can be divided into two main groups: the *N*-nitrosamines and the *N*-nitrosamides. Further, *N*-nitrosamines are divided into volatile and nonvolatile nitrosamines. This difference was made for practical purposes.

Volatile nitrosamines are a group of relatively nonpolar, low molecular weight nitrosamines with sufficient vapor pressure to be able to be removed from a food matrix by distillation and to be determined by gas chromatography.[1,2] The other nitrosamines, the so called nonvolatile ones, have a higher molecular weight, are more polar, and have a relatively low vapor pressure.

Nonvolatile nitroso compounds include long-chain dialkyl nitrosamines, *N*-nitrosoureas, *N*-nitrosopeptides, *N*-nitrosoamino acids, derivatives of *N*-nitrosothiazolidine acid, etc. and they differ widely in chemical and physical properties. The complexity of the composition of biological samples means that the determination of each individual N-nitroso compound is impossible and impracticable for a large number of samples, even if methods for their analysis were available.[3] So it was necessary to develop a universal method for the estimation of nonvolatile nitroso compounds as a group. The method employs the efficient splitting of the N-NO group.[4] It is used to estimate apparent total N-nitroso compounds (ATNC).

The basic kinetics and mechanism of the reaction with nitrite under acidic conditions has been thoroughly discussed elsewhere.[5-10] Nitroso compounds can arise from the nitrosation of many types of organo -N, -S, and -O compounds and nitrosating agents. The most frequent compounds are *N*-nitroso compounds. The most common reaction is the nitrosation of secondary amines or amides (Figure 1).

The effectiveness of the nitrosation depends on the nature of the Y_1 group. Figure 2 presents the catalysis of nitrosation, where Y_2-NO is a more active nitrosating agent than Y_1-NO. Figure 3, on the other hand, represents the inhibition of nitrosation. In nitrosation

0-8493-4623-1/95/$0.00+$.50

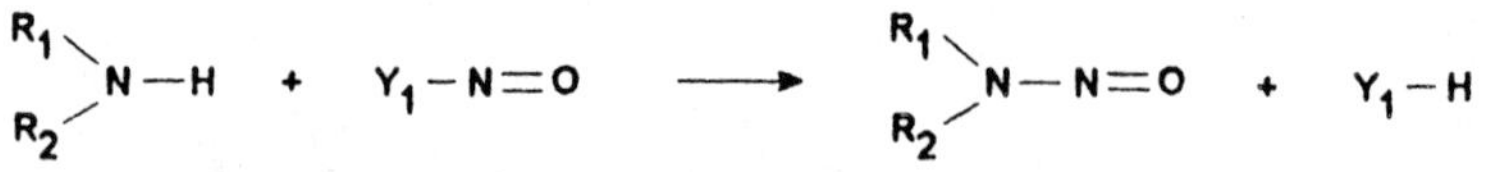

Figure 1 General mechanism of nitrosation of secondary amines. R_1, R_2 are alkyl, aryl, cycloalkyl.

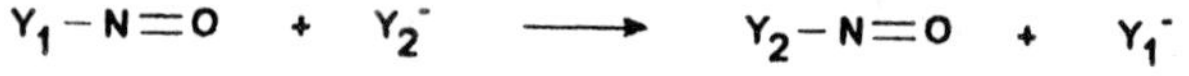

Figure 2 The mechanism of catalysis of nitrosation.

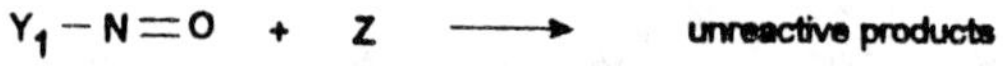

Figure 3 The mechanism of inhibition of nitrosation.

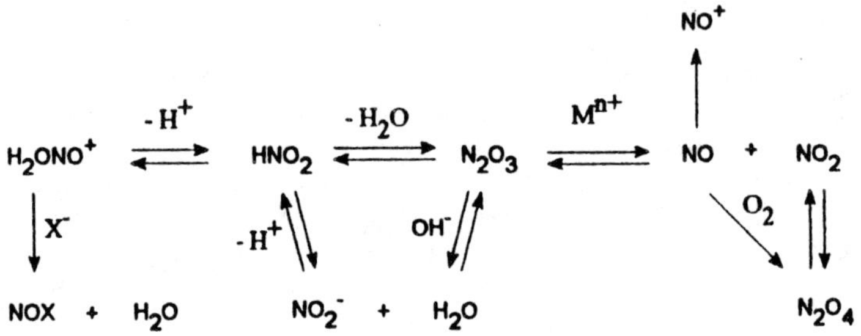

Figure 4 The interrelationship between active and inactive nitrosating agents. From Douglas, M. L., Kabacoff, B. L., Anderson, G. A., and Cheng, M. C., *J. Soc. Cosmet. Chem.*, 29, 581, 1978. With permission.

reactions a nitrosating agent Y_1-NO must be first generated from nitroso acids and a catalytic nucleophile. Determinations of the interrelationship between active nitrosating agents (N_2O_3, NO_2/N_2O_4, YNO, H_2ONO^+, NO^+) and inactive species (nitrous acid and nitrite ion) have been published[11] (Figure 4).

Catalysis occurs with certain anions Y_1^-. Of the anionic catalysts studied thiocyanate has the most powerful effect followed by halide ions in the following order:

$$SCN^-, I^- >> Br^- > Cl^-$$

In general, the stronger the nucleophile, the greater the catalysis. Bryant and Williams have studied the catalysis of nitrosation by dimethyl sulfide in m*M* concentrations; they found it to be an efficient catalyst.[12]

On the other hand, the nitrosamine inhibition is caused by substances which compete with the amine for nitrosating species. Certain inorganic and organic antioxidants are capable of inhibiting the formation of nitroso compounds under acidic conditions by reducing the nitrosating agent (Figure 5).

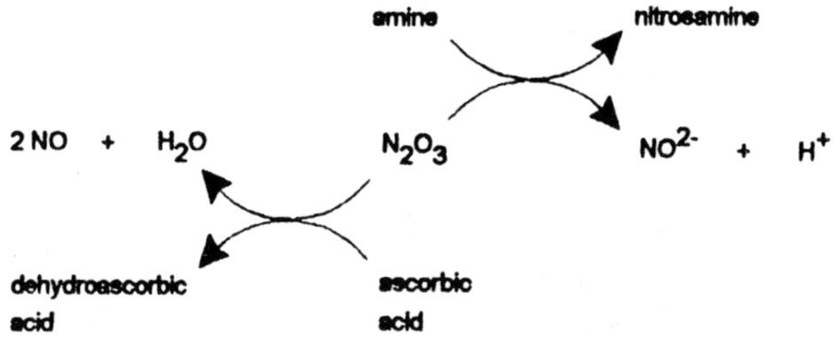

Figure 5 Inhibition of the formation of nitroso compounds under acidic conditions by reducing the nitrosating agent.

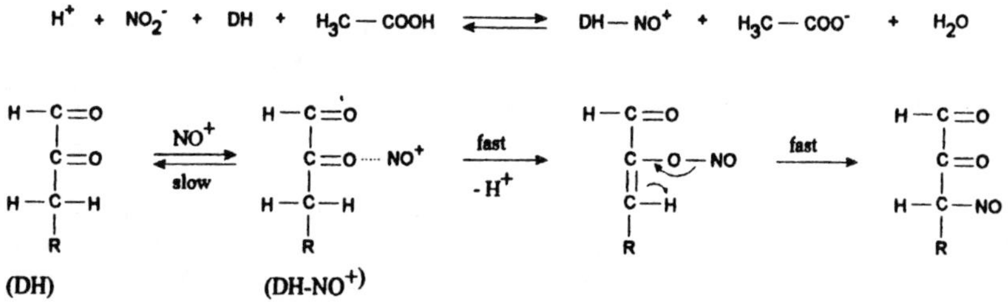

Figure 6 Mechanism of the reaction between 3-deoxyhexosulose and nitrite ion. R = $(CHOH)_2CH_2OH$. (From Wedzicha, B. L., and Tian, W., *Food Chem.*, 31, 189, 1989. With permission.)

Among organic antioxidants, ascorbic acid and tocopherols are found to inhibit the nitrosation in the concentration range from 500 up to 1,000 $mg.kg^{-1}$ (ascorbic acid) and from 100 up to 500 $mg.kg^{-1}$ (tocopherol). Douglass et al. have summarized the inhibiting influence of ascorbic acid in detail.[11] Lathia and Blum have published a review about the inhibiting role of tocopherols. They have found that tocopherols and ascorbic acid together have a stronger ihibiting effect on the formation of *N*-nitrosamine than each one alone.[13] Other inhibitors include sulfur dioxide, sulfamate, cysteine, and glutathione.[14] The ammonium ion, hydroxylamine, and retinol are nitrosation inhibitors.[11]

Phenols play an interesting role, since they can either inhibit or enhance the formation of nitrosamines, largely depending on the relative concentration of nitrite and phenol.[11] Kurechi et al. have found that alcohols in high concentration inhibited the formation of *N*-nitrosodimethylamine (NDMA) and *N*-nitrosodiethylamine (NDEA) from sodium nitrite at pH 3.0 but enhanced the reaction at pH 5.0.[15]

It is supposed that the 3-deoxyhexosulose (DH) and compounds derived from it are important intermediates in the formation of color in the Maillard nonenzymatic browning reaction. The kinetics of reaction between DH and nitrite ion in a model system was consistent with C-nitrosation[16] (Figure 6).

TOXIC EFFECTS

The nitroso compounds comprise a group of very potent mutagens and carcinogens. Haley has published an overview of acute oral toxicities of nitroso compounds in rats.[17] In general, these compounds have a relatively low toxicity.

N-nitroso compounds have been studied extensively with regards to their mutagenicity and carcinogenity. Mutagenicity of N-nitroso compounds is usually tested by using *Salmonella typhimurium* strains.[18,19]

The carcinogenic action of N-nitroso compounds has been tested in a large number of animal species.[20] These compounds in principle belong to the group of "multipotent" carcinogens which can have an ubiquitous carcinogenic effect.[21] Carcinogenic action may be related to a variety of organs and organ systems.[22,23] There are three different organotropisms, depending on the route of application of N-nitroso compounds. In contrast to *N*-nitrosamines, the organotropism of nitrosoamides like nitrosomethylurea depends on the method of application.[24] In many cases, N-nitroso compounds show synergistic effects when administered with other cancer-inducing or noncarcinogenic xenobiotics to experimental animals.[25]

There is very little known about carcinogenicity and mutagenity of C- and *S*-nitroso compounds,[26] cyclic *N*-nitrosamines containing sulfur (nitrosothiazolidines),[27-29] and N-nitroso derivatives of glycosylamines and Amadori compounds.[30]

Namiki et al. discovered that nitrite reacts optimally with sorbic acid, producing mutagens. Most mutagenic products of the reaction isolated were C-nitro and C-nitroso compounds.[26]

Very few ways of detoxifying final products are known. In some cases NDMA can be adsorbed onto charcoal or can be removed by ultrafiltration.[31] Some beverages, like whisky or other alcoholic beverages, show decreased levels of NDMA when illuminated with visible light or UV radiation.[32,33]

Generally speaking, the most effective method of detoxication is to prevent the formation of nitrosamines and their precursors during manufacture.

OCCURRENCE

The presence of traces of volatile *N*-nitrosamines in foods has been known for a relatively long time (about 30 years). Herman was probably the first (1961) who mentioned that human food contains N-nitroso compounds.[34] The great majority of papers list volatile nitrosamine levels in bacon, other cured meats, certain cheeses, nonfat dry milk, fish, beer, whisky and others. *N*-nitrosopyrrolidine (NPYR) was the major volatile *N*-nitrosamine found in fried bacon, *N*-nitrosodimethylamine (NDMA) is the one most frequently found in beer, beverages, and malt (Tables 1 and 2).[35-51] Over 170 samples of beer have been analyzed for NDMA and ATNC. The NDMA levels were found in the range from below 0.1 $\mu g.kg^{-1}$ up to 1.2 $\mu g.kg^{-1}$. ATNC were detected in concentrations of up to 562 μg (N-NO).kg^{-1}. No correlation was found between the amounts of NDMA and ATNC.[51]

Kellner et al. have determined concentrations of ATNC in 60 samples of beer up to 390 μg (N-NO).kg^{-1}. [52] The NDMA levels now are approximately 1 to 5% of what they were a decade ago.[50] Tricker and Kubacki have reviewed the occurrence and formation of nonvolatile *N*-nitrosamines occurring in foods and beverages. *N*-nitrosoproline and *N*-nitrosothiazolidine-4-carboxylic acid were the most commonly identified non-volatile *N*-nitrosamines in the diet [53] (Table 3).[54,55]

CHANGES DURING PROCESSING AND STORAGE

It is known that the NDMA in beer comes from malt. NDMA is formed during malt kilning by reaction between oxides of nitrogen (NO_x) in kilning gases and precursors of NDMA in the green malt.[56] Hordenine and gramine, two alkaloids found in barley malt,

Table 1 Occurrence of Volatile *N*-Nitrosamines in Food

Food	n[a]	NA found[b]	Range (μg.kg^{-1})	Ref.
Fried bacon	22	NPYR	7–139	36
Fried bacon	56	NDMA, NPYR	ND[c]–200	37
Cured meats	34	NDMA	ND–10	37
Fish	112	NDMA	ND–10	37
Cheese	58	NDMA	ND–15	37
Cured meats	64	NDMA, NDEA NPYR, NPIP	ND–8.6	37
Salt-fermented vegetables	49	NDMA, NPYR	ND–5	38
Cheese	209	NDMA	0.5–5	39
Cured meats	118	NDMA, NDEA, NPYR, NPIP	ND–55	40
Alcoholic beverages	50	NDMA	ND–4.9	40
Nonfat dry milk	57	NDMA	0.1–3.7	40
Fried bacon	20	NDMA, NPYR	ND–21	41
Microwave-cooked bacon	20	NDMA, NPYR	ND–1.2	41
Whisky	15	NDMA	ND–1.2	42
Tea	6	NDMA	ND–1.2	42
Fried bacon	68	NPYR, NDMA, NPIP	ND–56	42

Note: NDMA = *N*-nitrosodimethylamine; NDEA = *N*-nitrosodiethylamine; NPIP = *N*-nitrosopiperidine; NPYR = *N*-nitrosopyrrolidine.

[a] Number of samples analyzed
[b] Volatile nitrosamines;
[c] ND, not detected.

Most data adapted from Hotchkiss, J. H., *Adv. Food Res.*, 31, 53, 1987.

Table 2 Volatile Nitrosamines in Beer

n	NDMA range (μg.kg^{-1})	Ref.
260	ND–13	10
158	ND–68	11
18	ND–7	12
25	ND–14	13
75	ND–11	14
144	ND–56	15
22	ND–4.9	16
194	ND–0.6	17
258	ND–6.5	9
171	ND–1.2	18

Note: n = number of samples analyzed; NDMA = *N*-nitrosodimethylamine; ND = not detected.

are considered to be the main precursors of NDMA in barley malt[57] (Figure 7). These alkaloidal tertiary amines are products of germination in malted barley. Hordenin is found exclusively in the rootlets (in concentrations reaching up to 1,600 mg.kg^{-1}); gramine, in contrast to hordenin, is only found in acrospire (in concentrations reaching up to 600

Table 3 Occurrence of Nonvolatile *N*-nitroso Compounds in Food Products (μg.kg⁻¹).

Food sample	n[a]	NPRO	NHPRO	NHMTCA	NTCA	NMTCA
Unsmoked cured meats						
Pork luncheon meat[b]	3	0–40	—	—	—	—
Cooked ham[b]	3	0–40	0–100	—	—	—
Corned beef[b]	2	70–110	240–250	130–230	—	—
Bacon, raw[b]	3	—	0–30	0–40	0–30	—
Bacon, fried[b]	3	0–20	0–80	0–100	0–50	—
Smoked cured meats						
Icelandic mutton[b]	2	230–360	350–560	160–320	960–1070	—
Smoked sausage[b]	2	0–70	—	110–400	180–210	—
Bacon, raw[b]	5	0–20	0–60	0–1300	0–140	—
Bacon, fried[b]	5	0–40	0–90	0–2100	0–520	—
Bacon raw[c]	40	—	—	22–618	18–501	0–26
Bacon, fried[c]	25	—	—	14–72	5–136	—
Ham[c]	3	—	—	196–475	219–490	0–21
Beef[c]	3	—	—	129–255	328–570	0–28
Duckling[c]	3	—	—	409–462	829–1240	35–97
Pheasant[c]	4	—	—	24–75	901–1005	76–98
Cheese[c]	3	—	—	1062–1328	5–24	—

Note: NPRO = *N*-nitrosoproline; NHPRO = *N*-nitrosohydroxyproline; NTCA = *N*-nitrosothiazolidine-4-carboxylic acid; MTCA = *N*-nitroso-2-methylthiazolidine-4 -carboxylic acid; NHMTCA = *N*-nitroso-2-(hydroxymethyl)thiazolidine-4-carboxylic acid.

[a] Number of samples analyzed.

[b] Original data from Tricker, A. R., Perkins, M. J., Massey, C. R., Bishop, C., Key, P. E., and McWeeny, D. J., *Food Additiv. Contam.*, 1, 245, 1984.

[c] Original data from Mandagere, A. K., Ph.D. thesis, Michigan State University, Lansing, 1986.

Most data adapted from Tricker, A. R., Perkins, M. J., Massey, C. R., Bishop, C., Key, P. E., and McWeeny, D. J., *Food. Addit. Contam.* 1, 245, 1984.

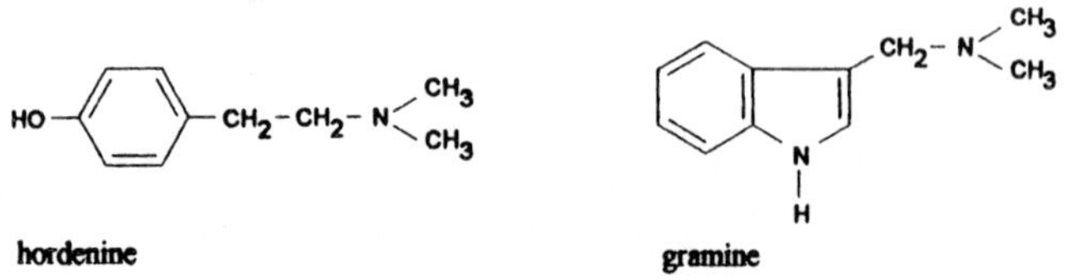

Figure 7 Structure of hordenine and gramine.

mg.kg⁻¹).[58] The chemistry of nitrosamine formation in malt is extremely complex (Figures 8 and 9).

There is no simple correlation between NO_x content of the drying air and NDMA formation. Nitric oxide, NO, does not form nitrosamines, but NDMA formation with N_2O_3 is more extensive than with N_2O_4.[59] Although dimethylamine (DMA) has been detected in green malt (in μg.kg⁻¹ levels) it does not seem to be the main precursor of NDMA.[60,61] DMA can be formed from other precursors during kilning [62] (Figure 10). The

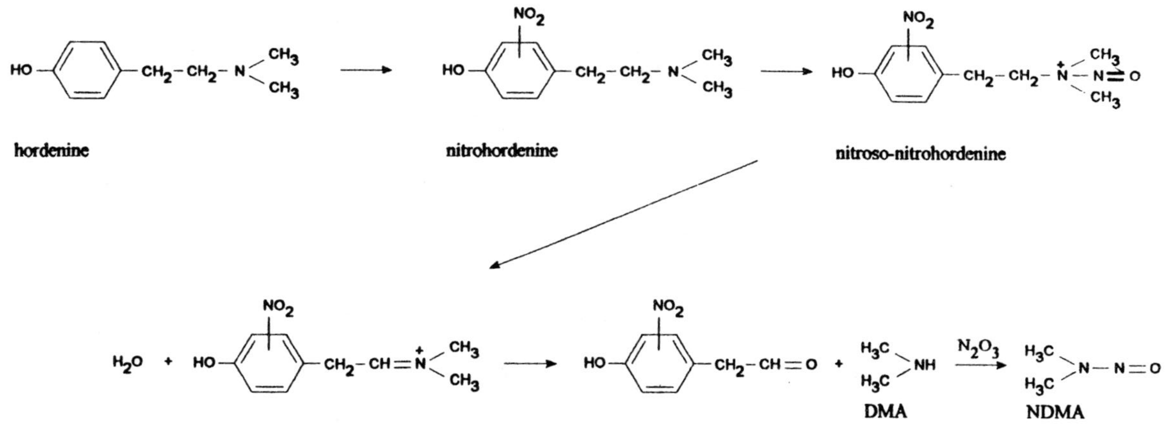

Figure 8 The chemistry of *N*-nitrosodimethylamine formation from hordenine in malt. (From Wainwright, T., *J. Inst. Brew.*, 92, 49, 1986. With permission.)

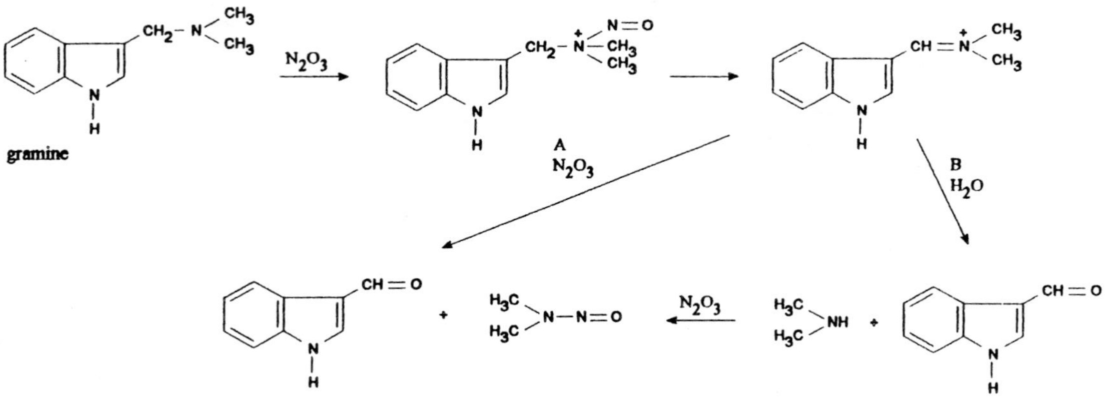

Figure 9 The chemistry of *N*-nitrosodimethylamine formation from gramine in malt. (From Wainwright, T., *J. Inst. Brew.*, 92, 49, 1986. With permission.)

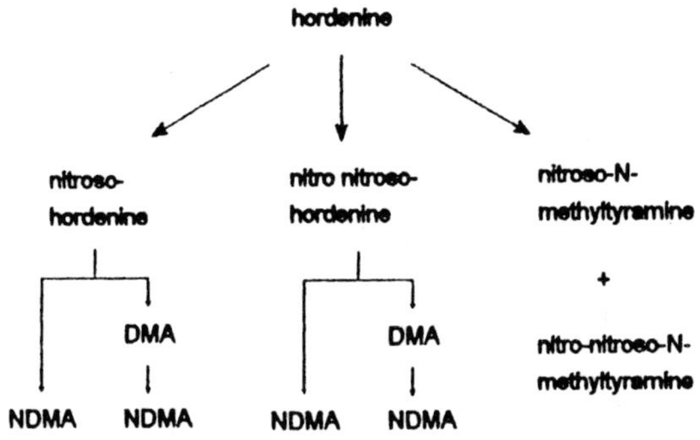

Figure 10 Possible ways of formation of *N*-nitrosodimethylamine in malt. (From Wainwright, T., *J. Inst. Brew.*, 92, 49, 1986. With permission.)

detailed study of the reaction mechanism performed by Wainwright confirmed that hordenine is decomposed during kilning with NO_x to give DMA at a stage when the NDMA is not completely removed. Other nitrogen-containing compounds, e.g., sarcosine, creatine, and choline, may also give low yields of NDMA[63] (Figure 11).

The concentration of NDMA in malt depends on conditions of germinating (temperature, moisture, and content of CO_2 in green malt) and kilning (temperature, moisture, and pH of malt and content of NO_x in the kilning air), and the formation of NDMA during germination and kilning can be affected[64,65] (Figure 12). It is known that malt contains a few $mg.kg^{-1}$ DMA, but there is usually no formation of NDMA during malt storage.[61]

The control of NDMA in malt can be achieved in various ways. One of them is avoidance of N_2O_3 and N_2O_4 which normally are present in kilning air, by using a heating system which uses indirect heating or low NO_x burners.[66-68] In this case, the content of NO_x in kilning air must be less than 0.07 $mg.m^{-3}$. The other way is to increase the content of SO_2 in kilning air by burning elemental sulfur or by direct injection of SO_2 into the kiln gas (doses of sulfur range from 100 up to 600 $g.t^{-1}$ of barley). Treating the malt with SO_2 resulted in NDMA levels from nondetectable to 5 $\mu g.kg^{-1}$.[69]

The NDMA content can be minimized by decreasing the formation of hordenine or DMA during germination (control of temperature and moisture, content of CO_2 in green malt, resteaping or application of bromate or ammonium persulfate before germinating).[62,64,65,70] Another way is to minimize transfer of hordenine before kilning from roots to husk or to prevent nitrosation of hordenine by spraying with dextrose (0.8%) or phosphoric acid (0.066%).[71] However, acidification of malt cannot prevent NDMA formation from gramine (Figure 13).

NDMA can be partially removed due to its volatility in steam during wort boiling or can be adsorbed onto charcoal, but this is not practical.[72]

In beer, the ATNC content seems to be important. Massey et al. have found that the maximum increase of the ATNC concentration during fermentation of the wort is caused by the presence of microbial species with nitrate reductase activity.[73] Smith has also confirmed that microbial nitrate reduction is the principal route of *N*-nitrosamine formation in brewing.[74] The nitrate-reducing organisms capable of growth during fermentation are normally Gram-negative bacteria, typically *Obesumbacterium proteus*.[73,74]

Although it is known that some meat products contain traces of various volatile nitrosamines, such as NDMA, NDEA, NDPA, NDBA (*N*-nitrosodipropylamine) and NPIP (*N*-nitrosopiperidine), NPYR is one of the most frequently found in cured meat

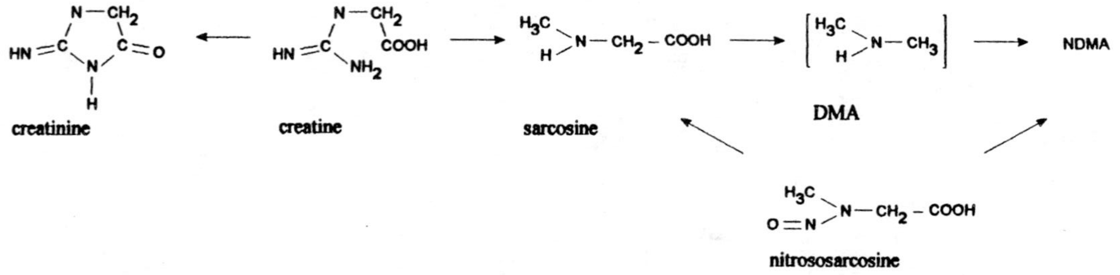

Figure 11 Proposed mechanism of formation of *N*-nitrosodimethylamine from creatine. (From Wainwright, T., *J. Inst. Brew.*, 92, 49, 1986. With permission.)

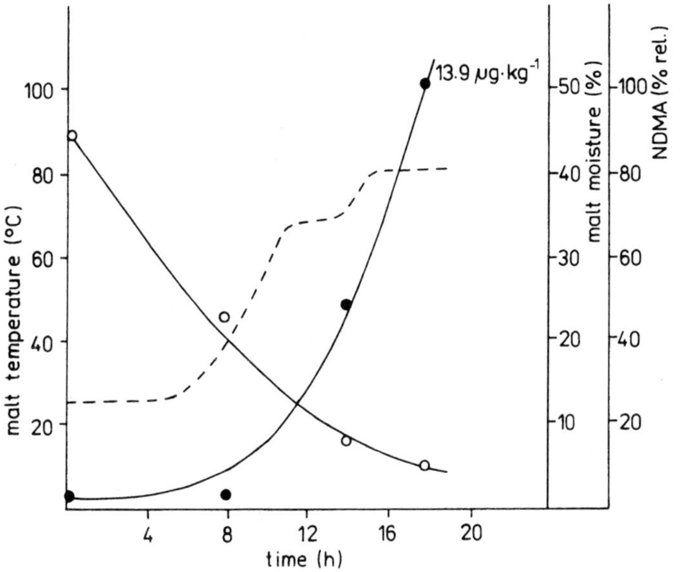

Figure 12 Influence of kilning conditions on formation of *N*-nitrosodimethylamine during kilning process. ○ = malt temperature, ● = NDMA. (From Čulík, J., Kellner, V., Špinar, B., Ilčík, F., and Basařová, G., *Kvasný Prům.*, 35, 353, 1989. With permission.)

products after grilling or frying.[76,77] Nebelin et al. studied the formation of NPYR and NPIP from proline, pyrrolidine, putrescine, spermidine, and cadaverine in a model system containing minced bacon and nitrite as a reaction medium. The results confirm that the formation of NPYR and other volatile nitrosamines is possibly due to acid-catalyzed hydrolysis during heating and that the formation of NPYR involves a decarboxylation step[77] (Figure 14). Sen et al. proved that NDMA, like NPYR, can be formed by thermal decarboxylation of nitrososarcosine.[78] The role of collagen, proline, *N*-nitrosoproline (NPRO), and N-nitrosated-prolyl derivatives of dipeptides, tripeptides, and tetrapeptides on the origin of nitrosamines was studied by Tricker et al.[79,80] As regards the NPRO in nitrite-cured products, 3 to 93% was protein-associated and only detectable after proteolytic digestion.[81]

Nonvolatile *N*-nitrosoamino acids, which were detected in 80% of the samples at levels of up to 0.4 $mg.kg^{-1}$, represent only a negligible part of the ATNC.[82,83] Nevertheless, a number of nonvolatile substituted nitrosothiazolidines and nitrosothiazolidine carboxylic acids and related compounds have been detected in smoked cured meats.[84-87]

It seems that the formation of *N*-nitrosothiazolidine (NTHZ) in cure-pumped bacon is linked to the heating-smoking step in bacon processing and that cysteamine is the most likely precursor of the NTHZ[88,89] (Figure 15). Decarboxylation of *N*-nitrosothiazolidine-4-carboxylic acid (NTHZC) does not seem, according both model system and frying experiments, to be the principal pathway to NTHZ formation in uncooked bacon.[90]

Some phenolic compounds, previously identified in hardwood sawdust smoke and smoked food may be nitrosated and compete with amines for available nitrite.[91] These reactions can lead to the formation of C-nitroso and C-nitro compounds, so that the formation of *N*-nitrosamines can be depressed[11,92,93] (Figure 16). Unfortunately, phenolic compounds which can potentially form C-nitroso derivatives by reaction with nitrite can

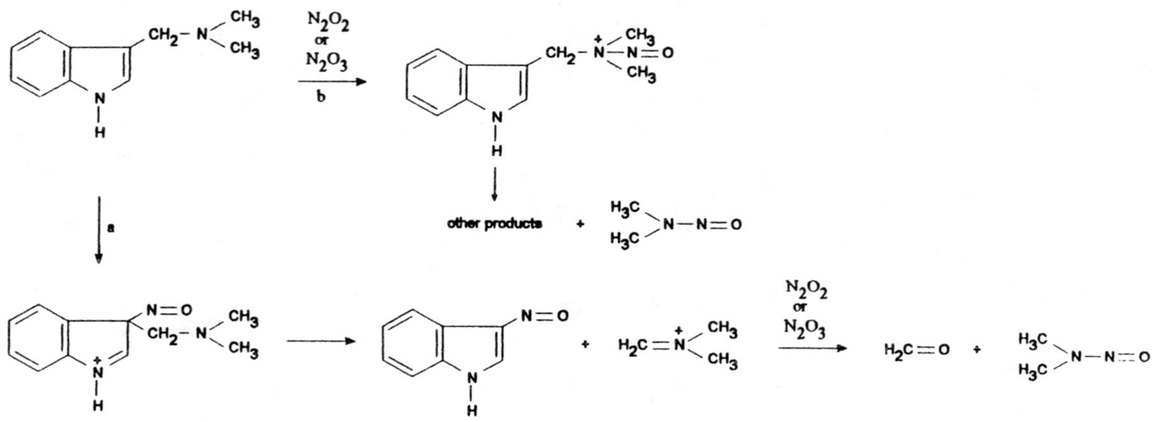

Figure 13 Two alternative pathways proposed to account for the high yield of *N*-nitrosodimethylamine in malt from gramine. (From Wainwright, T., *J. Inst. Brew.*, 92, 49, 1986. With permission.)

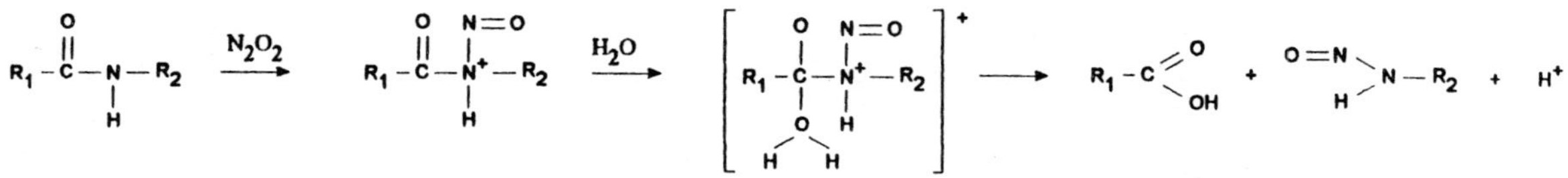

Figure 14 General mechanism for formation of nitrosopyrrolidine and nitrosopiperidine in a model system containing peptides and nitrite. (From Nebelin, E., Pillai, S., Lund, E., and Thomsen, J., *IARC. Sci. Publ.*, 31, 183, 1980. With permission.)

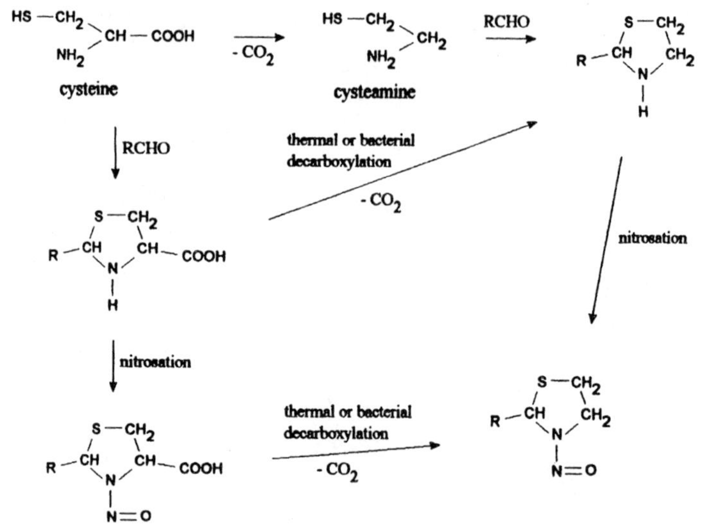

Figure 15 General mechanism for formation of various *N*-nitrosothiazolidine compounds in foods. R = H, CH_3, or CH_2OH, corresponding to formaldehyde, acetaldehyde, and glycolaldehyde, respectively. (From Sen, N. P., Baddoo, P. A., Seaman, S. W., and Weber, D., *J. Food Sci.*, 56, 913, 1991. With permission.)

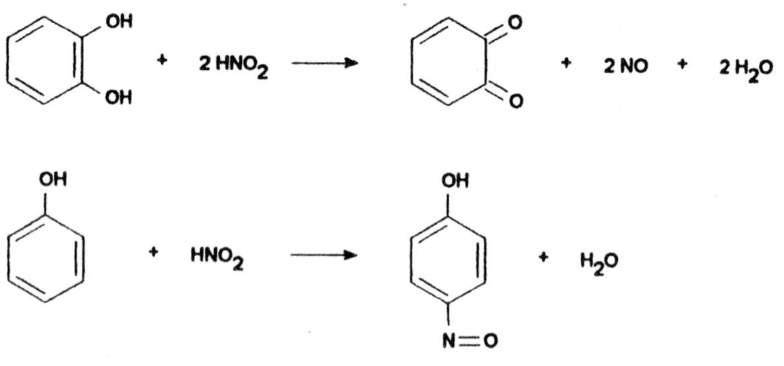

Figure 16 Formation of C-nitroso compounds from phenolic compounds.

act under some conditions as catalysts for the formation of *N*-nitrosamine from secondary amines and nitrite[94] (Figure 17). Knowles et al. proved that in the presence of nitrite, phenols under the appropriate conditions, undergo facile substitution reactions yielding the corresponding *C*-nitrosophenols and *C*-nitrophenols.[92]

Also, some *S*-nitroso compounds can take part in the transnitrosation and formation of *N*-nitrosamines.[95] *S*-Nitrosocysteine has been shown to be generated during the curing process of meat.[96] *S*-Nitrosocysteine can take part in transnitrosation, and the presence of the N-nitroso derivatives is the result of it.[97] This compound can act as an inhibitor of lipid oxidation, color development and as an anticlostridial agent in meat products.[98] Because transnitrosation occurs between *S*-nitrosocysteine and hemoproteins in meat products and there are some chances for nitrosamine formation, *S*-nitrosocysteine cannot be recommended as a substitute for nitrite.[99]

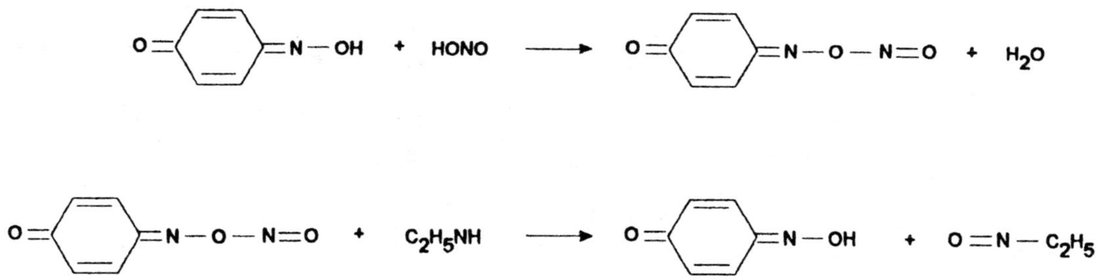

Figure 17 The role of phenols in catalysis of nitrosamine formation from secondary amines. (From Walker, E. A., Pignatelli, B., and Friesen, M., *J. Sci. Food. Agric.*, 33, 81, 1982. With permission.)

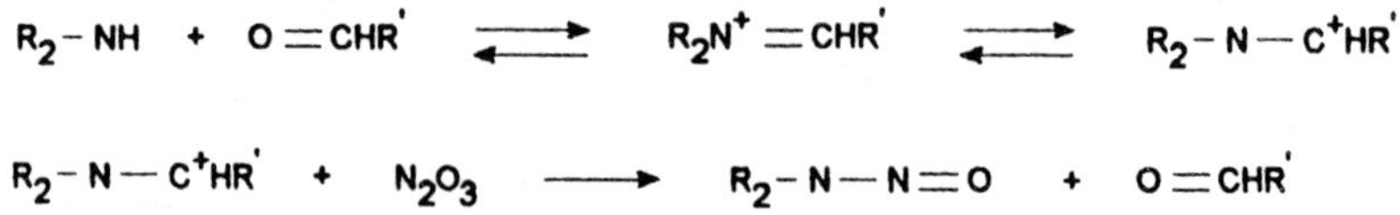

Figure 18 Catalytic effect of the formaldehyde on nitrosamine formation.

The level of *N*-nitrosamines in cured meats can be modified by choosing various pre-processing, frying, or curing methods.[100-102] Reduced levels of nitrosamines (NDMA, NPIP, and NPYR) can be achieved by using microwave cooking or by pre-cooking of nitrite-cured bacon (from 20 to 50%).[41,103] The effect of irradiation on reduced NPYR formation was also studied,[104] when it was found that the level of NPYR compared with the unirradiated control significantly decreases from 15 to 7.7 μg.kg^{-1}. The formation of nitrosamines during cooking can be inhibited by ethoxyquin and dihydroethoxyquin.[105] Various reducing compounds added to meat products for the purpose of improving NO_2- activity, e.g., α-tocopherol-coated-salts, ascorbic acid, L-cystein, sorbate, or propyl gallate act as efficient factors inhibiting nitrosamine formation.[106-110] On the other hand, formaldehyde has a catalytic effect on nitrosamine formation[111] (Figure 18).

Gough and Walters studied the effect of storage time and temperature on the level of NPYR in cooked bacon.[112] Data obtained after storage for 1, 21, and 36 d at 15 and 5°C showed that there was a tendency for the NPYR concentration to decrease with time, but there was no apparent correlation between NPYR concentration and storage temperature.

Volatile *N*-nitrosamines are rarely found in some fermented vegetable products, e.g., kimchi, a popular Korean traditional fermented product.[113] During kimchi fermentation, the level of NO_3- decreased, and NO_2- was detected in trace amounts. NDMA was the major volatile nitrosamine found in kimchi, but the levels were negligible. Sung et al. reported that the concentration of NDMA (range 1.6 to 10.4 μg.kg^{-1}) in soy sauce samples correlated with nitrate concentration, and that all samples contained large numbers of nitrate-reductase-containing organisms.[114] The level of NDMA in soy sauce can be reduced by using some additives like ascorbic acid (150 mg.kg^{-1}), sorbic acid (200 mg.kg^{-1}), and sodium benzoate (200 mg.kg^{-1}). Free amino acids, e.g., glutamic acid, proline, or histidine detected during fermentation proved inhibitory towards formation of NDMA.[115]

Massey et al. reported that ATNC were present in some cheese samples manufactured with added nitrate, including Edam and Gouda. ATNC were detected in most of those cheese samples in concentrations ranging from 30 to 210 μg(N-NO).kg^{-1}.[116]

Trace amounts of nitrosamines were observed in powered milk and milk proteins (1.3 to 67.0 μg.kg^{-1}, average level 7.4 μg.kg^{-1}).[117,118]

REFERENCES

1. Fiddler, W., The occurrence and determination of *N*-nitroso compounds, *Toxicol. Appl. Pharmacol.*, 31, 352, 1975.
2. Fine, D. H., Nitrosamines in the general environment and food, in *Nitrosamines and Human Cancer*, Magee P. N., Ed., Cold Spring Harbor Laboratory Press, Cold Spring Harbor, NY, 1982, 199.
3. Castegnar, M., Massey, R. C., and Walters, C. L., The collaborative evaluation of a procedure for the determination of *N*-nitroso compounds as a group, *Food Addit. Contam.*, 4, 37, 1987.
4. Walters, C. L., Downes, M. J., Edwards, M. W., and Smith, P. L. R., Determination of a non-volatile *N*-nitrosamine on a food matrix, *Analyst*, 103, 1127, 1978.
5. Mirvish, S. S., Formation of *N*-nitroso compounds: chemistry, kinetics and *in vivo* occurrence, *Toxicol. Appl. Pharmacol.*, 31, 325, 1975.

6. Mirvish, S. S., N-Nitroso compounds: their chemical and *in vivo* formation and possible importance as environmental carcinogens, *J. Toxicol. Environ. Health*, 2, 1267, 1977.
7. Fine, D. H., N-Nitroso compounds compounds in the environment, in *Advances in Environmental Science and Technology*, Vol. 9, Pitts, J. N., Metcalf, R. L., and Grosjean, D., Eds., Wiley-Interscience, New York, 1980.
8. Kellner, V., Ćulík, J., and Basařová, G., On problems of N-nitrosamine-origin and properties, *Kvasný prům.*, 28, 7, 1982.
9. Röper, H., Chemie und Bildung von N-Nitroso Verbindungen, in *Das Nitrosamin-Problem*, Pressmann, R., Ed., Verlag Chemie, Weinheim, 1983, 189.
10. Wainwright, T., The chemistry of N-nitrosamine formation: relevance to malting and brewing, *J. Inst. Brew.*, 92, 49, 1986.
11. Douglass, M. L., Kabacoff, B. L., Anderson, G. A., and Cheng, M. C., The chemistry of nitrosamine formation, inhibition and destruction, *J. Soc. Cosmet. Chemists*, 29, 581, 1978.
12. Bryant, T. and Williams, D. L. H., Catalysis of nitrosation by dimethyl sulphide, *J. Chem. Res. (S)*, 174, 1987.
13. Lathia, D. and Blum, A., Role of vitamin E as nitrite scavenger and N-nitrosamine inhibition: A review, *Intern. J. Vitamin Nutrit. Res.*, 59, 430, 1989.
14. Gray, J. I. and Dugan, L. R., Jr., Inhibition of N-nitrosamine formation in model food systems, *J. Food Sci.*, 40, 981, 1975.
15. Kurechi, T., Kikugawa, K., and Kato, T., Effects of alcohols on nitrosamine formation, *Food Cosmet. Toxicol.*, 18, 591, 1980.
16. Wedzicha, B. L. and Tian, W., Kinetics of the reaction between 3-deoxyhexosulose and nitrite ion, *Food Chem.*, 31 (3), 189, 1989.
17. Haley, J. T., An overview of chemical carcinogens, in *Handbook of Carcinogens and Hazardous Substances,* Bowman, M. C., Ed., Marcel Dekker, New York, 1982, chap.1.
18. Weng, Y. M., Hotchkiss, J. H., and Babish, J. G., *N*-Nitrosamine and mutagenicity formation in Chinese salted fish after digestion, *Food Addit. Contam.,* 9 (1), 29, 1992.
19. Umano, K., Shibamoto, T., Fernando, S. Y., and Wei, C. I., Mutagenicity of hydroxyalkyl-*N*-nitrosothiazolidines, *Food Chem. Toxicol.*, 22 (4), 253, 1984.
20. Magee, P. N., Montesano, R., and Preussmann, R., N-Nitroso compounds and related carcinogens, in *Chemical Carcinogens*, Searle, C. E., Ed., ASC Monogr. 173, American Chemical Society, Washington, D.C., 1976, chap. 2.
21. Schmähl, D. and Habs, M., Carcinogenicity of N-nitroso compounds, *Oncology*, 37, 237, 1980.
22. Schmähl, D., in *Maligne Tumoren*, Editio Cantor, Aulendorf, 1981, 130.
23. Krull, S. I. and Fine, D. H., N-Nitrosamines and N-nitroso compounds, in *Handbook of Carcinogens and Hazardous Substances*, Bowman, M. C., Ed., Marcel Dekker, New York, 1982, chap.6.
24. Druckrey, H., Preussmann, R., Ivankovic, S., and Schmaehl, D., *Z. Krebsforsch.*, 69, 103, 1967.
25. Habs, M. and Schmähl, D., Synergistic effects of N-nitroso compounds in experimental long-term carcinogenesis studies, *Oncology*, 37, 259, 1980.
26. Namiki, M., Osawa, T., Kada, T., Tsuji, K., and Namiki, K., Formation of C-nitro and C-nitroso mutagens by the reaction of nitrite with sorbic acid and its analogs and their inactivation with food constituents, *Carcinogens Mutagens Environ.*, 3, 109, 1983.
27. Lijinski, W., Kovatch, R. M., Keefer, L. K., Saavedra, J. E., Hansen, T. J., Miller, A. J., and Fiddler, W., Carcinogenesis in rats by cyclic N-nitrosamines containing sulfur, *Food Chem. Toxicol.*, 26 (1), 3, 1988.
28. Salvi, N. A. and Choughuley, A. S. U., Nitrosation of some food-related tetrahydro-beta-carboline-3-carboxylic acids, *J. Sci. Food Agric.*, 52, 537, 1990.
29. Lin, I. N. C. and Gruenwedel, D. W., Mutagenicity and cytotoxicity of N-nitrosothiazolidine-4-carboxylic acid, *Food Addit. Contam.*, 7, 357, 1990.
30. Pignatelli, B., Malaveille, C., Friesen, M., Hautepeuille, A., Bartsch, H., Piskorska, D., and Descotes, G., Synthesis, structure-activity relationship and a reaction mechanism for mutagenic N-nitroso derivatives of glycosylamines and Amadori compounds — Model substances for N-nitrosated early Maillard reaction products, *Food Chem. Toxicol.*, 25 (9), 669, 1987.
31. Zhukova, G. F. and Pimenova, V. V., Kantserog. N-nitrozosoedin.: Obraz. Opred. Mater., in *Proc. 3rd. Mater. Symp.*, Loogna, G. O., Ed., Institut Pitania, Moscow, 1978, 184.

32. Pollock, J. R. A., U.K. Patent Application, 2,071,692A, 1981.
33. Sharp, R. and Watson, S., U.K. Patent Application, GB 2,140,455A, 1984.
34. Herman, H., Identifizierung eines Stoffwechselproduktes von *Clitocybe sauveolens* als 4-Methylnitrosamino-benzaldehyd, *Hoppe-Seylers Z. Physiol. Chem.*, 326, 13, 1961.
35. Hotchkiss, J. H., A review of current literature on N-nitroso compounds in foods, *Adv. Food Res.*, 31, 53, 1987.
36. Havery, D. C., Fine, D. A., Miletta, E. M., Joe, F. L., Jr., and Fazio, T., Survey of food products for volatile N-nitrosamines, *J. Assoc. Off. Anal. Chem.*, 59, 540, 1976.
37. Gough, T. A., McPhail, M. F., Webb, K. S., Wood, B. J., and Coleman, R. F., An examination of some foodstuffs for presence of volatile nitrosamines, *J. Sci. Food Agric.*, 28, 345, 1977.
38. Kawabata, T., Uibu, J., Ohsima, H., Matsui, H., Hamano, M., and Tokiwa, H., Occurrence, formation and precursors of N-nitroso compounds in Japanese diet, *IARC Sci. Publ.*, 31, 481, 1980.
39. Spiegelhalder, B., Eisenbrand, G., and Preussmann, R., Volatile nitrosamines in food, *Oncology*, 37, 211, 1980.
40. Sen, N. P., Seaman, S., and McPherson, M., Further studies on the occurence of volatile and non-volatile nitrosamines in foods, *IARC Sci. Publ.*, 31, 457, 1980.
41. Österdahl, B. G. and Alriksson, E., Volatile nitrosamines in microwave-cooked bacon, *Food Addit. Contam.*, 7, 51, 1990.
42. Österdahl, B. G., Volatile nitrosamines in foods on the Swedish market and estimate of their daily intake, *Food Addit. Contam.*, 5, 587, 1988.
43. Havery, D. C., Hotchkiss, J. H., and Fazio, T., Nitrosamines in malt beverages, *J. Food Sci.*, 46, 501, 1981.
44. Spiegelhalder, B., Eisenbrand, G., and Preussmann, R., Contamination of beer with trace quantities of *N*-nitrosodimethylamine, *Food Cosmet. Toxicol.*, 17, 29, 1979.
45. Goff, E. U. and Fine, D. H., Analysis of volatile N-nitrosamines in alcoholic beverages, *Food Cosmet. Toxicol.*, 17, 569, 1979.
46. Scanlan, R. A., Barbour, J. F., Hotchkiss, J. H., and Libbey, L. H., N-Nitrosodimethylamine in beer, *Food Cosmet. Toxicol.*, 18, 27, 1980.
47. Walker, E. A., Castegnaro, M., Garren, L., Toussaint, G., and Kowalski, B., Intake of volatile nitrosamines from consumption of alcohols, *J. Natl. Cancer Inst.*, 63, 947, 1979.
48. Kann, J., Tauts, O., Kalve, R., and Bogowski, P., Potential formation of N-nitrosamines in the course of technological processing of some foodstuffs, *IARC Sci. Publ.*, 31, 319, 1980.
49. Sen, N. P., Seaman, S., and McPherson, M., Nitrosamines in alcoholic beverages, *J. Food Safety*, 2, 13, 1980.
50. Scanlan, R. A., Barbour, J. F., and Chappel, C. I., A survey of N-nitrosodimethylamine in U.S. and Canadian beers, *J. Agric. Food Chem.*, 38, 442, 1990.
51. Massey, R., Dennis, M. J., Pointer, M., and Key, P. E., An investigation of the levels of N-nitrosodimethylamine, Apparent total nitroso compounds and nitrate in beer, *Food Addit. Contam.*, 7, 605, 1990.
52. Kellner, V., Ćulík, J., Veselý, L., and Špinar, B., Problems of N-nitroso compounds, *Kvasný Prům.*, 37, 193, 1991.
53. Tricker, A. R. and Kubacki, S. J., Review of the occurrence and formation of non-volatile N-nitroso compounds in food, *Food Addit. Contam.*, 9, 39, 1992.
54. Tricker, A. R., Perkins, M. J., Massey, C. R., Bishop, C., Key, P. E., and McWeeny, D. J., Incidence of some non-volatile N-nitroso compounds in cured meats, *Food Addit. Contam.*, 1, 245, 1984.
55. Mandagere, A. K., Smoke-Related Nitrogen-Nitroso Compounds in Cured Meat Systems, Ph.D. thesis, Michigan State University, Ann Arbor, 1986.
56. Chappel, C., Current research on nitrosamines in beer, presented at the *Toxicology Forum*, Arlington, Virginia, March 1, 1980, 1.
57. Mangino, M. M. and Scanlan, R. A., Nitrosation of the alkaloids hordenine and gramine, potential precursors of N-nitrosodimethylamine in barley malt, *J. Agric. Food. Chem.*, 33, 699, 1985.
58. Ladish, W. J., Report on nitrosamines: studies on grains and the malting process, *MBAA Techn. Quarter.*, 17 (2), 96, 1981.
59. Challis, B. C., Shucker, D. E. G., Fine, D. H., Goff, E. U., and Hoffman, G. A., N-Nitrosocompounds: occurrence and biological effects, *IARC Sci. Publ.*, 41, 11, 1982.

60. Drews, B., Just, F., and Drews, H., Vorkommen und Bildung von Aminen in Bier, Würze, Malz und Gerste, *Brau. Wiss. Beil.*, 11, 169, 1958.
61. Sakuma, S., Ogawa, Y., Tezuka, T., and Katayama, H., Formation of N-nitrosodimethylamine during malt kilning, *Rep. Res. Lab. Kirin Brew. Co.*, 24, 15, 1981.
62. Wainwright, T., Slack, P. T., and Long, D. E., N-Nitrosodimethylamine precursors in malt, *IARC Sci. Publ.*, 41, 71, 1982.
63. Wainwright, T., The chemistry of nitrosamine formation: relevance to malting and brewing, *J. Inst. Brew.*, 92, 49, 1986.
64. Čulík, J., Kellner, V., Špinar, B., Ilčík, F., and Basařová, G., Volatile N-nitrosamines in malt. II. Effect of basic technological conditions of kilning on content of N-nitrosodimethylamine in malt, *Kvasný Prům.*, 35, 353, 1989.
65. Čulík, J., Kellner, V., Špinar, B., Prokeš, J., and Basařová, G., Volatile N-nitrosamines in malt. III. Effect of barley germination on the formation of natural precursors of N-nitrosodimethylamine in green malt and final malt, *Kvasný Prům.*, 36, 162, 1990.
66. Altemark, D., Hess, R., and Sommers, H., Wege zum nitrosaminfreien Bier, *Mschr. Brauerei*, 11, 415, 1980.
67. Flad, W., Minimierung der Stickoxid-konzentration beim Malzdarren, *Brauwelt*, 42, 2106, 1985.
68. Mutter, P. A., Indirect firing of malt kilns, *MBAA Tech. Quarter.*, 18, 180, 1981.
69. O'Brien, T. J., Lukes, B. K., and Scanlan, R. A., Control of N-nitrosodimethylamine in malt through the use of liquid/gaseous sulfur dioxide, *MBAA Tech. Quarter.*, 17, 196, 1980.
70. Wainwright, T., O'Farrell, D. D., Horgan, R., and Tempone, M., Ammonium persulphate in malting: control of NDMA and increased yield of malt extract, *J. Inst. Brew.*, 92, 232, 1986.
71. LLoyd, W. J. W. and Hutchings, S. J., Suppression of nitrosodimethylamine formation in malt, in *Proc. 19th Congr. of EBC*, London, 1983, 55.
72. Bärwald. G., Über die Adsorption von N-Nitrosodimethylamin an Aktivkohle, *Brauwelt*, 12, 391, 1979.
73. Massey, R. C., Key, P. E., McWeeny, D. J., and Knowles, M. E., An investigation of apparent total N-nitroso compounds in beer, *IARC Sci. Publ.*, 84, 219, 1987.
74. Smith, N. A., N-Nitrosamine in brewing, in *Proc. 23rd Congr. of EBC*, Lisbon, 1991, 68.
75. Caldebrank, J. and Hammond, J. R. M., Influence of nitrate and bacterial contamination on the formation of apparent total N-nitroso compounds during fermentation, *J. Inst. Brew.*, 95, 277, 1989.
76. Sen, N. P., Iyengar, J. R., Donaldson, B. D., Panalaks, T., and Miles, W. F., The analysis and occurence of volatile nitrosamines in cured meat products, *IARC. Sci. Publ.*, 9, 49, 1975.
77. Nebelin, E., Pillai, S., Lund, E., and Thomsen, J., On formation of N-nitrosopyrrolidine from potential precursors and nitrite, *IARC. Sci. Publ.*, 31, 183, 1980.
78. Sen, N. P., Seaman, S., and McPherson, M., Further studies on the occurence of volatile and non-volatile nitrosamines on foods, *IARC. Sci. Publ.*, 31, 457, 1980.
79. Tricker, A. R., Perkins, M. J., Massey, R. C., and McWeeny, D. J., N-Nitropyrrolidine formation in bacon, *Food. Addit. Contam.*, 2, 247, 1985.
80. Tricker, A. R., Perkins, M. J., Massey, R. C., and McWeeny, D. J., Characterization studies on insoluble total N-nitrosocompounds in bacon adipose connective tisue, *Food Addit. Contam.*, 3, 153, 1986.
81. Dunn, B. P. and Stich, H. F., Determination of free and protein bound N-nisoproline in nitrite-cured meat products, *Food Chem. Toxicol.*, 22, 609, 1984.
82. Sen, N. P., Baddoo, P. A., and Seaman, S. W., The analysis and significance of bound N-nitrosoproline in nitrite-cured meat products, *Food. Addit. Contam.*, 6, 21, 1989.
83. Tricker, A. R., Perkins, M. J., Massey, R. C., and McWeeny, D. J., Some nitrosoamino acids in bacon adipose tissue and their contribution to the total N-nitroso compound concentration, *Z. Lebensm. Unters. Forsch.*, 180, 379, 1985.
84. Mandagere, A. K., Gray, J. I., Skrypec, D. J., Booren, A. M., and Pearson, A. M., Role of woodsmoke in N-nitrosothiazolidine formation in bacon, *J. Food. Sci.*, 49, 658, 1984.
85. Massey, R. C., Crews, C., Dennis, M. J., McWeeny, D.J., Startin, J. R., and Knowles, M. E., Identification of major new involatile N-nitroso compound in smoked bacon, *Anal. Chim. Acta*, 174, 327, 1985.
86. Sen, N. P., Baddoo, P. A., and Seaman, S. W., N-Nitrosothiazolidine and *N*-nitrothiazolidine-4-carboxylic acid in smoked meats and fish, *J. Food Sci.*, 51, 821, 1986.

87. Sen, N. P., Baddoo, P. A., Seaman, S. W., and Weber, D., 2-(hydroxymethyl)-N-nitrosothiazolidine-4-carboxylic acid in smoked meats and bacon and conversion to 2-(hydroxymethyl)-N-nitrosothiazolidine during high-heat cooking, *J. Food Sci.*, 56, 913, 1991.
88. Pensabene, J. W. and Fiedler, W., N-Nitrosothiazolidine in cured meat products, *J. Food Sci.*, 48, 1870, 1983.
89. Pensabene, J. W. and Fiedler, W., Formation and inhibition of N-nitrosothiazolidine in bacon, *Food Technol.*, 39, 91,1985.
90. Pensabene, J. W. and Fiedler, W., Effect of N-nitrosothiazolidine-4-carboxylic acid on formation of N-nitrosothiazolidine in uncooked bacon, *J. Assoc. Off. Anal. Chem.*, 68, 1077, 1985.
91. Issenberg, P. and Virk, M., Inhibition of morpholine nitrosation by some phenolic wood smoke components, in *Abstr. Pap., American Chemical Society*, 168 AGFD, 53, 1974.
92. Knowles, M. E., Gilbert, J., and McWeeny, D. J., The potential formation of C-nitroso compounds in smoked, cured meats, *IARC. Sci. Publ.*, 9, 115, 1975.
93. Knowles, M. E., Gilbert, J., and McWeeny, D. J., C-Nitrosation products in food, in *Abstr. 4th Int. Congr. Food Sci. Technol.*, Papers 9a and 214, 1974.
94. Walker, E. A., Pignatelli, B., and Friesen, M., The role of nitrosamine formation, *J. Sci. Food Agric.*, 33, 81, 1982.
95. Dennis, M. J., Massey, R. C., and McWeeny, D. J., The transnitrosation of N-methylamine by a protein-bound nitrite model system in relation to N-nitrosamine formation in cured meats, *J. Sci. Food Agric.*, 31, 1195, 1980.
96. Kanner, J., *S*-Nitrosocysteine, an effective antioxidant in cured meat, *J. Am. Oil Chem. Soc.*, 56 (2), 74, 1979.
97. Dennis, M. J., Davies, R., and McWeeny, D. J., The transnitrosation of secondary amines *S*-nitrosocysteine in relation to N-nitrosamine formation in cured meats. *J. Sci. Food Agric.*, 30, 639, 1979.
98. Byler, D. M., Gosser, D. K., and Susi, H., Spectroscopic estimation of the extent of *S*-nitrosothiol formation by nitrite action on sulphydryl groups, *J. Agric. Food Chem.*, 31, 523, 1983.
99. Kanner, J. and Juven, B. J., *S*-Nitrosocysteine as an antioxidant, color-developing, and anticlostridial agent in comminuted turkey meat, *J. Food Sci.*, 45, 1105, 1980.
100. Ikins, W. G. and Gray, J. I., Mandagere, A. K., Booren, A. M., Pearson, A. M., and Stachiw, M. A., N-Nitrosamine formation in fried bacon processed with liquid smoke preparations, *J. Agric. Food Chem.*, 34, 980, 1986.
101. Pensabene, J. W., Fiddler, W., Miller, A. J., and Phillips, J. G., Effect of preprocessing procedures for green bellies on N-nitrosopyrrolidine formation in bacon, *J. Agric. Food. Chem.*, 8, 966, 1980.
102. Duxbury, D. D., Nitrosamines in bacon reduced by three alternative curing methods, *Food Process.*, 46, 113, 1985.
103. Miller, B. J., Billedeau, S. M., and Miller, D. W., Formation of N-nitrosamines in microwaved vs. skillet-fried bacon containing nitrite, *Food Chem. Toxicol.*, 27, 295, 1989.
104. Pensabene, J. W., Gates, R. A., Jenkins, R. K., and Fiddler, W., Effect of ^{137}Cs radiation on the formation of N-nitrosopyrrolidine in bacon, *J. Agric. Food Chem.*, 35, 192, 1987.
105. Bharucha, K. R., Cross, C. K., and Rubin, L. J., Nitroxides from ethoxyquin and dihydroethoxyquin as potent anti-nitrosamine agents for bacon, *J. Agric. Food Chem.*, 35, 915, 1987.
106. Buckley, D. J., Zabik, J. M., Gray, J. I., Booren, A. M., Orackel, R. L., and Beatty, E., N-Nitrosamine formation in Irish and US bacon as influenced by sodium nitrate concentration and the presence of alpha-tocopherol, *Irish J. Food Sci. Technol.*, 13, 109, 1989.
107. Bernthal, P. H., Gray, J. I., Mandagere, A. K., Ikins, W. G., Cuppett, S. L., Booren, A. M., and Price, J. F., Use of antioxidant-coated salts as N-nitrosamine inhibitors in dry-and brine-cured bacon, *J. Food Protect.*, 49, 58, 1986.
108. Bailey, M. E. and Mandagere, A. K., Nitrosamine analysis and inhibition studies, in *Lect. Proc. Eur. Meet. Meat Res. Workers*, 26, vol. II, M-8, 237, 1980.
109. Mirna, A., Untersuchungen über die Reaktion zwischen Nitrit und reduzierenden Verbindungen, *Fleischwirtschaft*, 65, 956, 1985.
110. Amundson, C. M., Sebranek, J. G., Rust, R. E., Kraft, A. A., Wagner, M. K., and Robach, M. C., Effect of belly composition on sorbate-cured bacon, *J. Food Sci.*, 47, 218, 1982.

111. Hauser, E., Gruber, E., and Mihalik, K., Zur Frage der Nitrosaminbildung in Bacon, Einfluss des Formaldehyds, in *Lect. Proc. Eur. Meet. Meat Res. Workers*, 27, vol. II, D-29, 480, 1981.
112. Gough, T. A. and Walters, C. L., Volatile nitrosamines in fried bacon, *IARC Sci. Publ.*, 14, 195, 1976.
113. Park, K. Y. and Cheigh, H. S., Kimchi and nitrosamines, *J. Korean Soc. Food Nutrit.*, 21, 109, 1992.
114. Sung, N. J., Klausner, K. A., and Hotchkiss, J. H., Influence of nitrate, ascorbic acid, and nitrate reductase microorganisms on N-nitrosamine formation during Korean-style soy-sauce fermentation, *Food Addit. Contam.*, 8, 291, 1991.
115. Sung., N. J., Hwang, O. J., and Lee, B. H., N-nitrosamine in Korean ordinary soy-sauce, *J. Korean Soc. Food Nutrit.*, 17, 125, 1988.
116. Massey, R. and Key, P. E., Examination of some fermented foods for the presence of apparent total nitroso compounds, *Food Addit. Contam.*, 6, 453, 1989.
117. Weston, R. J., Trace amounts of nitrosamines in powedered milk and milk proteins, *J. Sci. Food Agric.*, 34, 893, 1983.
118. Sen, N. P. and Seaman, S., Volatile N-nitrosamines in dried foodstuffs, *J. Assoc. Off. Anal. Chem.*, 64, 1238, 1981.

Part B

Ethyl Carbamate

Jan Velíšek

Ethyl carbamate, also known as urethane,[1,2] was identified about 20 years ago as a constituent of wines preserved with diethyl pyrocarbonate (diethyl dicarbonate)[3,4] and was later found as a by-product of fermentation in a variety of fermented foods and beverages. Research and review articles dealing with various aspects of ethyl carbamate occurrence in fermented foods and alcoholic beverages have recently been published.[5-8]

CHEMISTRY AND OCCURRENCE

Ethyl carbamate occurs in alcoholic beverages (beers, wines, liquors, fruit brandies) and even in commodities such as yogurt, bread, and soy sauce based on fermentation processes. The latter commodities contained ethyl carbamate at a level of up to 5 $\mu g.kg^{-1}$, whereas alcoholic beverages and especially spirits made from stone fruit such as kirsch (cherry spirit) contained variable quantities up to 13,400 $\mu g.dm^{-3}$ (ppb). No ethyl carbamate was found in unfermented foods or beverages.

Ethyl carbamate arises from several different precursors (Figure 1). Its formation from diethyl dicarbonate is well known and nowadays diethyl pyrocarbonate is not permited as a cold sterilant of wines and other alcoholic beverages in most countries. Wines treated with dimethyl pyrocarbonate, which was recently approved for use in wines,[9] contained methyl carbamate at a level of up to 10 $\mu g.dm^{-3}$.

The most important precursor of ethyl carbamate in fermented foods and beverages is urea, which is sometimes added to cultivation and fermentation media as a source of nitrogen for yeasts. Urea is also formed in the ornithine (urea) cycle from arginine. Its content in fermentation media (where it comes from microbial cells) rises with the ethanol content in the medium.[10] Fermentation experiments indicated that ethyl carbamate was not formed during fermentation, even in the presence of urea or ammonium phosphate. Heating at the end of fermentation broth, however, led to ethyl carbamate formation, but

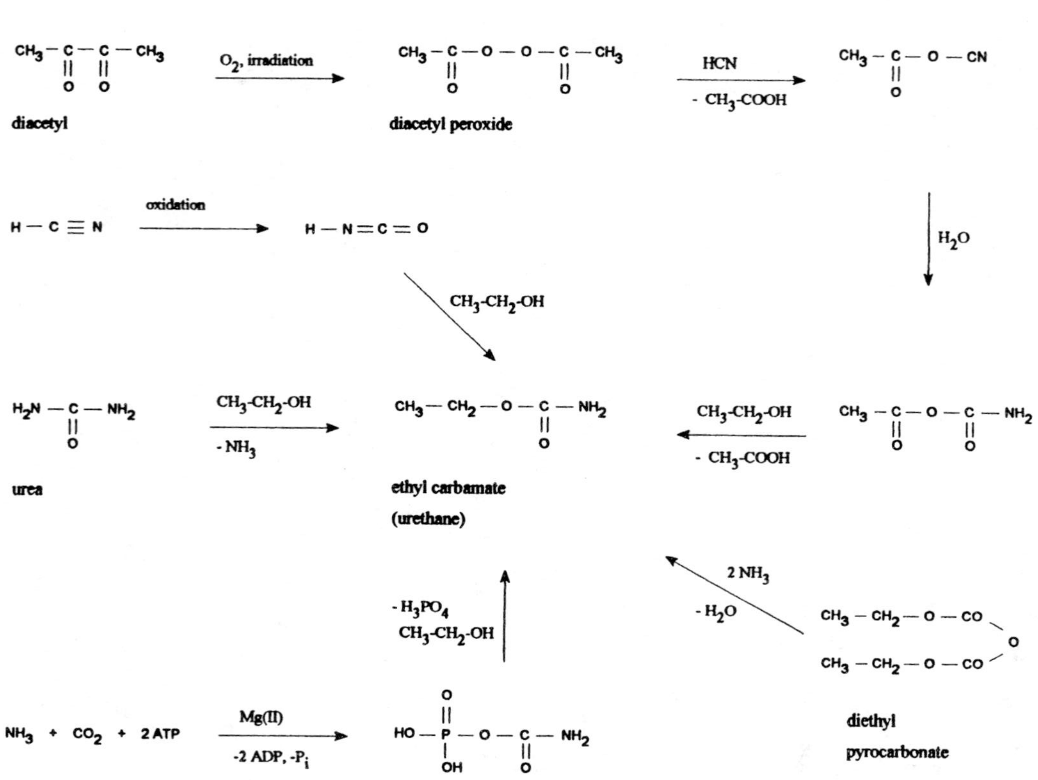

Figure 1 Formation of ethyl carbamate from various precursors.

only from fermentation supernatants where urea was used. In experiments with 0.3% urea as the yeast nutrient, resembling pasteurization conditions (60°C, 20 min), 176 $\mu g.dm^{-3}$ ethyl carbamate was formed. At 88°C/8 h (pot still) and 60°C/7 weeks (resembling a sherry) 82,700 and 122,000 $\mu g.dm^{-3}$ ethyl carbamate was found.[11]

At higher temperatures, ethyl carbamate arose even from L-ornithine, L-citrulline, allantoine, β-ureidopropionic acid,[4] ethylurea, and also from carbamylphosphate and L-carbamylaspartic acid (i.e., intermediate products of the biosynthesis and catabolism of pyrimidine nucleosides and purine bases, respectively) during their ethanolysis. It can possibly be formed from ethanol and cyanate which is formed by oxidation of cyanide and also from hydrogen cyanide and vicinal dicarbonyl compounds such as methylglyoxal, diacetyl, and 2,3-pentanedione (Figure 1).[12] In model experiments with 0.1% dicarbonyl compounds in 40% ethanol containing 20 $mg.dm^{-3}$ hydrogen cyanide, 200 to 1,300 $\mu g.dm^{-3}$ and 300 to 12,500 $\mu g.dm^{-3}$ ethyl carbamate was formed after 66 and 690 h, respectively. Higher amounts of ethyl carbamate arose when the solution was exposed to light.[5] In the presence of Cu(II), ethyl carbamate is formed even from proteins and ethanol.[13,14]

TOXIC EFFECTS

Ethyl carbamate is known to be carcinogenic, teratogenic, and mutagenic. Intensive health hazard assessment established permissable levels of ethyl carbamate in foodstuffs and beverages in most countries to 400 to 800 $\mu g.dm^{-3}$ for stone fruit beverages.[5,15,16] Removal of ethyl carbamate, especially from alcoholic beverages, or prevention of its formation is an urgent problem worldwide.

CHANGES DURING PROCESSING AND STORAGE

Several ways of lowering ethyl carbamate levels of alcoholic beverages have been used. The use of urea fermentation additives must be excluded from the manufacture of spirit ethanol. Very effective was the prior removal of Cu(II) ions by chelatation.[11] A decrease in the ethyl carbamate level in rice sake was achieved by the removal of urea using urease (EC 3.5.1.5), and urethanase decomposed the already formed ethyl carbamate.[17,18] Ethyl carbamate levels in spirits produced from stone fruit can be efficiently lowered using fruit without stones, because hydrogen cyanide originates as the breakdown product of cyanogenic glycosides occurring in the fruit seeds (page 61). The influence of light was also proved in freshly prepared distillates containing about 1,000 $\mu g.dm^{-3}$ ethyl carbamate. Its content rose to approximately 3,000, 5,000, and 7,000 $\mu g.dm^{-3}$ in a plum distillate after 35, 70, and 110 d of storage in light. Apricot distillate contained about 2,000, 2,500, and 3,000 $\mu g.dm^{-3}$ ethyl carbamate after the same storage period and exposure to light.[5]

Recommendations for minimization of ethyl carbamate concentration in fruit spirits also include use of fresh, sound, ripe fruit, use of a rapidly rehydrating dry pure yeast, acidification of the mash, fermentation in clean containers with a fermentation lock, fermentation at 18 to 25°C, holding the fermented mash for 4 to 5 months at 25°C, and slow distillation with careful separation of the potable fraction and use of a copper catalyst during distillation.[19]

REFERENCES

1. Schlatter, J. and Lutz, W. K., The carcinogenic potential of ethyl carbamate (urethane): risk assessment at human dietary exposure levels, *Food Chem. Toxicol.*, 28, 205, 1990.
2. Stoewsand, G. S., Anderson, J. L., and Munson, L., Inhibition by wine of tumorigenesis induced by ethyl carbamate (urethane) in mice, *Food Chem. Toxicol.*, 29, 291, 1991.
3. Lofroth, G. and Gejwall, T., Diethyl pyrocarbonate. Formation of urethane in treated beverages, *Science*, 174, 1248, 1971.
4. Fischer, E., Formation of carbamic acid ethyl ester (urethane) in beverages after treatment with diethyl pyrocarbonate, *Z. Lebensm. Unters. Forsch.*, 148, 221, 1972.
5. Baumann, U. and Zimmerli, B., Zur Bildung von Ethylcarbamat (Urethan) in Steinobstdestillaten, *Mitt. Gebiete Lebensm. Hyg.*, 78, 317, 1987.
6. Laugel, P., Bindler, F., and Grimm, P., Ethyl carbamate in fruit brandies, *Annu. Falsif. Expert. Chim. Toxicol.*, 80, 457, 1987.
7. Wucherpfennig, K., Clauss, E., and Konja, G., Beitrag zur Entstehung des Ethylcarbamat in alkoholischen Getränken auf der Basis der sauerkirsche Maraska. *Dtsch. Lebensm. Rdsch.*, 83, 344, 1987.
8. Battaglia, R. and Conacher, H. B. S., Ethyl carbamate (urethane) in alcoholic beverages and foods: a review, *Food Addit. Contam.*, 7, 477, 1990.
9. Sen, N. P., Seaman, S. W., and Weber, D., A method for the determination of methyl carbamate and ethyl carbamate in wines, *Food Addit. Contam.*, 9, 149, 1992.
10. Monteiro, F. F., Trousdale, E. K., and Bisson, L. F., Ethyl carbamate formation in wine: use of radioactive labelled precursors to demonstrate the involvement of urea, *Am. J. Enol. Vitic.*, 40, 1, 1989.
11. Ingledew, W. M., Magnus, C. A., and Petterson, J. R., Yeast foods and ethyl carbamate formation in wine, *Am. J. Enol. Vitic.*, 38, 332, 1987.
12. Ough, C. S., Ethyl carbamate in fermented beverages and foods, *J. Agric. Food Chem.*, 24, 323, 1976.
13. Riffkin, H. L., Wilson, R., Howie, D., and Muller, S. B., Ethyl carbamate formation in the production of pot still whisky, *J. Inst. Brew.*, 95, 115, 1989.
14. Riffkin, H. L., Wilson, R., and Bringhurst, T. A., The possible involvement of copper (2+) peptide/protein complexes in the formation of ethyl carbamate, *J. Inst. Brew.*, 95, 121, 1989.
15. Mildau, G., Preuss, A., Frank, W., and Herring, W., Ethylcarbamat (Urethan) in alkoholischen Getränken. Verbesserte Analyse und lichtabhängige Bildung, *Dtsch. Lebensm. Rdsch.*, 83, 69, 1987.
16. Conacher, H. B. S., The role of the Canadian health protection in the control of potentially hazardous chemicals in alcoholic beverages, *Can. J. Spectr.*, 34, 16A, 1989.
17. Kobashi, K., Takebe, S., and Sakai, T., Removal of urea from alcoholic beverages with an acid-urease, *J. Appl. Toxicol.*, 8, 73, 1988.
18. Kobashi, K., Ethyl carbamate in alcoholic beverages, *Eisei Kagaku*, 35, 110, 1989.
19. Pieper, H. J., Seibold, R., and Luz, E., Reduzierung von Ethylcarbamat bei der Herstellung von Kirschbränden, *Kleinbrennerei*, 44, 158, 1992.

Index

INDEX

A

B

C

D

E

F

G

H

I

J

K

L

M

N

O

P

Q

R

S

T

U

V

W

X

Y

Z